Making Informed Medical Decisions

Where to Look and
How to Use What You Find

Making Informed Medical Decisions

Where to Look and
How to Use What You Find

Nancy Oster, Lucy Thomas,
and Darol Joseff, MD

O'REILLY®

Beijing • Cambridge • Farnham • Köln • Paris • Sebastopol • Taipei • Tokyo

Making Informed Medical Decisions: Where to Look ar **362.1 OSTER** *hat You Find*
by Nancy Oster, Lucy Thomas, and Darol Joseff, MD

Copyright © 2000 O'Reilly & Associates, Inc. All rights re
Printed in the United States of America.

Published by O'Reilly & Associates, Inc., 101 Morris Street)5472.

Editor: Linda Lamb

Production Editor: Sarah Jane Shangraw

Cover Designers: Edie Freedman and Ellie Volckhausen

Printing History:

> July 2000: First Edition

Library of Congress Cataloging-in-Publication Data

Oster, Nancy.
  Making informed medical decisions : where to look and how to use what you find /
Nancy Oster, Lucy Thomas, Darol Joseff.
    p. cm. — (Patient-centered guides)
  Includes bibliographical references and index.
  ISBN 1-56592-459-2 (pbk.)
    1. Health—Decision making—Popular works. 2. Medicine—Decision making—
Popular works. 3. Physician services utilization—Popular works. 4. Consumer education.
I. Thomas, Lucy. II. Joseff, Darol. III. Title. IV. Series.

RA776.5 .O684 2000
362.1—dc21

                                                    00-036705

[M]

For Dave Oster, Bill Thomas, Janet Pickthorn,
Brian & Kate Joseff, Michelann & Shaun Oster, Brig Thomas,
and our parents.

In addition, this book is dedicated to the memories of those people whose
wisdom graciously lit the pathway for us. With strength, intelligence, grace,
and humor, these friends made difficult choices in the face of life-threatening
illness and shared their perspectives on the value of choosing your own path,
even when the final destination is uncertain.

JB Boggs	Ruth Gubits
Lisann Charland	Lauren Langford
Patti Flynn	Fred Rossi
Fred Glenwinkel	Lucy Sherak
Tairi Gould	and others

Table of Contents

Foreword

IN DECEMBER 1999 the nation's two leading medical journals delivered the same message: primary care doctors are being stretched beyond their limits and patients are being shortchanged in the process. A study in the *New England Journal of Medicine* determined that one in four primary care physicians feel that they are being asked to treat conditions that were previously handled by specialists and do not feel up to the job. A report in the *Journal of the American Medical Association* concluded that primary care physicians and surgeons frequently made decisions without discussing the intervention with their patients or seeking their involvement. In an editorial accompanying the JAMA article, Dr. Michael J. Barry suggests that "Physicians most likely would argue that there is simply insufficient time to adopt the shared decision making approach, particularly in the current managed care era in which most office based physicians feel pressured to see an increasing number of patients in the same amount of time."

The authors of both studies suggested the same solution: Give primary care doctors more training in treating serious diseases and in sharing decision making. This obviously will not work. How is the doctor who doesn't have enough time supposed to find more for additional training?

I suggest another model, a doctor-patient partnership. And the perfect vehicle for this partnership is the Internet. I am not recommending that we replace the physician with a computer, but rather that patients be encouraged to research their condition on the Internet. (I can hear my colleagues groaning that their patients are already coming in with stacks of printouts that they have no time to discuss adequately.)

But what if physicians and patients were to incorporate the Internet into the office visit in a systematic fashion? As I've learned from years of working with breast cancer advocates, no one is more motivated to become an expert on one disease than the person who has it. There is no question that a patient has much more time to spend at the computer screen than his or her doctor does. In fact, just the other day I heard about a colleague who admitted to his patient that he had *actually learned something* from the information on Paget's disease that she had downloaded.

Why can't doctors use this situation to their advantage? What if we consider the doctor-patient relationship a partnership where the doctor is a consultant? After the initial exam, patients are given the option of researching their condition, with certain web sites identified as being reliable. They then come to the follow-up visit and report what they found, and whether it has helped to shape their preferences for treatment. The patients are likely to have a much better understanding of their options and more realistic expectations for therapy. Together, doctor and patient can share both decision-making and responsibility.

This approach could be especially valuable for decisions affecting quality of life. The Internet has a discussion group, bulletin board, or chat about almost every condition known to man and woman. For example, tips for living with lymphedema—swelling of the arm after breast cancer surgery—are much more abundant on the Internet than in almost any medical textbook or consulting room. The power of the Internet is in the enormity of experience it encompasses.

The doctor's job is not to know everything but to come up with the treatment that is most appropriate for each patient. The Internet can be a great ally in this respect. It can help relieve the burden on the beleaguered primary care physician and give the patient more control over his or her medical destiny.

—Susan Love, MD
Author, *Dr. Susan Love's Breast Book* and *Dr. Susan Love's Hormone Book*
Founder, *SusanLoveMD.com*
Adjunct Professor of Surgery, UCLA

Preface

THE INSPIRATION FOR THIS BOOK came from the students in our classes for Santa Barbara City College Adult Education. The class is ambitiously entitled "Healthcare Information on the Internet." We learned a great deal from the wonderful students of all ages who have attended our classes over the last few years. We learned that the changes in healthcare delivery have made the traditional "patient" a more proactive consumer of healthcare. Some of our students are healthcare providers, some are dealing with serious illness, and a few just want to learn some new techniques for finding information.

Many of our students shared some new search strategies or brought perspectives to the class that enriched us all. Lawyers, chiropractors, nurses, retired and active physicians, veterinarians, and patients facing everything from stroke rehabilitation to bone marrow transplantation have attended our classes and shared their experiences. By sharing their experiences, they constantly added to our own points of view.

One thing that was really helpful for us was that we, ourselves, look at medicine and medical information from many perspectives. Darol, a physician, sees medicine through the eyes of a direct provider in an era of major changes in the healthcare system. Lucy, a medical librarian, sees medicine from the point of view of an information professional supporting both providers and consumers. Nancy, a medical writer and founder of a breast health resource center, sees medical information from the perspective of a patient advocate. All three of us have had experiences as the direct consumers of healthcare. All three of us have also embraced the Internet as a revolutionary tool in the dissemination of health information—and, unfortunately, health misinformation. We wanted to share our insights and offer some reliable resources and evaluation guidelines for a wider audience than we could reach in our small classes.

Why we wrote this book

In each class evaluation, the students consistently told us two things. The first was that the most valuable things they had learned were the critical skills for evaluating medical information. The second thing they told us was that they wanted a longer class with more information. Since all three of us had other full time occupations, our response to their requests was to write this book.

We wrote this book for anyone who needs healthcare information and/or who is facing a healthcare decision. We know from personal and professional experience that facing illness is one of the most difficult things you will ever do. As a consumer of healthcare you wish to understand enough about your illness to make clear decisions with your doctor's help. We offer you some tools and some guidelines so that you can be truly "informed" whenever you make a health decision.

In our classes and in our daily working lives, we hear stories of frustration with "managed" healthcare. We hear about disappointing experiences in trying to learn more about a diagnosis or variations in treatment. We also hear many questions about how to find information on new and experimental treatments. In this book, we share our insights and experiences about some basic skills we use for information gathering and for the evaluation of that information.

Many of the Internet megasites of medical information are very reliable, but the Internet seems to have as many sites making fraudulent claims as those with legitimate information. Whenever time permitted, we staged contests in our classes to find an Internet health site with the most impossible claims. Collectively we found some doozies. We include evaluation techniques throughout the book to help you discriminate between valid and proven healthcare information and some exaggerated claim.

We also give directions for finding medical libraries, journals and bookstores, because all of the information you may need is not yet on the Internet. The information you need may be in the printed medical literature or available through direct conversation with a knowledgeable expert.

What this book offers

This book presents an introduction to the world of medical information—in print, on the Internet, and through contact with medical experts and other patients. We direct you to the many places you can find medical information from bookstores and libraries to the Internet and support groups. We also offer you, the consumer of healthcare, some guidelines so that you can evaluate the information you find and participate more actively in your own healthcare decisions.

How this book is organized

The book is organized in four sections. The first three chapters deal with preparing for research, understanding your rights, accessing medical records, and special things you need to know about helping a family member or friend. The next three chapters list the types of resources that are available, where to find them, and how to use them. Chapters 7, 8, 9, and 10 cover the range of treatment options from standard to experimental treatment and from complementary and alternative treatment to learning coping skills and getting support. Finally, in the last three chapters, we cover how to decipher the statistics and risks related to various treatments, how to work with your doctor, and how to come to your own decision.

Throughout various sections of the book we have switched the pronouns "he" and "she" as well as "her" and "him." We've done this simply because we know that many doctors and other healthcare providers are women and many are men. This is also true of patients, of course. The use of "s/he" or other attempts to equalize coverage seemed too forced to us. Many of the conditions we discuss, such as prostate cancer, are gender specific, but most are experienced by members of both sexes.

The quotes

We interviewed many, many generous and wonderful people whose poignant stories are distributed throughout the book. The perspectives of those who have "been there" are invaluable to understanding the healthcare process. The information they share is also valuable as an example of how each person dealt with a serious condition. We, and they, hope that their experiences give you guidance if you are ever confronting serious healthcare decisions for yourself or for a loved one. The stories are genuine, moving, and from the heart of each of the people we interviewed. Those who shared their experiences are from all walks of life and all parts of the country—and even the world.

The quotes come from physicians and other healthcare professionals as well as those who have been patients. They have shared their advice and support. The healthcare providers offer valuable guidance on effective ways to get what you need in the changing world of healthcare.

A word about the Internet

While this book is about all formats for health information, we know that the Internet has become a major force in expanding access to all types of medical information. We assume our readers will have basic skills in accessing and using the Internet. We also assume that you can find a web site when you have the URL or web site address and that you understand how a search engine works. There are many classes and books that can help you acquire these basic skills. Some of the resources listed at the end of this book may also help. Current surveys show that a high percentage of the population now has access to the Internet. Based on these statistics, you can probably find a friend who can guide you to any of the Internet sites or search strategies mentioned in this book.

Acknowledgments

We wish to thank all of our reviewers, technical advisors, and all of those who generously shared their time and their stories:

Robert F. Anderson; Dianne Armitage; Kathryn Ball; Dell Barden; Albert Baroni; Judy B. Blanco; Barbara Brenner; David Broad; Loren Buhle; Donna Burr; Anne Cameron; Catherine Carpenter; Kate Carter; Mary Jane Caswell; David Culler; Kay Deeney; Rachel Doctors; Ron Doctors; Jo Duffy; Kirsti Dyer, MD; Stan Eisele; Barbara Essex; Lynn Fay; Rosemary Fitzgerald; Karen Frischmeyer, DVM; Patricia Funerton; Venkatesh Ganapathi; Bernard Glassman; Fred Glenwinkel; Pat Glenwinkel; Karen Grace-Martin; Nadine Greenup; Janie Grosman; Corinna Gordon; Ruth M. Gubits; Brother Lawrence Harms; Yashar Hirshaut, MD; Selene Hopkins; Stephen Hosea, MD; Marian Jean; Holly Principe Joseph; Nancy Keene; Charlotte Jurehn-Lewis; Frederick C. Kass, MD; Louise Keeler; Pam Laird; Molly Long; Tom E. Long; Susan Love, MD; Laurie Lyckholm, MD; Andrea Mankoski; Marilyn Chambers McEntyre; Steve McIntosh; Sara McKenna; Ann McKibbon; Rochelle Minchow; Sherry Morez; Kathleen Morgan; Joe Mortz; Laurie Moser; Sharon Multhauf; Sara O'Donnell; Julie Ohnemus, MD; Michelann

Ortloff; Dave Oster; Bill Pickthorn; Janet Pickthorn, MD; Cheryl Parrott; Isabelle Patton; Gary Ponto, MD; Cissy Ross; Heidi Sandstrom; TB Scanland; Gail Shannon; Marilyn Shaeffer; Lucy Sherak; Susan Shiras; Jef Short; Lou Smitheram; M. Steele; Mike Stephenson; Larry Stevens; Doug Sweet; Nancy Sweet; Betsy Thaggard; William R. Thomas; Katherine Trisko; Linda Walsh; Lyne Van Houten; Henry Weaver; Mary E. Weaver; Barbra Wiener; Nancy Wilczynski; Alison Okada Wollitzer.

We want to give special appreciation to Linda Lamb, our editor at O'Reilly, and Shawnde Paull, editorial assistant. We also have been grateful for the support and assistance from the Brothers at Mt. Calvary, Musa Mayer, Catherine Thorpe, and the staff of the Reeves Medical Library.

A final note

Our profound hope is that this book is useful and will assist you in finding the information you need. We understand that both the fields of medicine and that of information are changing constantly. We designed these guidelines with change in mind and with the expectation that they will accommodate change and remain a valuable tool.

We share our sincere encouragement and best wishes with you, our readers.

—Darol, Lucy, and Nancy

Disclaimer

The material presented in the patient vignettes represents those individuals' unique experiences. This information should be interpreted cautiously since their decisions may not be best for you. This book is not intended to replace discussion between you and your physician or caregiver.

CHAPTER 1

Preparing for Research

PERHAPS YOU HAVE BEEN TOLD that you have an illness or a condition that will require treatment; maybe you are experiencing some unexplained symptoms that have become worrisome to you; or maybe you have tried all the recommended treatments and nothing seems to have worked. Not every medical condition requires research, but there are some situations that prompt you to look further.

This chapter helps you plan and prioritize your search, increasing your chances of making the best use of your time and getting the answers you need. We discuss tips for effective listening and communication and talk about how to gather primary information from your doctors. This includes understanding the precise diagnosis, the time frame recommended for making specific decisions, and the range of options available to you. We also comment on getting information from other members of your medical team and reviewing your personal goals and resources.

Reasons to research

Regardless of your treatment outlook, when you are newly diagnosed with a medical condition, you are likely to feel yourself thrust into a world of medical jargon, tests, personnel, and processes that are unfamiliar and frightening. On top of being emotionally and physically stressed, you have to learn a new language and way of thinking about disease. Doing research can provide a way of gaining clarity and getting back some sense of control over your life. You may want to find out more about your condition, the range of treatments, or where to find the best doctor or treatment center for this condition.

Many medical conditions have well-tested, reliable treatments that work so well, further research is not necessary. A man diagnosed with diabetes talks about his initial response and treatment:

I started noticing a tingling and numbness in my feet. At first I didn't think anything of it, but I heard a radio ad about diabetes that mentioned that as one of the classic symptoms.

When I went in to see my doctor, I wasn't too surprised when it turned out that I was a Type II diabetic. In fact, I was relieved that it wasn't some nerve thing like paralysis in my legs. I knew diabetes was a controllable condition.

There really wasn't a whole lot of choice involved. He put me on medication and sent me to a dietician. The treatment worked right away.

I had confidence in the treatment because the condition is well understood. It's a success story for Western medicine. It's a matter of sugar levels, carbohydrates, and what you do to make the carbohydrates go away. In fact, after six months I was able to go off the medication and control it completely with diet and exercise.

Other conditions are not as easy to diagnose or treat successfully. A woman talks about her struggle to identify the cause of her daughter's abnormal development and behavior:

My daughter was a healthy, normal infant for about two or three months when she began losing milestones. She rolled over onto her back at two months and then never did it again for another eight months. She screamed all the time and didn't make contact with people like babies normally do. I would go to the pediatrician and read books and think, "This isn't right."

It wasn't until she was nine months old that the pediatrician agreed that her development was falling behind. He said he would watch her, but I wasn't comfortable with that so I got a referral to a pediatric neurologist. The CT scan and neurological work-up showed that she was developmentally delayed "for unknown reasons."

The severity of the problem and lack of clear-cut answers drove this mother to do more research to try to understand and help advocate for her daughter:

I quit my job to work with her full-time on sensory stimulation and motor development. We moved to Boston when she was 18 months old. A few months later she had her first serious illness of a metabolic acidosis. The team at the children's hospital decided to go back to the drawing board to look for the cause. They did metabolic tests to look for inborn errors of metabolism. Her phenylalanine came back elevated.

I went to the library and got some books. I knew right away from the descriptions that this was the problem. If any of the doctors had ever seen an infant with PKU [phenylketonuria], they probably would have known—blonde hair, autistic, pale skin, eczema, hyper-irritable, loss of milestones. It was all right there.

Only 1 in 14,000 newborns has PKU. All children are tested for it at birth, but the lab that did her test had not sent their techs to the training class. Most lab techs have never seen a positive result.

Within a week after starting her on the PKU diet, her personality changed and she was walking. It was like living with a miracle. Not all of the problems went away, but the day of her diagnosis was the happiest day of our lives because we finally knew what was wrong.

Your own reasons for wanting to research a condition might be less dramatic. Sometimes mild, but chronic conditions require you to be your own detective, looking for ways to alleviate the bothersome effects of an abnormal condition. A man with psoriasis talks about his search for ways to reduce the growth of calluses on his finger tips that crack and bleed frequently during normal daily activities:

Since my case is minor and unusual, I have not gotten a lot of help with it. The dermatologist couldn't even decide if it was psoriasis or eczema. He basically said, "It isn't cancer, here's some cortisone, go away." I feel like I'm on my own.

I get the National Psoriasis Foundation newsletter, but most of the research is on more acute conditions. The side effects of the drugs keep me away from trying them. The best thing I've found is a skin cream for women who have had radiation treatment for breast cancer. It's soothing but it doesn't cure my problem. I've learned to live with the bleeding fingers, but I keep reading and hoping I'll discover the cause and a way to treat it.

Asking your doctor for information

Researching your medical condition doesn't mean working alone. Your doctor has a lot of specific technical training, experience dealing with other people with similar conditions, and knowledge about other doctors and specialists. Your research will build on what your doctor tells you. (Chapter 12, *Reviewing Information with Your Doctor*, discusses how to work with your doctor to interpret what you find and decide on a course of treatment.)

Before you begin research, you'll want to make sure to communicate fully with your doctor on the following issues so that you have a clear understanding of your case:

- **Diagnosis.** What is it precisely? What does it mean? What assumptions are you making that might not be true?

- **Time frame.** Does this condition demand your immediate response? How immediate? What might you gain or lose by taking a little more time to research and decide?

- **Options.** What is the range of recommended treatment choices? What options are not recommended? Why? What would happen if you chose to do nothing?

Good doctor-patient communication is essential to successful research and informed decision-making. If you do not feel you are working well with a particular doctor, you may want to reconsider your choice of doctors. For help on that issue, Nancy Keene's book, *Working with Your Doctor: Getting the Healthcare You Deserve* (O'Reilly and Associates, Inc.), provides a complete step-by-step guide to finding the doctor that best suits your needs.[1]

Communicating effectively

Even if you are intelligent, knowledgeable about your health, assertive, and have an excellent relationship with your doctor, stress can impact your ability to understand what you are being told. If you are faced with a life-threatening or life-changing condition, the stress may be extreme. For example, many people report that upon hearing the diagnosis of cancer, they were unable to remember anything following the word "cancer."

A man explains his need to communicate more with his doctor about his emotional concerns:

> The biggest problem for me was that if I didn't communicate enough, I started imagining things—I'd get paranoid. Talking with my doctor and learning more about my condition has helped alleviate the paranoia.

Emotional responses are perfectly normal in stressful situations, so plan ahead for your doctor visits. Clarify what you want to know, and make sure that you understand what you hear.

One man has learned always to bring a written list of things to discuss with his doctor:

> A lot of times when I'm with the doctor, I kind of get into a fog. I don't have the presence of mind to ask the questions I should ask. I tend to be vague if I don't prepare. So now I write down the questions and the symptoms I have before I go in. I use this list to help me be more specific about what I want to know.

At first, you might not feel personally connected to that slide under the microscope, set of numbers on a blood panel, or image on a light box or computer screen. Bad news is not only difficult for you to absorb, but it is also difficult for your doctor to deliver. Not all patients want to be active partners in the evaluation and decision-making process. Your doctor may be waiting for a sign from you to indicate how much detail you want to hear and whether or not you want to take an active role in this process.

An oncologist (cancer specialist) describes his approach to the patient's first visit:

> I usually start off asking, "How are you?" I'm really impressed with the extraordinary range of responses. Cancer comes like a sledgehammer out of nowhere. We all have different ways of coping. Sometimes we want information and sometimes we really don't want information at all. We want a chance to talk out what we are feeling.
>
> My goal in that first visit is to give the patient an opportunity to ask a lot of questions. I create the space and time to talk. I try not to jump to conclusions about what a patient needs. If I do nothing else but allow somebody to set an agenda for himself, that may be all the help I need to give.

Preparing for doctor's visits

In order to use the limited time that you will have with your doctor as effectively as possible, here are some ways to prepare for your visit:

- Give your doctor a list describing your medical history, family history, all the medications (include nonprescription supplements such as herbs or vitamins) you are taking or that have caused negative reactions in the past, and any beliefs that might restrict your treatment choices. Ask if she would like this faxed to her office before the visit.

- Bring a list of questions you have about your diagnosis or treatment options, one copy for you and one for your doctor. The medical setting can be intimidating. A list will help keep you focused. List your questions in order of importance in case you run out of time at the end.

- Do preliminary research on your list of questions, if time allows, to become familiar with the medical terminology likely to be used in the answers.

- Ask a family member or friend to come with you to listen and take notes. Often an observer will pick up information that you miss. Discuss what you want to learn from the visit with the person you are inviting.

- Ask permission to use a tape recorder. Your emotional responses and preconceptions can alter what you hear. On a second listening the words the doctor actually used may not reflect what you assumed was being said. Often comments that did not seem important in the beginning become significant as you learn more about your condition and treatment options.

- Ask your doctor to spell words that are unfamiliar to you so that you can use them in your information searches later. Ask her for simpler explanations if the description is too detailed for you to grasp in the beginning.

- Be honest with your doctor. Let her know what you want to know and what you don't want to know. Express your concerns.

- Ask for help finding books, local libraries, support groups, organizations, and other resources where you can get more information on your condition or the options you are considering.

- Let her know all other types of practitioners you will be consulting, particularly nutritionists, herbalists, and other complementary therapists. Ask for recommendations to other professionals who might help expand your understanding and perspective.

- Give her a list of family and friends who will be helping you research so she will know whom you feel comfortable sharing your health information with.

- If you have copies of previous test reports that were not done through her office, take those with you.

- Ask her to indicate on any future lab requests that a copy of the results be faxed or mailed to you directly.

- Tell her you are giving her secretary your fax number or email address in case she comes across information that might be helpful to you.

- Thank your physician for taking time to talk with you.

Getting an overview

When you begin learning about your condition, you will do more listening than asking questions. Not all of what you hear will sound like plain English. Listen for keywords and overall concepts. As you hear words repeated, you will begin to understand some of them by the way they are used. If you are completely baffled by the jargon and technicalities, let your doctor know. She may be able to recommend some basic reading on the subject.

You may be worried about taking up too much of your doctor's time. During office hours, doctors often have patients waiting for them in multiple examining rooms. They understandably feel pressured to move efficiently through each visit. If your examination does not feel like it allows enough time for discussion, make an appointment for another visit. That way your doctor can concentrate on explanation and discussion without being distracted by the need to do a physical examination at the same time.

Some insurance companies will pay for treatment time, but not separate conference visits. You may be required to pay out-of-pocket for a conference visit. Check with your insurance company in advance to find out what their coverage includes.

Asking effective questions

Your first questions will probably be simple "what is" questions. As you gain a basic understanding of your condition, most of the "what is" questions will be answered through your own research.

The next set of questions are the "why" questions. These are the questions most likely to sound like a challenge to your physician's perspective. However, what might seem obvious to an experienced physician, is not always obvious to a newly diagnosed patient. You can soften these questions by asking "Why do you think that this option is preferred over that option?" Listen for the underlying assumptions. You may find that your physician is making an assumption about you that you would not make about yourself.

The third important set of questions are the "what if" questions. These are the planning questions. No one knows the ultimate answers, but professionals and other people more experienced with the disease or condition will have a well-developed intuitive sense of possible outcomes and can alert you to potential hazards. "What if" questions are especially valuable if you are thinking about trying complementary or alternative therapies.

Don't be surprised if the honest answer to a question is "I don't know." There are few clear-cut answers in medicine and lots of individual variations. Understanding the level of uncertainty is also part of the evaluation process.

Understanding your diagnosis

A diagnosis with a life-threatening disease or chronic condition can feel like a prison sentence: it's final and the door is slamming shut. However, a diagnosis does not tell you precisely what will happen to you. You may have been diagnosed with heart disease, diabetes, or a particular cancer. Each of those general categories includes a complex array of variations. It is important to ask your physician for a more detailed explanation of your specific condition.

The general category will help you find information in the popular press, but you will need specific details to sort through the studies and conclusions in medical journals or textbooks and determine which apply to your particular situation. For example, if you are diagnosed with breast cancer, you will want to know if it is lobular (in the milk sacs) or ductal (in the milk ducts).

Is it invasive or non-invasive (*in situ*)? How large is the tumor? What stage is it? How many stages are there and how are they determined? For diabetes, you will want to know if it is Type I or Type II. Will you need to take insulin or can you manage it with dietary changes?

Ask your physician for an overview of the subcategories used to identify variations in your type of disease or condition, with an explanation of which ones apply to you and which ones do not apply. As you begin your research, it's as important to understand clearly which characteristics your diagnosis does not include as it is to know those it does include.

Find out if there are specific disease characteristics that help guide the treatment recommendations for your individual case. For example, the hormone receptor status of a breast tumor (i.e., positive or negative) will help to determine whether or not a cancer is likely to respond to hormone therapy.

Questions to ask about your diagnosis

Your physician is one of your most valuable guides and resources as you begin your research. Through his own experience and training, he has developed a way of approaching and filtering information. He has developed his own understanding of how a particular disease affects the body and a mental map of the way the disease may progress with or without treatment. Ask him to share his perspective as well as answers to the following questions:

- What stage of development is the diagnosis? Is it advanced or early?

- Is this a mild or serious form of a specific disease?

- Is this a common form of the disease or will it be difficult to find information?

- Is this condition curable or just controllable. Is it chronic or life threatening?

- Is this a preliminary diagnosis? Are further tests needed or is this indisputable?

Medical terms

Don't be surprised if you feel overwhelmed and confused at first by medical language. Focus on the words your physician uses as he describes the specific characteristics of your diagnosis.

Some terms may be familiar to you from an experience with another disease. Do not automatically assume that terms used for one disease have the same implications when used to describe another disease. For example, breast cancer that has spread to the lymph nodes is not referred to as metastatic disease unless it is detected in distant organs of the body, whereas ovarian cancer is considered metastatic when it has spread to the lymph nodes. As another example, the word *communicable* may indicate to you that a disease is contagious. However, in the case of *communicating* hydrocephalus (water on the brain), *communicating* means that the cause of the hydrocephalic condition can be anywhere in the brain, not just limited to the ventricles as with the noncommunicating variety.

Prognostic significance of an event can also vary from condition to condition. For many cancers the fact that the disease has been found in distant locations—"spread to the bone" or "spread to the brain"—can be an indication of a less favorable prognosis. This is not true for all cancers. For example, the spread (*metastasis*) of non-Hodgkin's lymphomas (NHL) to multiple sites within the body does not necessarily mean that the disease will be fatal. However, you might easily assume that because of what you'd heard in the past about the prognosis for a relative's colon or pancreatic cancer.

Research without a diagnosis

Most of us experience health variations that might or might not signal the onset of long-term medical problems. Often a diagnosis provides the explanation for a string of suspicious symptoms. Sometimes a presymptomatic diagnosis is made as the result of routine screening tests. However, if the collection of symptoms does not form a recognizable pattern, it may be difficult to establish a medical diagnosis.

Lack of a diagnosis does not mean that your concerns about changes in your health are not valid. But it does mean that you will probably spend more time sorting through information on your own to identify the cause and significance of the changes you are experiencing. If you are looking for explanations for symptoms, you'll want to understand the medical terms for those symptoms, what conditions have already been ruled out by what tests, and what suggestions your doctor might have for further research and evaluation.

Researching a rare condition

Rare conditions can be especially challenging to research. Unfortunately, the rarer the disease, the less economic motivation there is for research and product development. You will need to identify the major category of disease it would fall under and try to find a knowledgeable specialist in that area. If the condition has a name, some research has been done on it, and other people have been diagnosed with it—but you may have to search extra hard to find them.

A man diagnosed in 1936 with narcolepsy (a sleep disorder characterized by involuntary periods of sleep during the day and disturbed sleep at night), talks about his lifelong search to find ways to manage his condition:

> I was 8 when my parents realized that something was wrong and took me to see the family doctor. After examining me and hearing about one or two incidences of cataplexy [sudden loss of muscle tone], he looked it up in his books and said, "Well, I think he has narcolepsy, but we don't know much about it." In those days there were no medicines, no treatment.
>
> I had to learn to handle it on my own. It was scary for me and for my family. When I was 20, I went to a psychotherapist who gave me my first medication. Those little white pills changed my life. In 1958, when I was 30, another doctor told me I didn't have narcolepsy. He diagnosed my problem as hypoglycemia, took me off the stimulant, and told me to eat lemon drop candies to increase my blood sugar. That was probably the worst year in my life.
>
> When I realized the hypoglycemia treatment wasn't working, I decided to go to a hospital in Chicago. They kept me there for ten days. A lot of doctors came in to see me. They must not have had many cases. I was rediagnosed with narcolepsy and given medication.
>
> I didn't meet anyone else with narcolepsy until 1979. Someone told me about a party for a group of patients at a sleep clinic. It was wonderful. I guess I really didn't believe that there was anyone else who had this condition. It isolates you. About that time, I also found out about the American Narcoleptic Association and joined it.

Now there is information on the Internet, but a doctor who has had experience with narcolepsy is still hard to find. I am my doctor's only narcoleptic patient. The good thing, though, is that doctors are getting to know more about these different kinds of diseases now and you can find specialists.

Prioritizing your research

"You have plenty of time to decide," is the phrase you would like to hear from your doctor, but that is not always the situation. Your physician may want to schedule more tests and urge you to make treatment decisions without delay.

Any diagnosis, particularly a life-threatening one, feels urgent as your life suddenly shifts focus and you struggle to put the changes into perspective. You may feel pressure to make life-altering decisions quickly. Talk with your doctor about the urgency of your condition. You might ask her the following questions:

- Which steps are time-sensitive and which ones allow time for research and careful consideration?

- What makes certain steps in the process more urgent?

- What is the specific range of time being discussed? (Urgent to you might mean tomorrow, while urgent to your physician could mean within the next couple of weeks.)

- What could I gain or lose by taking things slower?

Sometimes the next step will depend upon the results of the step preceding it. For example, a decision about whether or not you will have chemotherapy may depend on the extent and type of cancer found in the biopsy. Ask your physician to outline the expected sequence of events with an emphasis on the decision points that she foresees along the way.

An oncologist explains how he listens to his patients' concerns so they can work together to set an agenda for addressing them:

I make a lot of notes, handwritten and mental. Then we take a break to summarize and see if I can help them identify their top three concerns. There's a limit to how much information a person can address at one time.

In some cases, of course, there is very little time for research or deliberation. A man remembers his lack of time for any contemplation or research when experiencing severe pain from a pancreatic pseudocyst:

> My situation was so alarming that there wasn't much of a choice about what to do. It had to be done quickly. They would have liked to do surgery but it was too risky because I was underweight. They talked with me about it, but there was no choice. They had to put in a drain quickly, even though they weren't sure that it was going to work.
>
> A year later when I had a recurrence, surgery was an option and I had time to think about it before I made the choice.

Identifying your range of options

The purpose of your research is to develop a thorough understanding of the pros and cons of the options available to you. Your physician will give you an overview of the types of options that he expects you will want to consider. And in the course of learning more about those options, you may also come across additional options.

What if I do nothing?

The first question to ask your physician is "What if I do nothing?" Asking this question does not mean that you plan to do nothing, but a clear understanding of that option will underlie all future action.

Sometimes when faced with a myriad of choices, none of which seem clearly effective or desirable, the idea of ignoring the whole thing and doing nothing is appealing—especially when your diagnosis is not preceded by symptoms. Although inactivity may feel like a means of escape from an unpleasant situation, it has potential consequences. It is a choice, not an escape.

Doing nothing is certainly a reasonable choice when none of the available treatment options promise enough benefit to outweigh their potential adverse effects.

Insurance limitations

Beware of sentences beginning with "Your insurance will cover...." The question preceding this statement will usually be "What insurance do you have?"

This is an indication that the list of options being offered to you is limited by restrictions placed by your insurance company or managed care group on reimbursement.

Ask for the full list of options. Information on what your insurance will cover is important, but you are the one who will decide whether or not to pay the extra price for out-of-plan tests, procedures, or medications. Lack of pregnancy coverage has not stopped people from having babies, but treatment for chronic or critical diseases is often assumed to be limited by your insurance coverage.

Occasionally a patient who has been denied coverage by an insurance company will challenge the insurance company with a carefully researched case and will receive approval for compensation.

Experimental options

Ask about clinical trials. Let your physician know if you feel inclined to consider participation in a trial. He may already be familiar with an appropriate trial or may be able to suggest nearby treatment centers to contact.

In your readings you may come across some research that is so new that it is not yet in a clinical trial. If you are interested in exploring new research ideas, let your physician know to share that information with you as well. For more detailed information on clinical trials, see Chapter 8, *Researching Clinical Trials*.

When discussing an experimental treatment with your physician, you might ask if he would recommend it to one of his family members if they were in your situation. What would be his concerns?

Alternative and complementary options

Your view of what is an acceptable treatment may change over time. Sometimes after having exhausted the standard treatment options, patients will begin to look at alternative therapies or consider ways to complement standard treatment with less conventional therapies.

A woman with severe endometriosis explains why she began to consider alternative options:

> *As I become more familiar with what was available for treating endometriosis, I became frustrated with the lack of new information. I*

came to the same wall that everyone else does whether they are patients or doctors.

Some patients are more inclined to begin with a diet and exercise approach and then fall back on medical treatment if they are not satisfied with the results. For example, you might try to manage high blood pressure with dietary changes or a nutritional supplement to see if that works before you begin taking a medication to control your blood pressure.

Your doctor's medical training and expertise are focused on well-researched reliable forms of treatment. He may not be familiar with the broad spectrum of alternative and complementary approaches. These may require more research on your part to carefully weigh the safety and effectiveness of those options. See Chapter 9, *Complementary and Alternative Therapies*, for more information on how to research and evaluate these options.

Getting to know your medical team

Your primary care physician is the frontline person for a whole team of people working behind the scenes to evaluate your condition. When she gives you an explanation of your diagnosis, prognosis, and treatment recommendations, she is consolidating information from multiple sources. Each member of the team brings a special area of expertise to the evaluation process. For example, your primary physician will not go to the lab and watch your blood go through the analyzer; she will rely on the report from the lab technician who reads the test. Your oncologist will consult a pathologist for an explanation of your pathology report, and your surgeon will consult the radiologist for her interpretation of your x-ray films.

Don't be afraid to ask questions of the other specialists on your team. Some specialists normally have little contact with patients, so you might experience some initial reluctance, but if you ask concise knowledgeable questions that have a clear impact on your decision-making process, they will usually take the time to explain. Here are some examples of the people who might help you to understand your situation:

- **Pathologists and lab technicians.** Feel free to ask for a copy of your pathology report. You can even call the lab if you have questions about the range of values, if that is not explained on the report, or what distinguishes a normal result from an abnormal one. A man recounts his discussions with a lab technician who was drawing his blood in the hospital:

A senior med tech came in to draw my blood a couple of times. I asked her questions about the hemoglobin, the protein, and what it all meant. At that point no one knew if my intestinal bleeding had stopped or what might be the source. Understanding the blood tests helped me feel like at least I was in a little bit of control. We had no idea about the future, but this knowing more about what the blood tests were showing gave me comfort.

- **Radiologists and technicians.** You can ask to see your films. Often your primary physician or specialist will show them to you as she explains the findings. Although you may find it difficult to isolate the distinctions seen on a film, it can be helpful to have an experienced radiologist explain the characteristics she looks for and what those characteristics indicate.

- **Other specialists.** Depending on your condition, you will be referred to a surgeon, cardiologist, oncologist, neurologist, or other specialist. A specialist is comfortable talking with patients and usually has a passion for the specialty she is treating. She can give you ideas about what to expect, what leading-edge options to investigate, and direct you to recent medical journal articles that address your specific condition. Her experience gives her a well-developed intuitive sense about what options might be more likely to work successfully. Don't be afraid to ask for an opinion, with the understanding her answer will be based on her own general experience.

- **Nurses and nurse practitioners.** Nurses often spend more time with you and know you more intimately than your physician. The nurse's job is to help you prepare for the next step. They listen and they observe. Their perspective and full attention to your well-being can make them valuable liaisons in your initial understanding of the confusing and sometimes overwhelming information that is suddenly thrust on you along with a diagnosis.

- **Pharmacists.** A good pharmacist can keep you up-to-date on new medications for ongoing conditions, alert you to possible drug interactions (a good reason for having all your prescriptions filled at the same pharmacy), and help you learn more about how to take the medications you are using. A man with HIV talks about the role his pharmacist plays in his ongoing care:

> I see the pharmacist as a primary care provider for someone with HIV. I literally went shopping for a good pharmacist—it's what you have to do. The one I have now will tell me about medications to talk about with my doctor. When I had to do injections of pain medication, I was really scared it would trigger an addiction so I wasn't taking the medication. He went through the whole process with me and taught me about the appropriate use of pain medication.

Knowing your own interests and limitations

If two people set out to research the same condition, they might each have a different set of questions. The extent of your research depends on your energy level, how much time you have, your family situation, your confidence in your doctors, past experiences, prognosis, your perspective on quality of life, etc.

You might want to know:

- Everything—because knowledge is comfort to you
- All about the effectiveness of medical treatment options available to you
- What experimental or alternative treatments might offer you
- Just enough to competently make the decision just ahead of you at this stage of your condition
- Enough to know whether you can trust your doctor's recommendations for treatment (i.e., is this the standard treatment?)

Especially if you are having someone else help you research (see Chapter 3, *Helping a Friend or Family Member*, and Appendix A, *Patient Questionnaire*), you'll want to be very clear about what you are looking for.

Your beliefs

Although you may not be able to define clearly your philosophic or spiritual perspective, you will sense when that boundary is being crossed. You may believe strongly in mind-body connections or you may not. You may want to explore information that seems plausible to you, without feeling pressured to embrace it completely. If it takes cause-and-effect explanations to prove the validity of an argument for you, look for those and discard approaches that don't fit your criteria for consideration. You may also have spiritual beliefs that help guide you in your search and in your decision-making.

Be honest with yourself and with those around you about the approaches you want to pursue and the ones you don't. Your approach may shift in response to life changes and experiences. If it does, acknowledge it to yourself and communicate that to the people around you who want to help you.

When a well-meaning friend assumes that you share the same belief system or that you would benefit from adopting beliefs that you do not feel comfortable with, be honest with him. Assure him that you appreciate his concern, but your way of looking at things is different from his. Spend your time pursuing what feels right to you, not fulfilling an obligation to try out someone else's belief system.

Your boundaries

The goal of researching your condition is not to become an authority. It is to understand enough to evaluate the choices that you may need to make. You might not want to read about, hear about, or look at graphic illustrations of every possible outcome. Remember to ask yourself how much you really want to know before you dig deeper.

At certain times you may feel more vulnerable or suggestible than other times. Be alert to your feelings and don't go any further than feels comfortable to you at that moment.

Anxiety may build as you research and anticipate possible outcomes. You may feel fine during the day but wake up at night with your mind spinning through frightening scenarios. Those of us with vivid imaginations often give ourselves quite a workout. Recognize when you feel anxious, exhausted, or saturated with information and take a break. Often when you come back to your research refreshed, you will see it more clearly.

One of the best things a friend can do is filter information for you. When your anxiety level gets too high, but you need some specific answers, ask a friend to help. You can explain what you are looking for and what you would prefer not to read or see.

Hope is intertwined with your sense of well-being. If you don't want to hear about the negative aspects of a choice you have made or about someone else's bad experience described in vivid detail, let the people around you know and ask them to respect your feelings. Each person has a unique physical response to a particular treatment. We each make our own choices and then we work to achieve the best possible outcomes. If you feel uncomfortable hearing a story, ask the person telling it to avoid sharing the details with you. You can ask for more detail later if you decide it is relevant.

Managing your time and resources

In the perfect world we would all have plenty of time to spend doing research and all the choices would be clear-cut and easy to make. But jobs, family, and friends require your attention. Evaluate how much time, energy, and money you have to spend on research and pace yourself.

Jobs

If you are working a full-time job, your research hours may be limited to evenings and weekends, unless you have the freedom where you work to search the Internet during your workday. Medical libraries may be open only the hours that you are at work.

You may not have the vacation time or extra income to travel to distant cities to talk with specialists. However, if you identify resources or people whose perspective might be helpful to you, look at your network of friends and see if there is someone who might be able to visit that resource for you. You can also make contact by phone, mail, fax, or email to ask for and exchange information. Another option is to hire a professional researcher.

Family

Your immediate family will continue to need your attention, especially if you have young children. Your daily schedule may already be disrupted by frequent visits to doctors and treatment centers. Some family members may offer to help. If you can include them in the research process, it will help them understand what is happening to you and appreciate the complexities of the decisions you are trying to make.

Do not enlist research help from family members who already have a set of opinions about what they think you should do. If they offer to help, ask them to help with household tasks or errands to give you a little more time to work on health-related tasks.

Social life

Listen to your feelings. If a social outing sounds more appealing than a visit to the library or an evening in front of the computer, choose the social event and enjoy yourself.

Talking socially with other people is also a form of research. Informal, but sometimes valuable, contacts are often made through friends of friends. Or maybe someone you meet at a social gathering will mention an article she saw recently which will provide the clue that leads you to your next step.

Quiet time

If you are tired, rest. Allow yourself some quiet time to relax and slow down the pace of your thoughts. If you can find a distraction-free place, go there when you need to think.

Exercise, meditation, and prayer all bring your mind to a quieter place. Schedule them as a balance to periods of intense research.

CHAPTER 2

Knowing Your Rights

FACED WITH A DIAGNOSIS that may require extensive treatment such as surgery, ongoing medication, or anything requiring a hospital stay, you may sometimes feel confused or powerless. The very speed of treatment in a potentially life-threatening disease heightens this feeling of loss of control. Remember that it is your right to know and make choices about what is happening and that information will empower you.

This chapter deals with the rights you need to know about in order to make choices about your healthcare. We start with an overview of your right to participate. Then we look at the issue of informed consent when you are being presented with treatment options. The chapter ends with an extensive discussion of your rights to medical records, including why you might want or need access to your records and how to get it.

Your right to participate

Understanding your own diagnosis and participating in the decisions about your own treatment is one of your rights. You are the one person most concerned with the outcome of any treatment and you are most familiar with your own situation and preferences.

When the diagnosis is not known, the more you understand about the process, the more you feel you can cope with what is happening.

A patient with unexplained gastrointestinal bleeding said of the diagnostic procedures:

> Some of the people in the hospital were saying, "Oh, we're not sure what this is." It depended on who you talked with. The experienced staff members were easy to deal with. They were confident and reassuring because they had knowledge.

One nurse practitioner knew what she was talking about.... They
sent her to explain and answer my questions. I would ask about the
hemoglobin, the protein, the chemistry test, what was H-pylori? She
would knowledgeably discuss these things with me.

That's all I wanted. Knowledge made me feel like at least I was in a
little bit of control when I didn't know what was happening. I had no idea
of the future. Knowledge gave me comfort. I was in an information gather-
ing mode.... I would get as much information as I could from those people.

While some people can't get enough information about their diagnosis, others are not yet ready to face a diagnosis. It is also your right to absorb information as slowly as your emotions can handle that information, in order to
help you cope with these unwelcome changes in your health.

One patient looks back on her state of mind before back surgery:

After I checked out my surgeon and found out he was well-trained
and had a good reputation and then looked at the pictures of the knee sur-
gery, I didn't want to know any more. There was a whole section on the
complications of that knee surgery, but I couldn't even think about that. I
just prayed I wouldn't have any of those complications. I had to let go and
trust. Knowing too much would have made me crazy just then.

Another factor that impacts your right and need to get information about
your health is the advent of managed care. Managed care is most effective
when you manage your own care. You're probably all too familiar with many
changes in healthcare delivery in recent years. Increasingly we hear from the
media or friends of the problems patients have with denial of treatment,
postponement of treatment, or even receiving the wrong treatment. Individual physicians are often scheduled so tightly they only have only ten minutes with each patient. Often physicians cannot refer patients to specialists
outside of their own clinic or group, even if a particular specialist has the
expertise necessary and is exactly whom that patient needs to see.

One physician spoke of his own frustrations with managed care:

The phone call on Monday that makes my stomach sick is the phone
call from a patient who says, "I saw my doctor last Friday and they told
me to call you. They said I'd better see you sometime early this week."

That makes my heart sink because that's not her job to call the office in a panic, trying to set up her own referral.

Managed care has made things complicated because sometimes the person wants to be referred but doesn't have the authority in the system to make it happen. Sometimes the doctor will have to say, "I'd love to do this for you, but you'll have to go to your primary care doctor to get a referral." It becomes very complicated.

Another physician candidly commented:

If people think managed care is working or efficient, they just haven't been really sick lately.

With these and other changes, it becomes increasingly important that each individual act as her own advocate or have a friend or family member become that advocate. The body of law dealing with patients' rights is growing as health consumers demand to have some control over managed care, HMOs, hospital stays, and decisions about their own treatment.

You are probably quite comfortable and capable exercising your rights in most consumer areas such as automobile purchases, returning defective merchandise, etc. As a patient or consumer of healthcare, you also have many legal rights. These include:

- Right to see and copy medical records
- Right to obtain copies of tests
- Right to expect the privacy and confidentiality of your medical records
- Right to seek second opinions
- Right to register complaints
- Right to full disclosure if you are being asked to participate in clinical trials or research studies (more on this in Chapter 8, *Researching Clinical Trials*)
- Right to refuse treatment at any time
- Right to be informed about and consent to any treatment

Learning to exercise your rights can help you become a partner in your own medical care and to participate in treatment decisions. Exercising your rights will also help you avoid feeling like a victim of the healthcare system.

Informed consent

One of your rights and, in fact, the basis of patients' rights legislation is the concept of informed consent. The guideline for informed consent is that you, the patient, must understand three things about proposed treatment:

- Risks
- Benefits
- Alternatives

You must consent to treatment that involves touch or any invasive procedure. In order to consent, you must be informed about the specifics of each treatment or procedure and understand that treatment or procedure.

If you have not been informed of the risks, benefits, and alternatives for a procedure or drug regimen, and/or you have not consented to that procedure, the medical personnel treating you can be in serious legal trouble. If they have performed any procedure without consent, they may be legally committing assault and battery or criminal negligence. While informed consent policies and practices are generated by a combination of protecting patients' preferences and wanting to do the right thing, the motivation for these policies is combined with the very real fear of legal action.

It is no surprise that when consent guidelines are met, patient satisfaction usually increases and malpractice lawsuits usually decrease.

Hospital and physician consent policies

Hospitals establish structures and policies to support patients' rights. Hospitals and larger clinics have elaborate printed consent forms and policies. They also have requirements for advance directives, which is a legal document stating your healthcare choices and selecting someone to act on your behalf in case you are incapacitated. These consent regulations differ from state to state, but most states have similar provisions. All hospitals must actively exercise a formal consent process in order to be accredited by the Joint Commission on the Accreditation of Healthcare Organizations (JCAHO). The Patients' Rights section of the JCAHO's *Comprehensive Accreditation Manual for Hospitals* lists many specific standards that hospitals must meet to comply with the patients' rights requirements. One of these standards, RI 1.2.1, requires that informed consent must be obtained for every procedure and must be checked off or documented for every patient.[1]

Most insurers, including Medicare, will not pay for services in hospitals that do not meet the standards of the JCAHO and/or do not have JCAHO accreditation. With quality care, reimbursement, and their reputations at stake, hospitals take informed consent, accreditation, and patients' rights very seriously.

Physicians' offices are usually less formal than hospitals, but physicians, too, must inform you of the risks, benefits, and alternatives required by the doctrine of informed consent. Physicians are also at risk of losing reimbursement or even attracting malpractice lawsuits if they do not fully inform you of the risks, benefits, and alternatives for your treatment. They and their staff members will make a special effort to be sure that you have the information you need. You have every right to insist that you understand tests and any proposed treatment so that you can actively participate in decisions regarding your care.

Both in hospital and office settings, responsibilities to inform the patients and get their consent are often delegated to nurses, admitting personnel, and others. Only if it is the responsibility of a nurse or allied health professional to explain the risks and benefits of a procedure can the legal responsibility of informed consent be transferred. The ultimate responsibility for consent, however, still lies with the physician and hospital.

Can you modify a consent form?

If you enter a hospital for treatment, you are usually asked to sign a blanket consent form that will pre-authorize most procedures that can occur during your entire stay. You can ask to modify the form in several ways that may better reflect your wishes. For example, you can write your own modifications on the consent form to include some or all of the following limitations:

- You can consent only to procedures performed by a specific physician or surgeon.

- You can withhold consent to be treated by medical students, interns, or nursing and allied health students, even if you are in a teaching hospital.

- You can note that you consent only to the agreed-on procedure and not to any additional procedures that may be deemed necessary once the procedure has begun. (Of course, this might not be in your own best interests if this limitation causes riskier surgery at a later date.)

- You can specify that you do not consent to any transfusion of blood products.

Facing possible surgery, one woman who works in a large metropolitan teaching hospital made a notation on her consent form regarding surgeons:

Working in this hospital side by side with the surgical residents I know they are students—very bright students, but still students. I realize there are a few I would not want working on me if I needed surgery.

I decided if I do have to have surgery for my condition, I would specify in writing that I didn't want any of the residents doing any of the surgery, since you never knew who would be scheduled or on call. It was okay with me if they observed, or even assisted.

My surgeon assured me that this was a legitimate request and that many patients make this request. I felt much more relaxed making a medical decision, knowing that if I needed surgery, my own experienced surgeon would be doing the entire surgery.

You can simply write these or any other limitations in the margins of the forms before you sign. If you are told that you will not be treated at all if you modify the form, you could ask to speak with an administrator or to be transferred to a different hospital. It's best if you can clear up any misunderstanding early since it may be extremely difficult to exercise your option of changing hospitals or physicians when a time-sensitive surgery or procedure may save your life. You can also simply sign the consent form with the notation "signed under duress" noting that you requested changes that were not allowed. If you signed under duress, the consent form would probably be considered void in a court of law.

Medical records

As one part of the "informed" in informed consent, you are entitled to know what has been put into your medical record before agreeing to any procedure or treatment. You will be hearing treatment recommendations based on these medical records, and you may be able to make more effective and informed decisions if you see the actual medical records that contain your diagnosis and test results. Each doctor or medical professional may interpret your tests and records from the point of view of his own background and training. Interpretation can differ and it's best if you have the basic facts yourself.

As one patient put it:

> I had been an active jogger, running about 20 miles per week and entering the occasional 5K or 10K race. During one of those races I actually heard my knee "snap." An hour later it was swollen larger than a grapefruit! With ice I could keep the swelling down, but I knew I needed some kind of treatment if I wanted to run again—or even walk without pain.
>
> I went to a sports medicine doctor who took x-rays and recommended physical therapy and anti-inflammatory drugs. Luckily I got copies of the x-rays, because I took them to a surgeon who recommended surgery. Finally, I'd heard of a chiropractor who had success with knee injuries. I took the x-rays to him and he recommended chiropractic adjustments.
>
> I started out with the least invasive therapy that was the chiropractor but eventually had to have surgery. It fascinated me at the time that looking at the same knee and the same x-rays, each of the professionals recommended a different treatment. And then I thought, "Duh. of course. They'll always recommend what they are trained for."

Accessing older medical records

Each doctor visit or hospital stay generates medical records that are stored for some length of time—from a few years to over 100 years. Physicians usually keep records for at least 7 years or as long as the patients are still seeing that physician. Hospitals keep medical records much longer, often 25 to 30 years or longer. Each state regulates the length of time medical records must be kept.

If a physician retires, the records by law are transferred to another provider. Similarly, hospital records will be transferred if hospitals merge or close. So you may have to be a detective to find your records, but with diligence you can locate them and legally obtain copies. Some agencies that can help you locate doctors and merged or closed hospital records are:

- The American Medical Association, at *http://www.ama-assn.org*
- The American Hospital Association, at *http://www.aha.org*

Medical records laws vary

Currently US laws regarding access to medical records differ from state to state. In 1996 Congress passed the Health Insurance Portability and Accountability Act (HIPAA), which was intended to reduce administrative costs of healthcare by making possible the electronic transmission of administrative and financial healthcare records. In November of 1999 the Health and Human Services Department announced the proposed privacy standards for individually identifiable health information covered by HIPAA. These new privacy standards are law as of February 2000. While state laws address most medical records law, these new privacy standards for electronic transmission of medical records are federal law and impact all states. Until recently federal laws dealing with medical records and patients rights covered only federal government employees and those using VA hospitals.

Those aspects of medical records law that are not involved in electronic transmission of records are still covered by the laws of the state where the treatment is performed. More than half of the states have medical records access legislation, and there are currently over 30 bills in the US Congress dealing with the safety of and access to medical records. As insurers and hospital systems expand across state lines, many state laws will become subject to federal regulation. The technological innovation of the electronic medical record, which can be electronically transported across state lines, will probably lead to more federal regulation for medical records.

The web site at the American Medical Informatics Association, *http://www. amia.org*, provides one place to keep track of new and changing medical records legislation. Another web site for following medical records law is the . US Department of Health and Human Services web site at *http://www.dhhs.gov.*

Who owns your medical records?

All of the state laws basically agree that the medical records are the legal property of the healthcare provider or hospital, although it might seem that you are the one who would own your medical records. Sometimes insurance companies claim that the records are their property as well, since they paid for the services.

The information in the medical record, however, is the property of you, the patient. While you would not own the original medical record, you are legally entitled to copies of that record. You will usually be asked to pay a modest sum for copies, so it is best to look at your records and request only those pages that are relevant to your continuing care. For example, in California, AB610 establishes medical records access with charges not to exceed 25 cents/page or 50 cents/page if the records are on microfilm.

Why would you want your medical record?

You may neither need nor want copies of all of your medical records, but the most essential are those records dealing with insurance claims or ongoing conditions. Other useful records are those providing baseline information. These would include medical history, baseline EKGs and bone density screenings, all surgeries and treatments for serious conditions, prescriptions for current medications and eyeglasses, diagnostic tests including blood work and diagnostic imaging, immunizations, allergies and drug reactions, and copies of advance directives. All of these records can assist you in participating actively in your own care. Some of the reasons you would request copies of your medical records include:

- Understanding your medical condition more fully in order to participate in treatment decisions
- Acting as your own communications coordinator among the many different health professionals providing your care
- Having a legal document which describes any care you received, especially if there are questions about reimbursement or appropriate provision of care
- Verifying which services are covered by your health insurance
- Assisting you in preventing recurrence of the disease or condition in the future
- Maintaining continuity in your own healthcare if you move or if your health providers change (a real possibility in the managed care climate)
- Being able to ask your doctor to correct inaccuracies in the record that might have serious consequences at a later date (e.g., wrong blood type)

One woman who requested the results of her recent test was really surprised when she read the record:

> I had been going through tests for abdominal pain. My doctor
> thought it could be pancreatitis or a problem with my gallbladder. They
> recommended a CT scan.

I asked for the report as soon as it was available, because I was worried about the pancreatitis. When I read the report, I was immediately relieved to see the report said that I did not have pancreatitis. Then to my amazement I went on to read that my prostate was normal! Since I'm a woman and only males have a prostate gland, I wondered whose report I was reading.

When I went back to the radiology department, they had some confusion about who had dictated the report and said it was probably just a typo and to relax. I said no, and that I wanted another CT scan at their expense. They were going to perform gallbladder surgery based on this test and I didn't even know if it was I in the picture. Since the CT scan is expensive they tried to talk me out of it but I insisted. The second time around, they got the report right.

I think everyone should read all of their tests to make sure they are accurate. Also if a different doctor looks at your records and tries to tell you something you think is wrong, you will be able to say with authority, "That's not what the radiology report showed!" I was really lucky that I insisted on seeing my record—and getting it corrected!

One woman explains that keeping her medical records gives her a sense of control over her healthcare:

I can't imagine NOT keeping my medical records. Having my records gives me a sense of control in case there is ever a dispute or a question about when some test or treatment was given and what were the results. I want to know what the records say. Medical records are easy to keep—you can just put them all in a folder.

Without my records, I would feel less in control than I already do. We're at the mercy of the medical establishment. The doctors are so over scheduled they just don't have the time to look at my records even if they have them. I don't feel like I have a really personal relationship with my doctor, not like the family doctor in the small town where I grew up who just remembered my medical history. I've heard so many horror stories from people who were billed twice or for services they hadn't received. I also know people who were denied care or some test. If they had their records, they would have had a basis for demanding the care.

An emergency nurse shares some additional and very compelling reasons for keeping track of medications:

> *As an emergency department nurse and trauma coordinator, I found that people do not realize how important it is to know what drugs they are taking and what the doses are, including over-the-counter (OTC) drugs. Most often, when asked, the reply is "I take a pink one in the morning and half of a yellow one at noon and seven different ones at night."*

> *I try to educate on the importance of having all your information in one place so you are not delaying treatment for any reason. One of the techniques I offer is that of putting a list on the inside of the medicine cabinet, listing all the drugs, including OTCs, their doses, how often you take them, and the physician's phone number. This is applicable for each person in the family. This can be accomplished with the assistance of a family member or pharmacist.*

What information is contained in a medical record?

In a hospital setting many health professionals including nurses, physical therapists, dietitians, and educators as well as physicians contribute to the medical record of each patient. The Joint Commission on the Accreditation of Healthcare Organizations (JCAHO) and many other state and federal regulating agencies require that medical records include:

- Identification information about a patient (SSN, age, address, etc.)
- Medical history including family history provided by patient
- Physical examination reports
- Diagnosis and therapeutic orders
- Informed consent documentation or indication of the reason for its absence (i.e., patient not mentally competent)
- Observations of the patient including results of therapy
- Reports of all procedures and tests, and their results
- Conclusions at the end of a hospital stay or after evaluation and treatment and discharge instructions
- Evidence that the patient has received education regarding their medical situation and drug and discharge recommendations

Limitations to medical records access

While you are legally entitled to see and have copies of your medical records in most instances, there are a few limitations to this access, including:

- You must be an adult in order to access your records. You can see and get copies of only your own medical records, with very few exceptions.

- You would be limited in accessing the medical records of another person unless you are the designated patient's legal representative or conservator.

- As a parent and/or legal guardian, you may be denied access to the records of your children if the provider believes that such access would be detrimental to the child, as in the case of child abuse.

- You would be denied access to records involved with mental health, substance abuse, and HIV status. These are legally sealed to protect the patient from discrimination.

Most institutions allow access to medical records during certain business hours and recommend that you make an appointment to be sure someone will be there to assist you. Medical records departments are extremely busy places, so it's a good idea to make it easy for people to help you.

What should you do if you are denied access to your medical record?

To quote George J. Annas' excellent book *The Rights of Patients: the Basic ACLU Guide to Patient Rights,* if denied access to your medical records, you should "raise hell."[2] Some great ways to do this include:

- Calling the medical records department and asking for the supervisor or director

- Making formal complaints to the hospital ethics committee and/or governing board of the hospital

Formal complaints about any problems with medical records access, or any hospital services for that matter, should contain the following elements:

- Your full name and address and a way to contact you

- The names and addresses of the provider(s) and/or the hospital where the problem originated

- Specific details of the problem including dates and location

- Witnesses' names and their explanation of what occurred if you have this information

- Copies of medical records and any other information pertinent to the complaint

You can also contact your own state department of health, which controls medical licensure, as well as the office of consumer affairs, insurance, or department of corporations in your state. Usually the front pages of your local telephone book list these offices for each state. In most cases, informing hospital administrators that a request has been denied will be effective. As a last resort, you can seek legal representation, but this should rarely be necessary. Hospitals and clinics know that courts have consistently ruled in favor of the patients.

Resources for accessing medical records, tests, and reports

The American Health Information Management Association (AHIMA), formerly the American Medical Records Association, provides excellent information on medical records for consumers of healthcare. Their state chapters can assist you in finding the laws regarding medical records for your state. You can locate the AHIMA web site at *http://www.ahima.org.*

Each state has an attorney general's office that can also assist in determining patients' rights legislation and the medical records access law.

How private is my medical record?

Your medical records are protected by law. As stated earlier, legislation is being written to expand this protection due to the introduction of electronic medical records. Federal standards for the privacy of medical information have just been enacted since these records can now be transferred easily across many jurisdictions. Medical records, at least electronic medical records, can be obtained only under certain conditions from any and all insurance companies and healthcare providers for the following purposes:

- To allow health information to be used only for treatment and payment for healthcare

- To be disclosed while protecting individual identities without an individual's authorization for purposes such as research, public health and oversight in specifically defined situations

- To require written authorization from the patient for the use and disclosure of health information for any purpose other than treatment, payment, or national priority purposes

The guidelines have been adopted in order to create a set of fair information practices to inform people how their information is being used and disclosed. It requires providers to maintain safeguards to protect the confidentiality of individual health information.

Under the new guidelines, individuals are assured that they will receive written notice of information practices from health plans and providers and will be informed if those practices change. As always, individuals still have the right to obtain their own health records and to request amendment and/or correction of health information that is inaccurate or incomplete. Finally, individuals have the right to receive an accounting of the instances where protected health information has been disclosed for purposes other than treatment, payment, or healthcare operations. Some exceptions are still in force for disclosure of records essential to law enforcement and health oversight agencies.

Test results and your medical record

If tests are done while hospitalized, those tests and pathology reports will become a part of the hospital's medical record and would be accessible through the medical records department.

However, many tests are done in separate laboratories and you would need to access them separately. One strong recommendation is to ask your physician to request that a copy of any test, as well as copies of tests that are sent to other health practitioners, be sent to you, e.g., the tests your surgeon sends to your internist, etc.

Questions to ask about tests

As an aspect of the informed consent guideline, you are entitled to information on any test your physician prescribes. You should understand the following information before you undergo any testing:

- What is the purpose of the test? Is it used to diagnose a specific disease or to track the effectiveness of a given therapy? Some tests are part of routine physical examination and others are selected to diagnose a specific condition.

- Are any preparations necessary for the test? Do you need to fast or to drink fluids, etc? Should you wear a certain type of clothing? Will you need to arrange for transportation?

- How long will the test take and what is it like? Does the test take ten minutes or three hours? Will blood and urine samples be taken? Will you be given anesthesia or a sedative?

- Will the test cause any side effects such as swelling, headache, drowsiness, etc.? Which side effects are expected and which should be reported to your physician?

- Will I need special care or need to be under observation after the test or procedure? How long will this take?

- Will results of the test assist in diagnosis or selecting treatment modalities and is the test really necessary? Do you already have a clear diagnosis?

A retired healthcare professional was surprised at changes when she herself became a patient. She had always told patients about their rights, but found it difficult at first to exercise her own rights:

> After I went to UCLA, the doctor there sent a lengthy report, as they always do, to the doctor I've been seeing ever since. I was wise enough to ask a copy to be sent to me.
>
> One of the things he thought should be done was a muscle test. It's invasive and it's really painful. I remember feeling and saying to my doctor, that I didn't want to do that. I said it fearfully and he just looked at me like I was crazy and he said, "Sandy, no one is going to make you do anything you don't want to do."
>
> That had completely escaped me. I was in this mode. I was doing what I was told to do. It didn't dawn on me that, of course, I had some rights here. I ended up not having that test done. All it was going to do was say, "Yes, she has MS." I already knew that. That was a remarkable moment. It's so simple.

Tools for deciphering test results and medical records

Sometimes physicians worry that you may misunderstand the tests and reports, so you may have to reassure your physician that you will get assistance in interpreting the test results you don't fully understand.

There are several tools that can assist you in understanding your test results listed in Appendix B, *Resources*. Usually the laboratory tests indicate what the norm is for a certain test and whether your results are higher or lower than that norm. Also many pathologists and laboratories attach references so that a patient can understand their test results.

There are also many medical abbreviations, acronyms, and numerical designations for medical conditions and procedures that may make medical records difficult to comprehend. There are several information sources that can help clarify the language.

Often, when you request medical records and test results and/or billing information, you may get a piece of paper that is mostly numbers. The books listed in the next few paragraphs and others in Appendix B can help decipher these codes.

One useful book is *Current Procedural Terminology*,[3] or CPT, for physicians. This is a listing of codes for procedures, services and supplies. It is used for billing and for ordering tests and is updated annually by the American Medical Association and contains numerical designations for each procedure. Categories are listed in five-digit classifications.

While the CPT is used primarily for procedures, another important tool, the ICD, *International Classification of Diseases*,[4] is a numerical list of diseases or conditions requiring medical treatment. It is arranged with three-digit and decimal subcategories. The ICD is also updated frequently, but not necessarily annually.

Table 2-1 provides some examples of classifications.

Table 2-1. Classification Examples

ICD Category	CPT Procedure
540—Acute appendicitis	44950—Appendectomy
174.1—Malignant neoplasm of female breast	19160—Mastectomy, partial
410—Acute myocardial infarction	92950—Cardio resuscitation
718.85—Instability, hip	27130—Hip arthroplasty
584—Acute renal failure	90935—Hemodialysis

If you see a medical record or a bill with a long list of five-digit numbers, the CPT code book can help you decipher the specifics for the procedures in that record. If it is filled with three-digit numbers, look into the ICD. One web site that further explains the ICD numbering system is *http://www.cdc.gov/nchs/icd9.htm.*

Since these code numbers are nearly always required for insurance reimbursement, the ICD and CPT books are in most physicians' offices and clinics. Medical libraries and larger public libraries are also likely to have the CPT and the ICD.

Finally, it is useful to have a recent medical dictionary. Many medical dictionaries, such as *Mosby's* or *Taber's,* or even a reference like *The Merck Manual* are relatively small and reasonably priced. These are listed in Appendix B.

The pragmatic health consumer

When you need medical care, you select the best doctors and nurses and other health professionals available to you. You are relying on their professional training, skill, and experience. Then you literally trust them with your life. So, it is a good idea to give them reasons to work with you. While you want to be an active advocate in all matters concerning your own health, it is wise to be tactful and to avoid being confrontational.

Understanding your rights as a healthcare consumer brings with it the responsibility to guard and act on those rights. As your own healthcare advocate you are responsible for staying as healthy as you can and to keep track of your own health and health needs. In addition to keeping files of your medical records, you might want to keep a personal health log. Include in this log dates and length of illnesses such as pneumonia, flu, measles, mumps, chicken pox, etc. Also include lists of any drugs, foods, plants, or chemicals that cause allergic reactions. Other items may include travel to countries or areas that may have involved exposure to typhoid or other deadly disease and family health histories which may indicate you have a tendency towards developing some condition in the future.

Several free and fee-based health history programs are now available through the Internet. The free web sites are connected to some of the general health web sites. Two of these free sites are Medscape at *http://www.medscape.com*, where you would click on My Medscape, and WebMD at *http://www.webmd.com.* Be cautious with the amount of personal detail you use on a "free" web site, however. One of the ways the free web sites make their money is by selling mailing lists and their own products to users with identified interests. You might, for example, use a fictitious name or imaginary postoffice box. Three of the fee-based services which have programs for keeping health records on your computer are Healthminder, Life Form, and HealthProfiler. Each has a web site where you can download or order the software. The web sites for these services are *http://www.healthminder.com, http://www.lifeform. com,* and *http://www.healthprofiler.com.* The prices for the programs range from 10 to 50 dollars, but each has a free trial you can use to see if it meets your needs.

While it is important and helpful to have copies of your own medical records, your best ally in health is still your primary care physician, if you regard that physician as your partner. You gain only a short-term sense of satisfaction but lose a great deal by creating an adversarial role with your primary care physician. If you really feel that your physician is not working for you, you always have the right to change physicians.

A woman who coped with a painful chronic condition until a new surgery was developed for her condition gives this advice:

> *Toward the end, I had a very bad experience with a doctor. So I changed doctors. I always encourage people who call me to do that. If it's not working for you, if you don't feel supported, if you feel threatened or confronted, you don't have to deal with that. It makes everything worse. So I always encourage people to change doctors…that they don't have to have this doctor that's not working out for them.*

Most of those working in healthcare—the physicians, nurses, laboratory personnel and other healthcare providers—really want to provide good care and they really want to help you stay healthy. In reality, the ideal premise for managed care is based on preventive medicine, i.e., catching health problems early so that they have the best chance of being treated simply and successfully.

As a pragmatic healthcare consumer, you might want to be a bit creative in achieving your goals. For example, if you have trouble getting medical records from one source, find one of your doctors whose office will assist you in collecting records from all of the sources. One doctor's office can ask all of your other doctors and laboratories that your records be sent to you. Patient records access is usually easier when requested by a doctor.

Another creative solution is to do your own research if you are denied a second opinion. Later chapters in this book explain how to determine what the standard and alternative treatments are for given conditions. You can then ask intelligently why your recommended treatment options are different or why one particular option was omitted. Often physicians in HMOs are directed to propose treatments covered only at their specific facility or clinic. They sometimes can arrange but not recommend alternative treatment or treatment elsewhere. Sometimes the physician's problem is that he simply does not have enough time to research new procedures or drugs and you can add to his knowledge base while contributing to your own wellness.

So, be aware of your rights, and exercise them. Get the information you need to make decisions, and use this information so that you won't jeopardize your own healthcare needs.

CHAPTER 3

Helping a Friend or Family Member

IN CHAPTER 1, *PREPARING FOR RESEARCH*, we emphasized planning and prioritizing before you start researching for yourself. Taking the time to ask questions before starting research is doubly important when researching for another person. You can't assume that the other person will want to know what you'd want to know in the same situation. There may be considerations or facts of which you're unaware. Good intentions and diligent work will not necessarily translate into research that someone else welcomes. To avoid wasted effort and to reduce the potential misunderstandings and bad feelings, focus on what's really needed or wanted by the patient herself.

In this chapter, we cover talking with the patient to learn what she wants, identifying your role in the partnership, making sure your initial information is accurate, and the chapter ends with information on accessing medical records.

Talking with the patient

When a patient does ask for help gathering information, spend some time talking with her to identify what sort of information she would like, her personal values and goals, and financial realities.

Your goals may or may not be in sync with the goals of the patient. Some of the reasons you might offer information are:

- You have been asked to help because you are skilled at research or have the time to help out.

- You have certain training, access to information, temperament, or often fill this kind of role in a family group.

- You want to show support and caring for another person. (There are other ways to show support that you could also explore.)

- Knowledge is comfort for you (this might be true for you, but not true for the patient).

- You don't want to accept a disease/condition/treatment/prognosis as true. You want to fight it.

- You doubt the competency of the patient to do research, even if the patient thinks otherwise.

- You believe that a certain kind of treatment is superior to one already chosen by the patient.

- You believe that another treatment modality (Western, nonintervention, spiritual, mind-body, Eastern, nutritional, etc.) is superior to the modality which the patient has chosen or is likely to choose.

Be clear with yourself about your motivation and goals. If you have offered to help someone gather information, make sure that person wants your help.

The patient may not want your help. If so, you'll need to accept that. If she feels comfortable with her level of understanding and the treatment recommended by the physician, respect that decision. The process of going through the treatment may require as much energy as she cares to focus on this part of her life at this point. Help in ways that are supportive of the choices she has made. If she experiences side effects during treatment, you may be able to offer your help then, finding ways to reduce those discomforts.

A need for privacy may also prevent a patient from accepting your offer of help. When she is told that her body is not functioning properly, she may be feeling a sense of failure or embarrassment. She might not want to expose the details of the problem to someone else. Be compassionate; give her the personal space to decide the level of detail she wants to share with you. Offer to help, but don't push.

You can use the questions in Appendix A, *Patient Questionnaire*, to help you clarify the patient's feelings, values, and expectations so you can develop a research plan together. If you are reading this chapter as a patient, you can use the questions as guidelines for working with anyone who offers you help doing research.

Types of information

If the patient asks for your help, let her direct what information to gather. Is she looking for information on a specific type of treatment or is she looking for additional treatment options? Does she want to know how the disease affects her body and how the treatment works to correct the condition? Does she want to know more about the expected outcome or possible side effects of a treatment?

Try to gauge the level of detail that she is seeking. Does she want to read source material or summaries of the technical material? Have her identify what she feels she already understands and what areas of the diagnosis and treatment process still seem unclear.

Personal contacts

The patient might prefer to talk to people rather than reading books or articles. Does the patient want to talk with other people who have been diagnosed with a similar condition who might have insights to share with her? Does she want to find specialists or researchers who can offer her their perspective and who might be aware of other treatment choices?

Discuss beforehand which perspectives the patient is willing to explore and which she would prefer to avoid. Is she interested in a mind-body approach? Does she want to hear from people who have tried alternative or complementary therapies? Does she want to learn more about leading edge research? A woman explains that some personal contacts were helpful while others were not:

> Where I live, many people use complementary and alternative therapies. When people found out I had cancer, many would start, unasked, telling me how I should treat it. Some of the suggestions felt simplistic and unwelcome, almost an assault. They'd bring me ugly looking mushrooms in jars to grow and eat; they'd tell me of someone without insurance who had cured himself of a terminal cancer with Gerson therapy; they'd hand me audiotapes so I could visualize my white blood cells like hungry sharks.
>
> Everyone had an opinion and I endured many. I told myself they meant well. I very much appreciated the advice of the people that I did ask. I tended to ask people who had specific experience. For example, the

nurse who led support groups told me about a great yoga class for cancer patients.

Belief systems

Be clear with yourself about the patient's spiritual and philosophical outlook. Be sensitive to her response to options or approaches that she does not feel comfortable considering. Do not pursue those. Ask her before you invest time in researching an option or a perspective that she has not expressed an interest in pursuing.

A man talks about recognizing that his belief system was different from that of some of his friends:

> *One of my best friends has a degree in Oriental medicine. I purposely have never discussed my condition with this friend. I simply did not want to be arm-twisted into giving up on Western medicine and trying acupuncture and herbs. I have confidence in Western medicine, where the whole story of my condition is really well known.*
>
> *The people I told were people I knew would be supportive of my treatment choices. The people I did not tell were the people I pretty well estimated would try to manipulate me into some other path or simply make me feel guilty about the path that I was on.*

Deciding what to research can be a difficult call to make, especially if your belief system differs from that of the patient. If you recognize tension developing when you bring up a particular topic, make a note of it and ask if this is an area you should continue to explore.

Disturbing information

Does the patient want to know how dismal the picture may be? Some do, others don't. Discuss this before you dig into the information. Never begin a sentence "You probably don't want to hear this..." If she doesn't want to hear it, don't bring it up.

Some patients want to know about possible negative outcomes and understand the risks as part of their decision-making process. Few people want to dwell on the negative risks once the decision is made. Statistics, too, can be depressing and they are sometimes misleading. If the patient wants statistics, be sure that you also collect the criteria that describe the particular group being assessed.

Even a patient who does not want protection from disturbing information might want shielding from a graphic description or illustration.

Financial limitations

Talk with the patient about her financial limitations. Looking at treatments in Europe for a patient in the United States will not be helpful if she is not financially able to go to Europe or pay for the treatment.

Of course you should also not just assume that Europe is out of reach. Ask if she is willing to consider options that might be difficult for her to cover financially.

Determining your role

Your job assisting the patient may be to find resources, filter information, or summarize information in a way that will help to clarify the next step. If you are researching treatment choices for a child, parent, or someone too sick or not mentally alert enough to make complex decisions, you may also *be* the designated decision-maker. In that case, your role might be to help the patient understand the treatment process and/or to make decisions that represent what he would want if he were able to decide for himself.

However, a patient doesn't always want help with decision-making. He may just need help finding his sense of direction. If the larger picture is overwhelming, help him define a series of smaller incremental steps. Ask him what specific things are worrying him. Once his concerns are aired, you can help him figure out the steps to take to resolve them.

A man hospitalized for intestinal bleeding describes how his wife helped him gather information about a test that was being considered by his physician:

> My doctor was talking about doing a visceral angiogram. I'd never heard of it before. The doctors seemed more cautious in discussing it than they were with the other procedures. So my wife went to the hospital library to see what she could find out about the procedure and when it should be done.

It turns out that the angiogram looks for the source of the bleeding. It really isn't going to be useful unless you are bleeding. At that point, I was convinced that I was no longer bleeding. I discussed this with my doctor and we decided to do the colonoscopy instead. The information my wife brought me helped me discuss the procedure with my doctor.

The following sections describe individual tasks you might perform for a patient. You might want to explore these suggested tasks with the patient as you work together on his research agenda.

Finding the best sources of information

If the patient wants to do his own reading, you can help refine the research process by identifying resources such as books, articles, or Internet sites that will yield the kind of information that he is seeking.

A woman inexperienced at using the Internet talks about the help she got looking for information from a more experienced friend:

When I got shingles, a friend searched the Internet for me. I know there are volumes of information out there you can access, but I don't know how to get to it. He does. He helped me find a couple of things that I hadn't been told by anyone else. One of them my doctor told me not to try, but the other one seemed to help.

Research requires a lot of sorting through the chaff. Probably more time is spent discarding inappropriate information than is spent reading helpful information. You can provide a valuable service if you help to identify sources for finding the best-documented, well-balanced information.

When giving resources, remember that less is more. Reduce a long list of possibilities to the several best resources—books, web sites, etc.—aimed precisely at issues the patient wants to consider. Consider the quality of the content and the reputation of the author or organization behind it.

Identifying questions

Time spent with the patient's doctor and other specialists is limited and needs to be used well. You can help the patient compile a list of questions for his doctor to increase his understanding of his condition and the options available to him.

Research will produce more questions than it answers in the beginning. As the patient's understanding grows, however, his questions will become more focused. You can work together to develop focused questions.

Finding specialists

Insight can be gained from speaking with specialists and researchers who have experience treating or studying the condition you are researching. These are the people who are most likely to know about promising new treatments.

You can help by identifying those experts, gathering their writings on the subject, and finding contact information for them.

Filtering information

Popular media often use sensational attention-grabbing headlines to get viewers for their program or to sell their magazine. Discoveries can be less important than they appear or fleeting in impact. For example, nationwide television newscasts might trumpet news of a treatment advance for Parkinson's that is really just preliminary results from a small study with mice. The treatment advance may well have some impact in scientific circles as indicating a promising future direction for further research; however its practical impact for a patient with Parkinson's—aside from offering hope that research is ongoing and may someday result in treatment advances—is very little.

Or, media might report particular studies without the context of other studies on the same condition or effect. Individual studies show only a small part of the total picture. You might well want to filter out the sensational "story of the day" or look for follow-up information to clarify the details.

Accounts of a disease that appear in medical literature can also be frightening to a newly-diagnosed patient who has not yet developed an overview of the prognosis for his particular situation. Medical journals tend to chronicle uncommon or severe cases, not the average case.

Prescreening contacts

Meeting another person who has been diagnosed with the same illness and faced with some of the same treatment choices can provide the patient with hope and perspective, but only if the attitude of the survivor is understanding and compassionate. The experience of meeting someone who has an angry or bitter attitude can be emotionally unsettling, as this woman explains:

> I have learned that I need to be careful who I talk to. When someone begins telling me in graphic detail about the problems they had with a treatment I am considering, I need to cut them off. One woman asked me if I was sick from my chemotherapy. When I said I wasn't, she told me that I would be, and then went on to tell me exactly how sick she had been.

An angry survivor may have valuable information, but you might want to make the initial contact yourself. Then you can ask the patient whether or not he would like to meet or talk with the person.

Summarizing information

A patient might not want to study the research materials himself, but would prefer a summary of the information. This is not an easy job, especially if you, too, are learning as you go.

If you are helping an aged parent or a child, it will be especially important to be able to translate what you find into reassuring and/or age-appropriate terms. After spending some time immersed in the subject yourself, you will begin to recognize the materials that offer the clearest explanation and can use them to help you with the overview.

Acting as an advocate

If you are a designated decision-maker, you will also be acting as an advocate. Sometimes a patient will want you to come along as an advocate or for support even though you are not an officially designated agent.

An HIV patient describes his search for an AIDS buddy to help him during visits to the doctor:

> I take someone with me to my appointment sometimes, especially when I'm scared. The first thing I did when I moved down to San Diego was look for an AIDS buddy. I go to AA. So I stood up at an AA meeting and said, "I need a professional healthcare person who is extremely aggressive but very obedient who will be my patient advocate."

Afterwards, this guy comes up to me and says, "I am HIV-positive but I have never been sick, so taking care of you will help me understand the disease better." It turns out he is a nurse, has extra nursing experience, like being an ER nurse and a trauma care nurse, and he is HIV-positive! I knew he was the right person—if it's not mutual, it's no good.

An oncologist observes that this is an area that you really need to explore carefully to be sure that you have a clear understanding of what exactly the patient would like you to do:

It takes reasonably good communication between the patient and her advocate so they know their roles before they get to the doctor's office. Some women have come in to see me and all of a sudden felt their advocate was much more of an advocate than they wanted.

A daughter explains how important this role became when her mother became too sick to take charge:

Normally if my mom was sitting here with us, her cognitive functions would be equal to ours. She takes care of all her own bills, she shops, and she knows what she needs. But she was really, really sick and by herself. Her main focus was on breathing and how to get to the bathroom and to the bed. Food was even out of her mind. No one would be able to keep it all together in that state. At that point, she needed our help to figure out what to do.

I talked with her doctors and one of my sisters researched the drug that they were suggesting. We all agreed the drug was worth trying. Now, she says the best thing she ever did was raise intelligent daughters.

Forming a partnership

You will want to develop a sense of partnership with the patient. If the patient is making the decisions, her concerns will be the focal point in the partnership. If you are acting as a healthcare agent, you will be the decision-maker, but the patient's needs and feelings remain the focus of that process.

Knowing that she has someone else working alongside her to find the best possible course of action gives the patient a sense of strength that she might not feel working by herself. You can be an even more effective partner by focusing on listening, observing, and brainstorming with the patient.

Listening

As well as being an information gatherer, you need to be an attentive listener. There are times when the patient just needs someone else to hear what she is thinking so that she can hear it herself. One woman describes how the listening process helped her mom make decisions:

> My mom would sometimes call me up to ask my opinion on a decision she was trying to make and then start arguing with me about the choices before I even had a chance to say anything. At the end of the call, she would hang up feeling confident that she knew what she wanted to do and I would hang up wondering what my opinion would have been if I'd had a chance to express it.

As you listen, you can note the recurrent concerns and the areas of resolution. The areas of concern will direct the next brainstorming sessions and future research.

Observing

The patient's doctor doesn't have much time to spend with the patient. A doctor generally has to rely on written reports from nurses and other medical personnel who come into contact with the patient during treatment or tests. The patient will be able to provide subjective information, but a third person, paying attention, can also offer valuable information. The mother of a young child describes how her observations changed the course of her son's treatment:

> When my 3-year-old son had leukemia, I kept charts of his response to the medications he was taking. I noticed that after one particular medication he always experienced a setback. The doctors were not happy with his progress. I mentioned my observation and showed them my charts. At first they discounted the possibility it was that particular medication causing the problem. Later, when their solutions didn't work, they came back to my charts and decided to change the medication. It worked. After that, they listened to what I had to say.

A woman talks about contacting her mother's doctor after realizing that the doctor probably wasn't aware of how sick her mother had become:

I drove to San Diego and stayed with my mom. I could see that she was getting weaker and weaker. I woke up in the middle of the night thinking, "My mom's dying and her doctors don't know it. Nobody's in charge and nobody's talking to each other." The next morning I got on the phone and called her doctors. Her primary care doctor called back in the evening. I explained the situation that I was seeing with my mother. The doctor said she would call the pulmonary specialist and agreed that we needed to speed up the diagnostic process.

Brainstorming

Brainstorming about difficult questions is invigorating and often helps to identify another way of looking at a problem or a new place to look for a possible solution.

As you get involved in the research and evaluation process, you will begin to develop a sense of what you think you would do if you were in the patient's position. This is natural. But for the patient, getting advice and opinions from friends and family is often the opposite of help. The patient, not the advice-giver, will have to live with the consequences of the choices she makes. A woman explains watching a friend struggle with advice from his wife:

I have a friend who was diagnosed with prostate cancer. His highest priority was making sure that he survived; second was avoiding side effects such as potential impotence or incontinence. He wanted to find out what was the best that Western medicine had to offer. His wife, however, was very concerned that he would consider methods like surgery and radiation instead of first trying nutritional changes, stress reduction, and healing rituals. She tried to talk him out of his treatment philosophy. Although she meant well by giving him articles about changing his diet, this difference of approach caused a lot of tension at first. Finally he put his foot down. This was his cancer and he was going to handle it his way. Then things calmed down. (After deciding on radiation seeding, he also added some of the changes she advocated.)

While you may or may not agree with the patient's beliefs in all areas, to be an effective research partner, you must recognize and respect her viewpoint. Be aware of your own inclination toward certain solutions and try to avoid letting that influence your research or overshadow your relationship with the patient.

Think of yourself as an information-gathering assistant and research strategist. You are helping to free the patient to focus on finding the solutions that make the most sense to her.

Talking with the doctor

Now that we have talked about how to identify what kind of help the patient wants and how to clarify your role in the process, we will discuss some of the logistics. Depending on your role in the relationship, you may or may not accompany your friend or family member on his visits to the doctor.

The following sections describe some ways to be sure that information from the doctor is shared accurately.

Going to appointments

You will accompany a child or incapacitated parent to medical appointments if you are expected to make medical decisions for him, but going to the appointment can also be helpful if you are helping a friend do research.

The patient's doctor is an important original source of information. Accuracy is lost as information is passed from person to person. The closer you get to the source of the information, the less likely it is to be distorted by interpretation.

Being with the patient at an appointment will give you an opportunity to meet the doctor and will let the doctor know that the patient feels comfortable sharing his medical information with you.

Taping the discussion

Most doctors, if asked, will agree to let you tape the discussion of the diagnosis and treatment choices. It's surprising how often listening to the tape later reveals information that you missed in the initial hearing. A tape is also helpful when you disagree with others on exactly what was said.

A woman who had teamed up with her sisters to help their sick mother explains her need to pass on complete information:

*The doctor said I could record the visit. I wanted to be able to tell my
sister exactly what she had said. If you have more than one person helping out, you really want to be sure that you communicate accurately.*

If you are not able to accompany the patient, listening to a tape of the discussion is the next best thing.

Calling the doctor directly

If you are the patient's parent or guardian, talking with the doctor directly is
not a problem. The adult child of an aging parent usually has easy access to the
doctor, as does a spouse. Access is more limited if you not a family member.

A doctor will probably not give you information about his patient unless the
patient is present and has given his permission or gives the doctor permission in writing beforehand to share that medical information with you.

Understanding the timeline

In addition to learning about the specific diagnosis and prospective treatment options, you need to get a clear understanding of the urgency of the
situation. How much time is available for research and decision-making?
Which decisions need to be made first? Which can be made later? What is
the expected sequence of events? For example, if the patient has a tumor,
will he have chemotherapy before or after surgery? Which steps are dependent on the results of the previous steps?

Asking for copies of reports

Test records and pathology reports are helpful to have in your possession
when you begin researching. Test and pathology reports identify markers
that are used to predict the aggressiveness of the disease and what types of
treatment it will respond to.

Family members might be able to get the doctor to request copies of reports
be sent directly to them, but if you are researching for a friend, ask your
friend to request the written results and give you a photocopy.

Accessing patient records

In the previous chapter, we discussed a patient's right to access her own medical records. The following sections describe issues that relate to accessing the medical records of another person.

Patient protection

Medical records contain potentially sensitive personal information. Computers permit the storage of large amounts of information and make that information more accessible. While the ease of access to information in an emergency situation can save a life, ease of access for less ethical reasons can ruin a life.

Concerns are being raised at both the state and federal levels about the need for more regulations restricting access to and use of information in medical records. Permission for access to those records, while sometimes up to the discretion of the record-holder, is gradually becoming more regulated. This means that direct access to another person's records will usually be restricted to family members and even that access is limited. See "Limitations to medical records access," in Chapter 2, *Knowing Your Rights*.

Finding the records

If the patient lived in one town all of her life and always went to the same doctor, gathering records will be relatively easy. Her doctor will have copies of all lab, imaging, surgery, and hospitalization reports in the patient's file. More often, however, the patient's records are scattered around town or even around the country.

The reports directly related to the current medical problem would be in her current doctor's records. That is the best starting place. If the patient had a previous related illness or procedure done somewhere else, the doctor's records will contain copies of those reports, if she has requested them.

Sometimes older records contain information on how the patient responded to treatment for some other condition that can help to evaluate how she might expect to respond to a treatment she is considering now. If you are researching for an aged parent who is not able to remember or communicate previous problems, such as reactions to particular medications or surgical complications like excessive bleeding, it would be especially helpful to know about them and alert her doctor. Previous history will also help to evaluate how the patient's body might react to the proposed treatments.

Finding older records will be more difficult. Ask the patient or other family members to help you make a list of her previous medical problems and treatments. You need approximate dates and specific places of treatment to find the records. The length of time that records are held varies. Records more than ten years old may not be available.

Getting permission to see the patient's records

Rules about access to medical records vary from state to state. Talk with the receptionist in a small office or the medical records department in a larger institution. Unless you are a parent, guardian, or conservator, you will need the signed consent of the patient to see her records.

If you are not a legal guardian or conservator, but have accompanied the patient to appointments with her doctor and it is clear that you are an active participant in the research process, the doctor may give you access to information in the patient's records. Labs and hospitals, however, will not be familiar with your relationship to the patient. They will require written proof that you are a legal agent or written authorization from the patient. Check with the staff to find out what paperwork they require.

You should not expect immediate access to the records. You may be given or mailed copies of the records if they are brief, or mailed a summary if they are extensive. Usually you will be charged a fee for the record copying service. You can ask to have the record faxed to speed up the process, but remember that sensitive information might be accidentally sent to the wrong fax number.

Whenever possible, the simplest approach is to have the patient request the information herself and give you copies. If you feel you are unfairly denied access, refer to Chapter 2 for suggestions on how to respond.

Becoming a healthcare agent

If the patient that you are helping is unable to make her own decisions, the medical personnel treating her will look for a family member or close friend to act as a surrogate decision-maker. As a healthcare agent, the designated person will be given the rights and responsibilities of the patient. This includes access to her medical records.

Many states allow advance directives so a patient can designate a specific family member or friend as her healthcare agent should she become incapacitated sometime in the future. In New York this is called a Healthcare Proxy. In California it is called a Durable Power of Attorney for Health Care. It does not take effect unless the patient has become incapacitated.

If a designated healthcare agent is not available or the patient or court has not designated one, the medical personnel treating the patient will need a surrogate to make informed consent decisions. The usual order of preference is legal guardian, spouse, adult child, adult parent, adult sibling, adult relative, and close personal friend.

Medical genealogy

The search for medical records does not always stop with the patient. Now that medical research has begun to uncover specific genetic links to certain diseases, more doctors and patients are looking back through the family tree for family patterns of disease.

Family medical background can be a decision-making factor in whether or not to choose more aggressive treatment or prevention options. For example, a family history of breast cancer and prostate cancer, might make a man with an elevated PSA more likely to follow-up this blood marker test with a biopsy of his prostate rather than opt to watch-and-wait. Multiple cases of these diseases in his family would indicate that he could have a BRCA gene mutation, which would make him more at risk for prostate cancer.

When a family member is diagnosed with a disease, family stories of grandparents, aunts, or uncles who had the same disease may emerge. If the family history will affect treatment choices, it is useful to try to verify the stories, which are often vague. The family might describe a cancer that affected some part of a woman's reproductive system as "woman problems," which isn't too helpful.

Some hospitals keep their medical records longer than the customary seven years (a standard used by doctor's offices). Teaching hospitals and institutions doing research may have older records. It may be worth contacting the facility where a family member was treated to find out how far their records go back and who is allowed to access them.

These records can help to validate the patient's family history. A woman with an unexplained condition describes what she did and didn't find in her mother's hospital records:

> When my CT [computed tomography] scan showed multiple cysts on my pancreas, the radiologists and gastroenterologist told me they had never seen anything like this before. There was some concern that it might be a pancreatic cancer. My mother died from a metastasis to the lung after having had endometrial cancer. But since endometrial cancer doesn't usually metastasize to the lungs, the doctors looked elsewhere for another primary cancer.
>
> I contacted the hospital where she died to get copies of her records. They had done a CT scan of her pancreas, but nothing of significance was noted. However, the records contained detailed information about her condition as well as her medical history and her account of other members in the family who had had cancers and lung problems.

If you contact a facility to request past family records, be prepared with the following:

- **Death certificate of the relative.** You will not be allowed to access the records of a living relative unless you are a legal agent of that relative.
- **Proof of your relationship.** The death certificate or an obituary may list you as a relative. If the patient was your parent, you can use your birth certificate.
- **Proof of your identity.** A driver's license or passport will be sufficient.
- **Approximate date of treatment or hospital care.** An exact date is not necessary, but a date range will help to identify the records you are requesting.

If the patient's doctor requests the records, the copying fee is usually waived.

CHAPTER 4

Identifying Information Resources

YOU NEED TOOLS AND SKILLS for any project. In this chapter, we identify the tools available to you for gathering medical information. The Internet has expanded access to these tools, many of which are available electronically as well as in print form.

This chapter covers the formats of medical information, including medical textbooks, medical journals, consumer health books and magazines, newsletters, pamphlets, audio and videotapes, computer databases and CD-ROMs, and news reports. Understanding these formats can help you decide on what sources you want to consult for a particular search and help you select a starting point.

Range of resources

You might use several resources in your search for information, depending on your needs. For example, when you first research a life-threatening condition, you might want to first get an up-to-date medical textbook and a reliable consumer health book on the condition. With that background, you might do more focused research, e.g., into newest treatments.

Table 4-1 shows the benefits and limitations for a range of resource types.

You can find information in most of these formats at your local library, a medical library associated with a hospital or medical school, at bookstores, through organizations, or by subscription to printed publications. A computer with a modem will provide you access to much of this information in electronic format. We will talk more about accessing libraries and other sources in Chapter 5, *Gaining Access to Information Resources*.

Table 4-1. Benefits and Limitations of Resource Formats

Format	Content/Availability	Limitations/Biases
Medical text-books	Basic information; standard treatments; well edited and reviewed	General in scope; biased against alternative medicine; only a few online texts truly current
Medical journals, peer-reviewed	Current information; review articles; update medical textbooks; indexed	Treatment breakthroughs too new to evaluate; often discuss unusual cases
Medical journals, not reviewed	Current information; medical opinion	May discuss untested remedies; not reviewed
Physician guidelines	Represent consensus on best and/or most cost-effective treatment; include flow charts	Represents one point of view; best to compare several guidelines, if possible
Consumer health magazines and books	Popular topics; easy to understand; easy to obtain in stores, newsstands	Not reviewed for accuracy; often biased towards alternatives; endorse products for profit
Newsletters	Easy to understand; well-written; reliable if information is from a reputable source; indexed	Simplify some medical situations; must subscribe to obtain
Pamphlets and booklets	Easy to understand; basic information; readily available	Simplifies most diseases and treatments; biased towards producer
Programs and abstracts	Good information; very current	New and untested therapies; narrow in scope; difficult to understand
Audiotapes and videotapes	Easy to listen to and view; learn things a different way	Quality varies; may be bias from producer
Computer databases and CD-ROMs	User-friendly electronic access; locate up-to-date & complicated facts quickly; some free on Internet	Some expensive to access or obtain; often must use library
News reports	Very current information; keep abreast of latest drug and treatment options	Incomplete information; often hype for company or organization; difficult to find supportive data

Medical textbooks

Medical textbooks, published by professional medical publishers, are updated frequently. Many of the most general textbooks, such as *Conn's Current Therapy*[1], are published annually, but most are updated every three to four years.

Textbooks are published for every field of medicine and surgery and for every aspect of each field. Because of the complexity of modern medicine, numerous authors, under the direction of one or more editors, produce a medical or surgical text. Each contributor is a specialist who writes the section on his particular area of expertise within the larger subject area. For example, the classic medical textbook, *Harrison's Principles of Internal*

Medicine, 14th edition, 1998,[2] lists 8 editors and 375 contributors. It is published in two volumes containing 2,569 pages with a 170-page index. This much information might seem overwhelming at first, but the index guides you to specific concepts and the scope of each chapter is clearly defined.

You would look in a medical or surgical textbook to find a good overall discussion of a medical topic and to find generally accepted treatment(s) for that condition. While textbooks tend to be conservative in scope, they provide an excellent starting place. They are invaluable for giving you a basis for asking further questions and doing more in-depth and current research. Most textbooks take over a year to publish after they are written, so the most recent information, such as new medications or clinical trials, will not be included. Medical texts that are updated annually will be the most current, of course.

When you are researching a medical condition, use medical textbooks as a basis for finding further information. Note the date of publication of the book and the dates of the references in the bibliographies. Look to medical journals for information on newer therapies and discussions of the effectiveness of the therapies being advised.

You would not expect to find alternative medical approaches to treatment in a medical text unless the book itself is about alternative medicine. Some of the classic medical texts do mention time-honored folk cures such as calamine lotion for poison ivy, etc., but most textbooks only describe treatments that would be performed by a mainstream medical professional.

A notable feature of Harrison's text and many other classic medical textbooks is that Harrison was the first editor in 1954, but is no longer living. This textbook became a classic under Harrison and so the title includes his name to help differentiate this book from others. The practice of using a known physician's name in the title, even if that person is no longer living and no longer the editor, is very common in medicine but can be confusing when you are searching for a book by a particular author.

An evaluation guide can help you to identify which medical, nursing, and allied health textbooks are considered the most authoritative. Three sources are: "Brandon/Hill Selected List of Books and Journals for the Small Medical Library," "Library for Internists," and "Doody's Rating Service." These guides are discussed in more detail in Chapter 7, *Understanding Standard Treatment Options*.

Medical journals, peer-reviewed

The most respected medical journals are peer-reviewed journals. This means that before the journal is published, all articles in that issue have been read and evaluated by one or more physicians or scientists with expertise in the field covered in the article. Often the reviewer will write an evaluation or further discussion of the article. These discussions or reviews will either be included at the end of the article or listed separately as an editorial in the same journal.

Even if a review is not included in the issue containing the original article, letters to the editor in subsequent issues will often discuss a given author's findings, especially if the findings are unusual. Unlike letters to the editor in popular magazines, these letters or comments are researched, indexed, and often include extensive references.

Medical associations and organizations such as the American Medical Association (AMA), the American College of Physicians (ACP), or the American College of Surgeons (ACS) publish most medical journals. Universities and major scientific and medical publishers also publish medical journals.

Look to medical journals for the following kinds of information:

- Current discoveries regarding treatment and clinical outcomes
- Updates of the basic information found in medical textbooks
- Clinical trial information for certain drugs or therapeutic options
- Unusual cases or unusual patient reactions to a given therapy
- Guidelines from medical boards and associations, and standards of treatment for specific medical conditions
- Review articles written by known experts in a given field and which include a historical review of treatment and a description of currently accepted modes of therapy, often accompanied by reviews of specific cases

The reference *Medical and Health Care Books and Serials in Print*[3] has a very complete listing of medical journals. In this listing, a peer-reviewed journal is designated as a *Refereed Serial*.

It's always wise to be cautious even when you read peer-reviewed medical journal articles. Much of the information reporting new therapies or alarming side effects is as yet not corroborated. Early positive studies of a new drug or therapy may involve only a handful of subjects in a specialized setting that may not yet have been duplicated anywhere else. Statistical reporting errors and experimental biases do occur and may show up later when the study is repeated or subjected to further review.

Case reports in medical journals may include reports of individual severe or even fatal reactions to a drug or surgical intervention, even though the vast majority of patients respond well to that same treatment. You can avoid unnecessary panic if you remember that most case reports represent only a single notable case.

Medical journals may reflect a particular bias. Some medical journals are more conservative in what they print than others. The *New England Journal of Medicine* publishes only a fraction of the articles submitted. Don't expect to find many articles on very controversial approaches in the more conservative or established medical journals. Also, journals rarely report negative findings and this represents a different type of bias. On the December 19, 1999 television program, *60 Minutes*, two medical researchers who were prevented from publishing negative drug findings because of "gag clauses" in their contracts with the pharmaceutical companies supporting their research were interviewed.[4]

Peer review is meant to help balance the perspective presented in an article, but reviews may also reflect adherence to traditional or popular thought on a particular therapy.

Occasionally, exceptionally biased reviews slip past the editorial staff. In November 1997, a very negative review of *Living Downstream*[5], a book about chemical and environmental links to cancer, appeared in the *New England Journal of Medicine*. It turned out that the review was written by a researcher with affiliations to a chemical company. In this case the journal did not do a thorough background check. To their credit, the *New England Journal of Medicine* later printed a correction and wrote an article discussing their own investigation of conflicts of interest that they had discovered.[6] When opinion is involved, it's wise to look into the affiliations of the author.

Non-reviewed medical journals

Some medical journals are designated "throwaway" by physicians because they are free and totally subsidized by advertising. Some of these may have articles of interest to the consumer, because the articles are written in an easy-to-understand format and often give summaries of current approaches to diseases in the news such as Lyme disease or carpal tunnel injuries. One "throwaway," *The Cortlandt Forum*, has wonderful cartoons. Another, entitled *Physician's Travel and Leisure*, has interesting travel articles and medical meeting dates along with medical information. You may come across these journals in a doctor's office or medical library, but they are not indexed and seldom kept for any period of time.

Physician guidelines

Guidelines, or Clinical Practice Guidelines, are formally developed statements and plans of treatment including flow charts to assist healthcare practitioners and their patients in making healthcare decisions. Many guidelines are produced by professional organizations such as the American College of Cardiology or the American Association of Respiratory Care. Other guidelines, such as the Prevention Guidelines from the Centers for Disease Control and Prevention (CDC) or the guidelines published by the Agency for Health Care Policy and Research (AHCPR), are produced by the US Government. Many guidelines are also produced by individual HMOs, hospitals, and clinics.

The goal of a Clinical Practice Guideline is to obtain consensus on the most effective course of treatment for a given condition or disease. Since their inception, the guidelines have been seen as a method of reducing costs and improving outcomes for various treatments. Insurers and HMOs often mandate that a practice guideline exist for all covered procedures.

As a consumer of healthcare, you may find it very helpful to locate clinical practice guidelines for any therapy recommended for you. The professional medical associations seem to have the "best treatment" recommendations as guidelines for a high standard of care, while the insurers may have the most cost-efficient guidelines. Both groups may have similarities in the format of their guidelines, but the details may also differ widely. It is good to find several guidelines, if you can, and compare them. For example, there could be a difference in the time recommended by physicians' groups and insurers for the length of a hospital stay after surgery. Often it is in the patient's best interests to send him home as soon as possible, but this would not be true in every case.

You can find clinical practice guidelines and standards of care published by the professional medical associations in their journals, on their web sites, and often in books or monographs. You can ask your hospital and/or HMO for the clinical practice guideline for any procedure recommended for you as a patient. "Practice guidelines" are searchable index terms in MEDLINE and Cinahl, two medical databases, so you can often locate guidelines published in a variety of journals representing many points of view. The guidelines endorse a coordinated care plan that is usually beneficial to the patient. One government web site posts new guidelines at *http://www.guidelines.gov/index. asp*. There is more on physician guidelines in Chapter 7.

Consumer health books

Consumer health books are written by authors with a wide variety of backgrounds and expertise. The credentials of the author(s) are usually on the title page or in the biographical information at the end of the book. Consumer health books are written in language for the non-medical person and often include personal stories of individuals who are dealing with an illness or tragedy. Some consumer health books include information on alternative or holistic treatments as well as criticisms of conventional medicine. Others, written by medical doctors and other health professionals, will provide explanations of conventional medical practices.

Most traditional publishing houses and a few specialized publishers include consumer health books in their range of publications. Some consumer health books are *self-published*, meaning published by the author rather than a commercial publisher. The information contained in a self-published consumer health book is not necessarily questionable, but you should be alert to the fact that an established publisher didn't print it. The content of such a book might interest such a small audience that the publishers didn't see any possibility of profit.

Consumer health books add an important dimension to the literature of medicine. They add the personal and human stories that accompany any medical odyssey. They also provide a watchdog function, often questioning the most conservative treatments, especially those with poor or mixed results. They may offer alternatives from Eastern and folk medicine, nutritional therapies, exercise therapies, and even laughter therapy as in the case of Norman Cousins' popular book, *Anatomy of an Illness as Perceived by the*

Patient.[7] Most of these books will have a distinct point of view. Be alert to biases that support a particular author's point of view.

Another essential contribution of consumer health books is that they help patients and their families become active participants in choosing a course of treatment and managing their own care. The well-written consumer health book will discuss medical conditions and treatment options in clear under-standable language and is often the first place to turn in understanding a complicated diagnosis. Look for consumer health books with good bibliog-raphies that include references to medical textbooks and journals as well as to other consumer health publications. Avoid books that offer only opinion or are so general that they offer nothing new or useful. Many of the medical books published by *Consumer Reports* are excellent.

Finally, consumer health books offer support and even guidance from peo-ple who have experienced serious illnesses. They share their experiences in dealing with the medical establishment and making critical decisions. Many of these books help patients and families dealing with life-threatening illness cope with the roller coaster of emotions that takes them from hope to despair and back again.

Evaluation and recommendation rating systems are not as clearly defined for consumer health books as they are for more formal medical textbooks. Some reviewing guides for consumer health books include Rees' *Consumer Health Information*,[8] the December issue of *Library Journal*, and special reference editions of *American Libraries*. The Consumer and Patient Health Informa-tion Section (CAPHIS) of the Medical Library Association publishes a news-letter called *Consumer Connections* and also maintains a web site at *http:// www.njc.org/caphis/caphis.html*. Both review consumer health materials.

When determining the reliability of information in a consumer health book, consider the writer's credentials as well as the credentials of any reviewers who have evaluated it. Remember that consumer books are fashioned to sell. Miracle cures and medical breakthroughs attract book buyers.

Consumer health magazines

Consumer health magazines are usually published by regular trade publish-ers and alternative health publishers. Mainstream trade publishers of con-sumer health magazines include Cowles, publisher of *Vegetarian Times,* and *Conde Nast*, who publishes *SELF* and *Women's Sports and Fitness*. One well-known alternative health publisher is Rodale Press, publisher of *Prevention, Men's Health, New Woman,* and many other titles.

Consumer Health magazines such as *Prevention* may be general in nature, or they may cover a specific health practice such as yoga, acupuncture, or vegetarianism. The magazines provide important information about mainstream and alternative medical therapies in a readable format.

Prevention of illness and the emphasis on maintaining a healthy lifestyle is one of the greatest contributions of the consumer health magazines. While the more conservative peer-reviewed medical journals occasionally mention diet, herbal remedies, exercise, and lifestyle factors in preventing and overcoming illnesses, these topics are the backbone of the consumer health magazines. Consumer health magazines also contribute information on coping strategies for disabling conditions such as arthritis and chronic pain.

Another strength of the consumer health magazines is that they act as a watchdog on the medical establishment. Some consumer health magazines actively question the overuse of some of the more heavily prescribed drugs such as Prozac or potentially dangerous therapies such as radiation treatments. They also question long-term prescription and nonprescription drug use. Typically, articles in these magazines recommend treatments that involve very little expenditure on traditional drug therapy, but may instead recommend expensive vitamins and herbal products.

Unfortunately no evaluation tool for assessing the reliability of a consumer health magazine has been developed. An article can make impossible claims or recommend discontinuing a lifesaving mainstream therapy, even when there are no scientific facts to support these recommendations. Readers of consumer health magazines should be careful in their evaluation of the information presented, realizing that the authors can, and sometimes will, write whatever will sell.

Exercise caution regarding the advertising in the consumer health magazines as well. Advertisers are the primary source of income for these publishers, and they may have an article praising a certain product in the magazine that has several ads for that same product.

The audience for consumer health magazines is made up of health-conscious adults, alternative health practitioners, and patients using alternative regimens to treat specific conditions. There are consumer health magazines for those dealing with breast cancer, prostate cancer, or other diseases as well as magazines dealing with psychological issues such as eating disorders.

You will not always find a full spectrum of medical treatment approaches in consumer health magazines, but many of these magazines do provide well-balanced coverage of some of the popular mainstream and alternative therapies. Consumer health journals will continue to make their contribution by bringing new medical information to the public in a readable format.

Medical newsletters

Newsletters are published by associations of medical professionals, support organizations, advocacy organizations, local and national treatment centers, and manufacturers of medical products. Most newsletters are included as part of a membership or given out free to clients. Some newsletters are available by subscription.

A newsletter published by an organization, such as the National Psoriasis Association, is used to distribute information on the latest studies and new treatments for those living with this chronic condition and to provide members with a calendar of upcoming events.

Treatment centers, like Memorial Sloane-Kettering Cancer Center and the Mayo Clinic, use newsletters to keep clients and donors informed about their services and upcoming events. They also focus on advances in medical treatment, especially research advances made by their facility.

A commercial entity uses a newsletter as a marketing tool to highlight information about the company's products or showcase its services. A pharmaceutical company might publish a professional newsletter which provides timely information for medical professionals or for the consumers who use their products. This is smart marketing because it shows that the company is knowledgeable, professional, and really cares about the consumer. For example, *Innovations in Oncology Nursing* is an informative newsletter produced by Zeneca Pharmaceuticals.

An increasing number of newsletters are being offered to the public by subscription. Some, like the *University of California at Berkeley Wellness Letter, Harvard Health Letter,* or *Surviving* from the Department of Radiation Oncology at Stanford University Medical Center, are published by university medical schools. Others are compiled by commercial publishing companies. The *New England Journal of Medicine*, for example, publishes summaries of articles from the journal in its consumer newsletter, *HealthNews*. Boardroom Inc. publishes a newsletter called *Bottom Line Health*, which gives short abstracts of recent medical articles they feel might be of interest to their readership.

New information can usually reach publication more quickly in newsletter format than in a magazine, where it passes through a more complicated editorial and production process. Since a newsletter addresses the interests of a particular group, the articles will be more tightly focused around a specific condition or advocacy issue. Space limitations force articles to be more concise. Often a newsletter article will direct you to a larger article or book where you can find more detail.

Newsletters offer a transitional platform presenting information from medical journals to the consumer public. Newsletters like Harvard's *Women's Health Watch* translate articles from medical journals—which often contain a plethora of academic medical terms, jargon, and abbreviations—into an article that includes enough background information and explanation of terms to make it readily understandable to health consumers.

Medical newsletters do not contain advertisements like magazines or newspapers. Editorial pressure from the advertisers is less of a concern. You can, however, expect newsletter articles to be written from a particular perspective. In fact some newsletters, particularly advocacy newsletters, are written primarily to promote a particular cause. This does not mean that the perspective is not valid, but be aware that newsletters seldom offer conflicting views. If you want a balanced perspective, you will want to do your own follow-up work. Generally a newsletter article will refer to the original source of the information. You can look up source material and read it in its original context if you need to depend on the accuracy of that information.

Pamphlets and booklets

Pamphlets and booklets are sometimes published by nonprofit organizations such as the American Heart Association. Pamphlets usually provide a brief overview of a particular condition or some aspect of a condition. Booklets will go into more detail, often including illustrations.

Drug companies and medical device manufacturers also produce pamphlets and booklets. While the purpose of the material may be to sell you on why they think their product works, they often give a well-written overview of the condition and how a particular treatment is expected to work. Some of these will be written for physicians and some for patients. Both can be useful, although you might want to have a medical dictionary handy if you plan to read the versions written for professionals.

Often you will see pamphlets in your doctor's office. A dermatologist will have a rack of information on conditions like psoriasis, eczema, and skin cancer. The doctor purchases these pamphlets to help explain these skin problems to his patients. Sometimes they are published by an association such as the American Academy of Dermatology and sometimes by a commercial entity such as a drug company or a publishing company.

You can expect booklets and pamphlets to offer statistical information, glossaries, tips for prevention or early detection, step-by-step guides on the treatment process, notes on possible side effects and how you might avoid them, and lists of local and national resources.

You should not expect to find a detailed overview of a condition. Booklets and pamphlets tend to be written to illustrate and support a particular choice of action and may be biased. They are not designed to offer a complex or carefully balanced explanation.

Programs and abstracts

National organizations and professional associations frequently hold conferences and symposiums. These events are expensive to attend and participation is often limited to people working in medical professions. However, the speakers and poster presentations at these events reflect leading-edge research.

Sometimes it will be months or even years before research presented at a conference is published in a medical journal. Smaller studies might never even make it into a medical journal.

A book of abstracts is often published after a conference or it may be given out at registration to entice participants to attend the talks, workshops, and poster presentations. Each abstract gives an overview of the research being done by the presenter and the conclusions the presenter has drawn from the results. The book of abstracts provides summaries of the presentation that the participant will have for reference. Usually abstracts include information on how to contact the presenters.

If you cannot attend the event yourself, try to find someone in your community who will be attending the conference and ask if you can scan through the book of abstracts afterwards. You can also check to see if a nearby university has cataloged the abstracts or if they have been published in the journal published by the organization holding the conference. While you may uncover a small unpublished study, look critically at the information. Abstracts are less comprehensive than a full research paper and material that has not yet been published has not passed through the editorial gauntlet used to filter out less reliable data.

Audiotapes and videotapes

Audio and videotapes offer a non-text format for presenting educational information. Videotapes are especially effective for demonstration. Watching a videotaped demonstration of exercises to relieve back pain or techniques for lymphedema massage is much more effective than reading a how-to explanation in a book. This kind of audio and videotape is often made by an organization selling a product or a program.

Video and audiotapes are sometimes used to record interviews, lectures, and panel discussions. This format offers an individual perspective from an authority on a specific topic, often a notable person in that field who might be difficult to contact personally. Such tapes may be made as part of a commercial information series or might be recorded at an educational conference or symposium and sold to the participants. Both nonprofit and for-profit groups make use of audio and videotapes as a means of distributing information.

As a teaching tool, a videotape may use animation and other visual effects to illustrate the process of a disease, treatment, and healing. The video and audio formats might offer an overview of a condition or a detailed explanation of a particular aspect, but not a detailed overview.

The scope of information will be limited by the amount of explanation that can be presented in an hour or less. This does not allow enough time for a fully balanced perspective or detailed explanation. Most video and audiotapes promote and support a specific point of view or choice of action.

The marketing of this format is dependent on sales to large audiences, so you will find the topics are usually focused on areas of general interest rather than unusual conditions. The approach might be unusual, but the condition it addresses will probably be common.

Look to video and audiotapes for overviews, step-by-step demonstrations, and insight into new approaches and perspectives.

Computer databases and CD-ROMs

Databases are available online. Some, such as MEDLINE, produced by the National Library of Medicine, at *http://www.ncbi.nlm.nih.gov/PubMed* are freely available to the public. Other databases are produced by companies or research services which index information from many sources, database the information, and offer access to the data for a fee based on the amount of usage. Many of the fee-based databases also have minimum monthly charges. The largest group of these can be accessed through Dialog, which maintains access to over 900 fee-based databases. The medical databases in this group include Embase, a European medical and drug database; Chem-line; and other pharmaceutical, business, patent, and scientific databases.

Since it takes training and skill to use subscription databases efficiently, it is usually more cost-effective to hire a researcher who has experience in using these databases rather than beginning "cold" to subscribe and try to find information instantly. We talk more about when it is appropriate to hire a researcher in Chapter 6, *Effective Search Strategies*.

Many databases are also available on static CD-ROM format as well as through the Internet. You might encounter health information on CD-ROM either if you make your own purchase or in a library or resource room. By buying the information on a CD-ROM, the user is able to obtain a fixed price for searching a given database. A CD-ROM is usually more user-friendly than a dial-up database. The information is the same, with the exception that it is usually less current because of the time it takes to produce and distribute the CD-ROMs.

In recent years, CD-ROMs have been marketed to support a particular medical specialty such as orthopedics or radiology. The producers combine selected indexes from MEDLINE with some key medical and drug textbooks to create a specialized product for a select group.

The transfer of medical textbooks onto CD-ROM has grown to a point where most major medical textbooks are now offered in this format as well as in print. The benefits to the user of such a CD-ROM are that it takes little space, makes searching by keyword easier than by using an author's index, and provides a faster speed in searching through a particular body of information. The drawbacks are that many CD-ROMs are very costly, and you need a relatively new computer with lots of memory to read them efficiently.

Publishers of medical journals have also begun to market their journals in the CD-ROM format. Many give the CD-ROM free to subscribers of the journal. All of the eleven American Medical Association journals are on CD-ROM, and you can get a disk that contains all the issues for an entire year. The savings in space and the portability are very desirable features of these CD-ROMs. As with the medical textbooks and databases, these journals are also accessible through the Internet, but usually for a fixed subscription fee.

Some CD-ROMs were created to take advantage of the interactive format and are not copies of existing databases, journals, or books. There are CD-ROMs such as the famous *A.D.A.M.*,[9] designed to teach anatomy, or those produced to support interactive medical decision making, such as *Be a Survivor*, produced by Lange Productions.[10]

News reports

Late-breaking medical news bombards us daily. Most of our familiarity with a disease, prior to being diagnosed with it ourselves and learning about it in more detail, comes from what we read and hear in these formats. Breakthrough news sells newspapers and keeps viewers' and listeners' attention.

Media news accounts will also prompt phone calls from caring friends who suspect that this new advance just might be the answer to your problems. Sadly, medical information on the news is often more hype than help.

Newspapers

Newspaper editors and reporters monitor the national newswires for exciting new stories. Readers want the latest news from the front in the War on Cancer, AIDS, or an outbreak of infectious disease. Much of this news on advances comes to newswire in the form of press releases and statements from press conferences.

Press releases are written and press conferences are held by medical researchers reporting on the outcomes of their studies and by companies developing medical products. These are not unbiased reports. It is the role of the reporter to look deeper, ask educated questions, and search out other perspectives. Newspaper reporters are not often given the leisure to spend more than a few days or sometimes even a few hours gathering and evaluating the information and writing a balanced report.

Many of the headline reports are taken directly from the newswire, and few newspapers have the research staff to verify each medical announcement. An in-depth report will come days or even weeks after a medical breakthrough hits the headlines. You will need to do your own follow-up in most cases, so note the details—especially who released the information and where the work was done.

Television and radio news

Again, newscast information comes from the newswire and is formed into soundbites. Most of the supporting information will be in the form of anecdotal human interest stories. Radio and television reporters have even less time than newspaper reporters to gather the background information needed to give a balanced report.

Often when you hear a report, the information flies by before you have a chance to write down the important details. Don't be hesitant to contact the radio or television station to ask for the details you missed or to ask about the source of a report.

Television documentaries

When a breakthrough, a particular approach to treatment, or a type of disease has achieved a high level of audience interest, a television network may produce an in-depth report or documentary focused on that topic. In Bill Moyers' documentary *Healing and the Mind*, he interviews physicians, scientists, therapists, and patients about their experiences and research on the physical influence of emotions on health and healing. This is a five-part series with a clear focus on exploring multiple perspectives.

Local stations can usually direct you to a network or network affiliate where you can purchase a copy of the written transcript or a video of the program. Networks like the Public Broadcasting Service, *http://www.pbs.org*, that produce primarily documentary-type programs often have catalogs of documentary videos for sale. Even a copy of an in-depth report produced locally can usually be purchased from the station.

While some documentaries may be produced to highlight a particular perspective, most try to address questions likely to be raised by those who disagree. A documentary usually starts from scratch to provide both background and an easy-to-understand overview.

CHAPTER 5

Gaining Access to Information Resources

IT'S NOT ENOUGH TO KNOW the different formats for medical information and the kinds of resources you would like to access. You also need to know where to find what you need.

Even if you already know where there is a great medical center library, patient resource center, or have access to the Internet, you can benefit from knowing what kinds of centers specialize in what kind of information, and how to get access if it is restricted.

In this chapter we will talk about the following information centers:

- Libraries
- Bookstores
- Government agencies
- Professional associations
- Nonprofit organizations
- Patient resource centers
- Medical research centers
- Medical product manufacturers
- Virtual information centers—the Internet and other online services

We will describe how to find each of these information clearinghouses, how accessible they are to the patient community, and what to expect to find at each.

Libraries

There are basically three types of libraries: public libraries, academic or school libraries, and special libraries. Medical school libraries are considered academic libraries, but in reality they are distinct in that their collections are so focused. Each type of library is supported by some constituency or group, and it is the library's mission to serve the information needs of that group. Understanding the differences between types of libraries can help you more effectively use their holdings and possibly gain access to some libraries not typically open to the general public.

Public libraries serve the information needs of the community that supports them through local taxes. Larger public libraries will most likely have computers with Internet access and excellent indexes to information in periodicals and magazines. They will also have some excellent medical reference materials such as directories of physicians and drug information.

Even the smallest public library usually has an interlibrary loan department that facilitates borrowing books and getting reprints from other libraries and library networks. Through these networks, libraries throughout the United States and the world share resources. So, if you can locate an item held in a library somewhere else, your public library can probably borrow it for you for a set amount of time. You can often find titles through library catalogs on the Internet and then request them. The library staff members will be very helpful in locating materials. No library loans materials from its reference collection—those have to stay physically in the library. Certain medical books may be quite difficult to obtain since many of them are considered reference books, especially those that are the most current.

Public libraries are open to all in the community and usually have convenient evening and weekend hours. Because of ease of access, the public library is a good starting point for finding medical information. If your public library does not have much medical information, the reference librarians can usually recommend other nearby places to find information. Since no single library can have all information, networking among libraries and information providers has long been a part of library services.

If you are not a student at a college or university, the public library is your primary library.

Academic libraries

Academic library collections will reflect the courses taught at the colleges and universities they serve. Most private colleges and universities are open only to their own faculty and students. Public colleges and universities, however, are usually open to the entire community since they, like public libraries, are supported with public tax funding. In most cases you will not be allowed to check any materials out of a college or university library unless you are a registered student, but you can read and make photocopies of materials in their collections. Some college and university libraries allow community members to purchase a borrower's library card for a specified time period.

Colleges and universities usually will have excellent serials or journal collections and have strong coverage of scientific information, sociological issues, and often psychology and medicine. Since the library supports the courses taught at the university, you can expect to find a strong science collection in a university that offers advanced degrees in the sciences. Universities and colleges that have medical, nursing, and dental schools will have the best medical collections. Many community colleges have nursing and allied health programs and these, too, will have strong health collections.

Medical school libraries

Medical schools are divisions of academic institutions, but they are often in separate locations from their parent university and their library is usually separate from the main campus library. This is because the information and many of the services in a medical school library are unique to medical libraries. Another reason that medical schools and their libraries are separate from a main campus is that medical students need to have experiences with the medical needs of a large and varied population base. Medical schools, for this reason, are usually located in the larger metropolitan areas of the country.

Medical school libraries have the largest collections of medical information, second only to the National Library of Medicine. There are 125 accredited medical schools in the US and all have excellent libraries for medical information. The medical school libraries will have thousands of medical journal subscriptions, access to electronic and paper indexes to information, and a strong collection of medical textbooks and CD-ROMs on every possible medical topic.

If the medical school/medical library is tax supported, you can usually gain access to the information in their comprehensive collections. If you do not live near a medical school, you might consider traveling to the closest university medical library if you are doing a great deal of medical research and wish to complete it quickly. The information from these libraries is often available through interlibrary loan services at smaller hospital and public libraries, but it can take weeks to get some information and it is sometimes best to travel to the source. A web site giving the locations of all of the medical schools in the United States and Canada has been created by the American Association of Medical Colleges (AAMC). The address of that web site is *http://www.aamc.org*.

You can go to the AAMC web site, click on "medical schools," and determine which school may be closest to your location. Medical schools are listed alphabetically in order of the state or province in the United States or Canada. Since you know that all medical schools MUST have a medical library, you need only determine how much access to that library will be available to you. The National Library of Medicine maintains a directory of the National Network of Libraries of Medicine. A call to them at (800) 338-7657 will assist you in locating a medical school library with community access.

Special libraries

Special libraries are private libraries that serve the information needs of the organization supporting them. Thus a hospital library is a special library that will have information supporting the clinical departments and services of that hospital. A children's hospital will have a strong collection of information on children's diseases, while a cancer center will have excellent resources for information on cancer. Many special libraries are departments of nonprofit hospitals and often have certain hours for public access.

Many hospital libraries allow access for the general public, but some do not have the staff or materials to extend access beyond their own employees. Not every hospital has its own library. Teaching hospitals are the most likely to have strong medical libraries with extensive journal collections. Teaching hospitals are the hospitals that have residency programs for physicians training in medical specialties such as surgery, internal medicine, primary care, medical oncology, radiology, pediatrics, etc.

There may be a separate consumer health library or patient education center in a hospital or consumer health materials may be incorporated into the collection in a hospital library. If access is not generally open to the public, you may be able to access the library through a written request from your physician or through some hospital staff member. When you feel you need access to a hospital library, it never hurts to ask. Many previously inaccessible hospital medical libraries are now offering some public hours because of high demand as well as mandates for patient and family education from the Joint Commission on the Accreditation of Healthcare Organizations. Section P.F.4 of *The Comprehensive Accreditation Manual for Hospitals* states that hospitals provide and support resources for patient and family education to maintain their accreditation.[1]

In a hospital library you can expect to find physician directories, drug references, and current textbooks for every area of medicine. You would also find medical journals not available elsewhere in the community as well as staff who are knowledgeable about researching medical questions. You also usually find pamphlets or clipping files on current medical topics. If you do gain access to a medical library, ask which resources are available, since there may be some items that are limited to use by the physicians and hospital staff.

Many communities are starting consumer health libraries. These may be in a corner of the public library or hospital library or they may be free standing and supported by member donations. Consumer health libraries are growing in numbers as people are becoming more concerned about healthcare and becoming fully informed about treatment options for themselves and their families. Many of these consumer health libraries are specific to one type of disease such as cancer or arthritis, and some are general in scope and cover all aspects of medical treatment. Consumer health libraries are usually listed in local telephone books. Many of them are also listed on a web site organized by the Consumer and Patient Health Information section of the Medical Library Association. The address for this web site is *http://www. mlanet.org.*

Bookstores

A familiar local bookstore might be your first stop after the diagnosis of a chronic or potentially life-threatening disease. It is unlikely that your local bookstore will stock highly detailed medical books, but you will find plenty of introductory books on the major diseases, medical dictionaries to help you understand the medical jargon being used to describe your situation, and books that offer biographical insights into the ongoing process of adjusting to the life changes that may accompany such a diagnosis.

University and medical school bookstores

In addition to browsing local bookstores, you can visit the bookstore at a nearby college or university or look for a bookstore that specializes in medical texts. A college or university bookstore may carry textbooks for nursing and premed classes.

Medical schools also have bookstores. The texts available at a medical school bookstore will be geared toward a student who already has a basic understanding of the medical science concepts taught in premed classes. You will need to be more knowledgeable on the topic you are researching to be able to understand the explanations provided in these books.

A bookstore that specializes in medical books will be more difficult to find. Try the phone book in a large city for a specialty bookstore. An Internet search on "medical textbooks" will find medical bookstores in other cities that might have mail-order services.

Medical textbooks are expensive. The average price of a medical textbook in 1999 was $119.[2] Some of the more popular books have lower prices, however. The 1999 "centennial" edition of *The Merck Manual*, for example, is about $35. *The Merck Manual* is a classic reference book that describes many diseases and conditions and their treatment.[3] If you find a book that looks useful, check to see if it is available at your nearest medical library or if the book can be borrowed from your local public or medical library on an interlibrary loan.

Bookstores may have more convenient hours or locations than libraries, but are not as well-suited for research. Bookstores are seldom designed with comfortable couches, chairs, and tables for reading and taking notes. The staff may not be as knowledgeable about the books as the reference staff at a library, particularly a medical library.

Bookstores are the best place to find current popular books and magazines. What they don't have on the shelves, you can special order if the book you want is still in print. There is usually no extra charge for a special order, but it may be a few weeks before you will receive it.

Internet bookstores

Many bookstores are beginning to sell their books over the Internet. They are essentially mail-order bookstores, but you shop and place your order via the Internet. Some are actually "virtual" bookstores that have no traditional storefront.

Amazon.com, *http://www.amazon.com*, is probably the best known of these new electronic bookstores. They have both in-stock and special-order books available by mail, and even sell some out-of-print books. Powell's bookstore, *http://www.powells.com*, in Portland, Oregon has a strong collection of used and out-of-print books as well as new and current books. You can access their catalog and place an order over the Internet.

There is an online site that compares prices on the Internet, which might be especially useful for more expensive books at *http://www.dealpilot.com*. There is also a site for used/out-of-print book searches: *http://www.mxbf.com*.

Medical book distributors also have Internet web sites, but again, the cost of a professional medical text may be prohibitive. Most of these are focused on sales to bookstores, libraries and to medical professionals. Login Brothers Book Company, *http://www.lb.com*, is an example. Browsing their online catalog can give you an idea of what professional books are currently available on the subject you are researching. Login sales are usually limited to libraries and bookstores, however.

Government agencies

Government agencies offer health information to consumers at all three levels, federal, state and local. To locate various government agencies, check your local library for a copy of the *Directory of Healthcare Agencies and Associations*. Yearly almanacs also often list current addresses and phone numbers for federal and state government agencies.

You can expect these government agencies to offer public health information and statistical reports. For example, the National Cancer Registry collects cancer statistics and reports them by cancer type, gender, and ethnicity. Regional branches of the Registry collect and publish statistics for a particular part of a state.

Many government agencies offer special programs for low-cost access to screening and disease prevention. Some also publish fact sheets and treatment guidelines. Most agencies have a range of booklets and pamphlets. You can use these agencies to direct you to other, more specific sources of information.

At the national level, the US Department of Health and Human Services, *http://www.hhs.gov*, oversees eight national agencies that provide services essential to the protection of the health of all Americans, especially for those who are least able to help themselves.

Three Health and Human Service agencies are especially familiar—the Food and Drug Administration (FDA), the National Institutes of Health (NIH), and the Centers for Disease Control and Prevention (CDC). The FDA, *http://www.fda.gov*, assures the safety of food, cosmetics, pharmaceutical, biological products, and medical devices. The NIH, *http://www.nih.gov*, includes the National Library of Medicine, the National Center for Human Genome Research, and seventeen institutes which each focus on research on diseases such as Alzheimer's, diabetes, cancer, arthritis, and heart disease. The CDC, *http://www.cdc.gov*, monitors and works to prevent outbreaks of disease and also maintains national health statistics.

At the state level, the state Department of Health oversees state health concerns such as patient rights, health statistics, public health education, and subsidized access to health services. Each state also has a Medical Board that licenses physicians and investigates complaints.

At the local level, a network of agencies is usually housed under the county Department of Health or Health Services. County health agencies offer medical services, public health information, health assessment, education programs, and monitor environmental health concerns.

Traditionally, access to national, state, and local agencies has been by phone. Some phone books list county, state, and US Government offices at the front. You can also look in the white pages under the name of your county, state, or "United States Government" for health agency listings. Some of these offices are primarily administrative and are not set up for walk-in visits, but you can call ahead to find out, ask questions, and have information sent to you.

Some of these agencies are starting to provide information via the Internet, particularly at the state and federal levels. This gives you access to information more quickly and in greater depth than you are usually able to get by phone. The federal government provides some of the highest quality health information web sites. The National Cancer Institute, *http://www.cancernet. nci.nih.gov*, provides cancer diagnosis, staging and treatment information, fact sheets for patients and physicians, as well as up-to-date treatment and prevention progress reports and clinical trial information.

State departments of health are building web sites that provide health information beneficial to people living outside their states as well. For example, the New York State Department of Health, *http://www.health.state.ny.us/nysdoh*, publishes a collection of Infectious Disease Fact Sheets on their web site at *http://www.health.state.ny.us/nysdoh/consumer/commun.htm*.

Internet access to county Department of Health information is less likely, but some counties are beginning to put consumer health information online. Marion County, Indiana, publishes information about their communicable disease program, healthcare services, and environmental health factors on their web site at *http://www.mchd.com*.

Professional associations

Professional associations serve the interests of their members. Some of the well-known professional medical associations are the American Medical Association (AMA), the American College of Physicians (ACP), and the American College of Surgeons (ACS). Most provide consumer health information as one of the services for their members. Professional medical associations publish journals, pamphlets, treatment guidelines, and position statements that can be very useful to patients.

Professional medical associations serve physicians and other medical professionals worldwide, and they reach their members through the mail, the Internet, and at annual meetings. Except for the largest organizations, the offices of a medical organization serve primarily as a clearinghouse providing information and support for their members.

There are many ways to access the information available from professional associations. The easiest point of access is usually through the web site of that organization. One particularly good list of medical associations is at the Yahoo web site. The address is *http://www.yahoo.com*. At the time of this writing, these are listed under "health," "organizations," then under links to "professional" and "medicine." A list of links to hundreds of medical associations will come up. Select the one that would cover a topic of interest and click on that link. Most of these have a consumer section, guidelines, and even the full text of their recent journals. Often the web site of the association will have an email address or telephone number so that you can contact the association and ask questions not covered on the web site.

If the medical association you are trying to contact does not have a web site, you can find their telephone number and address in the *Medical and Health Information Directory*,[4] a reference found in most medical libraries.

Nonprofit organizations

Organizations are gold mines of information. Many have hotlines to answer your questions and help you find local treatment and support resources. Branch offices and larger local organizations will have offices that you can visit in person. For smaller organizations you will need to find the name and phone number of a contact person who can send you a newsletter and literature about what the organization has to offer.

Many organizations have small libraries of books, videos, and audiotapes. Most offer educational booklets, pamphlets, and fact sheets. Some organizations can help you find published treatment guidelines and match you up with another person who has had an experience similar to yours.

Disease-specific organizations keep their client-members informed about the latest research and treatment options through their newsletters and educational events, such as conferences and symposiums. Some organizations focus on mainstream medical treatment, while others like International Association of Cancer Victors and Friends or the Cancer Control Society explore complementary and alternative treatment options.

Most nonprofit organizations identify a particular community whose needs they serve. Health-oriented nonprofits serve the patient community through education, support services, updates on research findings, and advocacy for public and political recognition of the needs of patients. They also publish pamphlets and newsletters and provide contacts to local support groups, etc. For example, the American Cancer Society, *http://www.cancer.org*, is a nationwide community-based voluntary organization dedicated to eliminating cancer through research, education, advocacy and services.

Many health-oriented groups are disease specific. For example, the American Heart Association is dedicated to preventing heart disease and to supporting those people who have heart disease. Other well-known health organizations include the Arthritis Association and the American Lung

Association. Some, like the National Women's Health Network, are gender-specific or reflect the health needs of a particular cultural heritage such as the National Latina Health Organization, the African American Breast Cancer Alliance, or the National Asian Women's Health Organization. Some nonprofit health organizations focus primarily on education, publishing, and support services, while others promote political policies to increase research funding or raise money to fund research.

Many of the national organizations have local branch offices. Some nonprofits are strictly local organizations. Often a person or group of people who have personal experience with a particular disease and want to help others starts these local groups.

Large national organizations can be found through the *Directory of Healthcare Agencies and Associations,* a reference book in most large libraries. Local branches and local nonprofits can be found in the phone book. Check the white pages if you know the name or look under "Associations," "Human Services Organizations," "Social Service Organizations," or "Support Groups" in the yellow pages. Almanacs usually list the addresses and phone numbers of national organizations.

Call your county health department to find out about local nonprofit health organizations. Some county health departments or local information and referral agencies publish a community resource directory or offer a resource line to help you find community organizations. The reference desk at the public library is another good place to ask about both national and local health organizations. If your physician specializes in your disease or condition, the office staff can probably direct you to local and national organizations.

Another way to find local nonprofits is through your United Way. The number will be in the white pages of your local telephone book, or you can check through the national web site, *http://www.unitedway.org.* The goal of United Way is to help local organizations help people in their own communities. They will have a listing of most local nonprofits.

Again, don't forget to check the Internet. Most national groups have web sites with educational information, event calendars, and contact information. Even small local groups may have contact information online.

Patient resource centers

Patient resource centers are scattered around the country. Some are disease or condition specific, such as the Community Breast Health Project in Palo Alto, California or the Alzheimer's Resource Center in Brooklyn, New York. Some are gender specific, like the Minneapolis Women's Cancer Resource Center, and some provide a wide range of health resources such as Planetree Health Resource Center in San Jose, California.

Some resource centers are part of a medical treatment facility, and some are developed as independent nonprofit organizations, specifically to address the information needs of health consumers, patients, and their families.

Ask your physician or his office staff for information on nearby resource centers. You can also try looking under "Social Service Organizations" in the yellow pages of your phone book or the name of a particular disease in the white pages. Often, county health departments or information and referral services can direct you to local resource centers.

To find resource centers in other communities, you can get the name of information and referral agencies in out-of-town telephone directories in your local library. You can also try doing a search on the Internet. A national organization might also be able to direct you to resource centers throughout the country.

Resource centers run by volunteers are likely to have more limited hours than those that are part of a medical facility and run by paid staff. Some resource centers may be open some weekday evenings and on weekends, and many schedule private appointments for visits during unscheduled hours. Most resource centers are open to the public, although those housed in a medical facility might be provided expressly for patients of that facility. Check to be sure.

A patient resource center usually houses a specialized library of books, videos, audiotapes, newsletters, and clipping files and provides public access to the Internet for information searches. Most resource centers offer a telephone hotline for support and information about other local resources. They also collect flyers and brochures from local healthcare providers, complementary therapists, and appropriate national groups. Volunteers and staff will be available to help you with your search for information.

Often a resource center will develop a network of people willing to share their personal experiences on a particular aspect of the disease or treatment. The center will also have a schedule of educational programs, symposiums, and ongoing drop-in support groups.

As with other health-specific nonprofits, the people who work in resource centers spend a lot of time sifting through information on the condition(s) which is the center's focus. The staff will be familiar with current treatment issues, where to look for specialists, and where to contact researchers working on new treatments.

A resource center that combines information with patient support offers a good starting place for anyone who is newly diagnosed.

Medical research centers

Medical research is divided into basic research and clinical research. Basic research is conducted in a lab setting, in test tubes and petri dishes or lab animals. Experimentation done in test tubes or petri dishes is called *in vitro*. Experiments done on living tissue, such as in lab animals, is called *in vivo*. Medical schools and universities are good places to look for basic science research.

When a new insight in biology or the development of a new agent is applied to therapeutic studies, it becomes clinical research. Clinical research studies are done in hospitals, medical clinics, and physician's offices. We will talk about these in more detail in Chapter 8, *Researching Clinical Trials*.

Medical research is funded by a mixture of sources. Medical companies seeking approval for new products fund research as well as privately-funded grants offered by large organizations. The largest entity funding medical research is the federal government through agencies like the National Institutes of Health (NIH). In 1994 the NIH estimated that industry money accounted for 52 percent of $33 billion spent on US medical research.[5]

Look for centers that specialize in a particular disease. For example, the Center for Narcolepsy Research at the University of Illinois at Chicago would be a good place to find information about the latest studies on narcolepsy. Sansum Research Foundation in Santa Barbara, California, is a diabetes research center. You can contact them for diabetes information and research updates.

To find a listing of medical research centers, check with your nearest large medical library for a copy of *Medical Research Centers: A World Directory of Organizations and Programmes*, published by Stockton Press.[6]

The experts in a specific field of medicine write individual chapters of a medical textbook. Usually the authors are also doing research at their facilities. You can follow up by using the Internet to find the web site for the facility for more information about the work being done at a specific facility. You can also look for journal articles by that researcher in MEDLINE.

Medical journal articles are direct links to research studies. Most articles list affiliations and contact addresses on the first page of the article. Contact the authors to be kept up on further advances in their ongoing research. You can also look at the bibliography in a medical article for information on additional documented studies.

The Internet is an efficient way to find information on recent studies. Some sites and email newsletters specialize in medical news. Breast Cancer Net, *http://www.breastcancer.net*, has daily links to press stories on breast cancer. The web site, Doctor's Guide to the Internet, can be found at *http://www.psl-group.com/MEDNEWS.HTM*. It offers, among other things, current medical news. When reading or hearing a medical news announcement, note the source of the study. Supporting information will often be available on the web site of the facility or agency supporting the research for the study cited in the news story.

If you find a research center working on an area of interest to you in a location close enough for you to visit, let them know that you are interested in their work and would like to visit. Some research facilities are part of clinics and some are research labs. A lab would be less likely to welcome a walk-in visitor. Laboratory facilities, however, may have a newsletter or annual report they can mail you giving you more detailed accounts of their work. Media kits and original press releases of promising research are often available from research centers or can be accessed is on their web sites.

Personal contact with the researcher may be more difficult, but is not impossible. If an email address for the lead researcher is available at the facility or listed in a published article, a brief, well-composed question may elicit an answer and could even lead to further discussion. Researchers tend to be passionate about their area of interest and many are willing to share their experience, theories, and expectations with interested listeners.

Medical product manufacturers

Companies that sell medical products are an often undervalued source of medical information. In addition to drug and medical device companies, look for companies that are devising new diagnostic and treatment techniques and equipment. These are companies doing research on new biomarkers for identifying diseases or identifying the genetic risk of developing a disease or condition.

While you can expect to find some bias and marketing spin when reading about effectiveness of a product, you can also expect to find some leading-edge research and well-written overviews of the conditions the products are designed to treat or diagnose. To get a fuller picture, collect information from competitive companies. The quickest way to find out about the limitations of a product or treatment is to read the competitor's explanation of why his product is better.

Most medical school libraries will have a current copy of Dorland's *Medical and Healthcare Marketplace Guide*, edited by Robert Smith, published by Legal Communications. This reference is too expensive for most small libraries, but the reference librarian at your public library can help you look for the nearest library that has this directory. Another directory to look for is the *Health Devices Sourcebook* published by Emergency Care Research Institute.

For the names of companies that make a particular drug, check the *Physician's Desk Reference*, which is available at nearly all libraries and can also be purchased at many bookstores.

News articles and reports often highlight new treatments, procedures, and devices. Note the name and location of the manufacturer of the product. Contact the journalist or reporter if that information is not included in the report.

The Internet is an excellent place to find information on commercial products. An Internet search on a drug or product name will usually lead you to the manufacturer's web site. From that you can get product information, press releases, and contact information.

Stock market investors search for companies making exciting new advances in medical treatment. Business directories like *Dun & Bradstreet Publicly-Traded-Companies*, *http://www.CompaniesOnline.com*, *Moody's Handbook of*

Common Stock, Value Line Investment Survey, and *Standard & Poor's Stock Reports* direct stock investors to companies in the healthcare industry group (i.e., biotechnology, biologicals, pharmaceuticals, medical products). You may find research that is in progress, but not yet conclusive enough to have reached the press release stage. Keep in mind that stock information targeted toward stimulating investment will always emphasize the positive outlook for that company's research and resulting products and rarely mention a problem.

The best place to meet and talk with company representatives is in the exhibit hall at a major conference. Access to these, however, will probably be limited to the professional medical community. One place to find listings of conferences is *http://www.pslgroup.com/MEDCONF.HTM*. If you know the name of the sponsoring organization, you can probably get a listing of exhibitors and contact the ones that interest you directly.

A small company might not be prepared for a walk-in visit, but they are accustomed to dealing with potential investors by phone, mail, and by appointment. Many companies have a person on staff who handles investor relations. A larger company may have a public relations representative. Mentor, a prosthetics manufacturer in Santa Barbara, California, for example, has a Patient Information Coordinator whose job it is to educate the public about the company's product. A drug company will have scientific researchers on staff. Some medical device companies and biotech companies will have medical professionals such as physicians and pathologists as well as basic scientific researchers on staff who may be willing to answer any detailed questions.

Ask about written materials such as the company's annual report, pamphlets and booklets on a medical device, and overviews of the condition it addresses. They may also have videos. These are marketing tools, but they will include useful basic information. These companies educate medical personnel about how their products work and how to use them. Sometimes a monograph, or scientific explanation, of the product is written to educate physicians about the product. If the company has a mailing list, you can ask to have them include your name.

Since medical products must receive approval from the Food and Drug Administration, the FDA at *http://www.fda.gov* will have approval information on any medical product marketed in the United States.

The Internet and electronic subscription services

You've seen Internet web site addresses or URLs used as references throughout this chapter and throughout the entire book. The Internet has revolutionized the way we access information and offers the computer user access to the largest collection of information in the world. The Internet, however, has no central catalog and no review or oversight process to control the quality of information you'll find.

To access the Internet, you need a computer, a modem, and an Internet account through a local or national Internet Service Provider (ISP). Small ISPs offer Internet services in most communities. Larger companies like AOL, Netcom, and Earthlink offer services in most communities. One company, AltaVista, that produces the largest search engine, is also an Internet Service Provider. Many phone companies and, more recently, cable TV companies also offer Internet service to individuals.

If you don't have a computer, you can access the Internet on computers at a nearby college, the local library, patient resource center, or sometimes even the local coffee shop. You might also ask a friend who has a computer to show you the Internet and help you to do some searches.

If you're already familiar with the Internet, you've probably used various search engines such as altavista.com and yahoo.com, that help you locate the information you're seeking. There are also many excellent "multiple" search engines. These search engines simply search many other search engines, since no one search engine even comes close to locating everything on the Web. Three of these useful multiple search engines are *http://www.dogpile. com, http://www.infind.com* and *http://www.37.com,* which searches 37 different search engines at the same time. Another search engine allows the user to ask a question, *http://www.askjeeves.com.*

There are also web sites that evaluate information on the Web and provide a subject index to many useful sites. One of the best known of these sites is The Librarians Index to the Internet, *http://www.lii.org,* maintained by the Berkeley Public Library in Berkeley, California.

What you will find on the Internet

Go to the Internet for the latest news, press releases, recent journal articles, drug information, patient guides and current research information from clinics, hospitals, medical schools, and universities, and a connection to people who study or have experienced the condition that you are researching.

Information posted to newsgroups, mailing lists, and web forums appears almost instantly after it is posted to the Internet. The information on a web site can be updated within a few minutes. This information passes through no filter or approval process. A scientist can post his findings to the Internet immediately, without passing them through the peer-review process required for journal articles.

One professor was especially excited when he found such quick feedback to his research and lectures when he posted them on Internet:

> I'm a professor at UC Berkeley. Often, after I give a talk I post the text of my talk to the Internet. To publish the text as a journal article might take months. When I post it to the Internet I have feedback from people around the world in my email box the next day.

This does not mean that all information on the Internet is always the most current information on a topic, particularly on the Web. Newsgroup postings expire and mail lists and web forums postings are dated. Information posted to a web site remains on that site until the web site owner decides to replace it. Many web site owners give a date for the most recent update of the page.

This lack of restrictions and hierarchy is why the Internet is the source of such a broad wealth of information. Look to the Internet for guidelines, advice, and current research information, but remember to examine these for information on the credentials and experience of the author.

What you won't find on the Internet

The Internet is a new medium. The information you will find on it usually has been published in the last ten years. Even MEDLINE, the most complete database of medical journal articles, does not offer articles that date back before the mid-1960s.

View the Internet the way you would a newspaper or magazine, rather than a textbook. It is a dynamic forum where information can be updated quickly, but sometimes at the expense of accuracy.

Advertising on the Internet is not as clearly identified as it is in a newspaper or magazine. It is always a good idea to verify the accuracy of anything you read when making health decisions, but especially when you read it on the Internet. Compared to other ways of publicizing a product or service, producing a professional looking web site is inexpensive. You will see web sites for new products or treatments that look quite professional. Always look for research studies, not anecdotal studies, which support the claims being made. A few basic guidelines for evaluating health information on the Internet are the following:

- If the treatment or product being advertised on a web site cures a multitude of unrelated conditions, it is probably hype or exaggeration.

- If the results of a study have not been reproduced or duplicated elsewhere, they are suspect.

- If there is a request for money on the web site, or an offer to start a franchise to sell the products on that site, look at the information as an advertisement.

- If the treatment or product is listed with personal but incomplete endorsements by individuals, but little actual scientific fact, it is suspect.

There is an additional list of health information evaluation criteria entitled "Red Flags" in Chapter 9, *Complementary and Alternative Therapies*. There is also an excellent review article in the *British Medical Journal (BMJ)* entitled "Published criteria for evaluating health related web sites: review."[7] Table 5-1 (from that article) summarizes the evaluation criteria from 29 rating tools for Internet based health information follows:

Table 5-1. Frequency of Explicit Criteria for Evaluation of Health-Related Web Sites by Criteria Groups.[a]

Criteria Groups	Frequency (%) (n=165)
Content of site (includes quality, reliability, accuracy, scope, depth)	30 (18)
Design and aesthetics (includes layout, interactivity, presentation, appeal, graphics, use of media)	22 (13)
Disclosure of authors, sponsors, developers (includes identification of purpose, nature of organization, sources of support, authorship, origin)	20 (12)
Currency of information (includes frequency of update, freshness, maintenance of site)	14 (8)
Authority of source (includes reputation of source, credibility, trustworthiness)	11 (7)
Ease of use (includes usability, navigability, functionality)	9 (5)
Accessibility and availability (includes ease of access, fee for access, stability)	9 (5)

Table 5-1. *Frequency of Explicit Criteria for Evaluation of Health-Related Web Sites by Criteria Groups.[a] (continued)*

Criteria Groups	Frequency (%) (n=165)
Links (includes quality of links, links to other sources)	5 (3)
Attribution and documentation (includes presentation of clear references, balanced evidence)	5 (3)
Intended audience (includes nature of intended users, appropriateness for intended users)	3 (2)
Contact addresses or feedback mechanism (includes availability of contact information, contact address)	2 (1)
User support (includes availability of support, documentation for users	2 (1)
Miscellaneous (includes criterion that lacked specificity or were unique)	33 (20)

[a] Of five authors who assigned weights or priorities to their proposed criteria, four cited content and one cited peer review (categorized as miscellaneous) as most important criterion. Percentage total does not equal 100 due to rounding-off.

Unless you are looking for information on a very rare condition, the amount of information available on the Internet will probably be overwhelming. Do not expect to be able to read everything that is available on your health topic. It may take some searching to find the most accurate, up-to-date information.

A professional researcher shares this tip for coping with huge numbers of hits on an Internet search:

> One guideline use for searching the Web is that I never look at more than the first 40 listings from one search engine on a given topic. If I don't find what I'm looking for in the first 40 references, I try a different search engine or one of those multi search engines. No one search engine accesses the entire web.

Online services

Online services such as Prodigy and America Online (AOL) offer access to the Internet in addition to areas for live discussion and access to specialized databases. The Internet service is only part of what they offer. These companies have developed software that makes it very easy for a new user to set up their computer and understand how to use the Internet or their other services. The software to set up your computer is usually available free. You may already have a collection of disks that have been sent to you in the mail or with subscription offers. These services are comparable in cost to a standard ISP account. Their ease of setup makes them an easy way for a new user to learn about the Internet.

Subscription services

Subscription services, such as Ovid, *http://www.ovid.com*, Lexis-Nexis, *http://www.lexis-nexis.com*, and Dialog, *http://www.dialog.com,* have been used for a long time by medical professionals for access to medical journal articles. Subscription to these services is expensive, but worth the cost for a library or a professional researcher for the access to over 1,000 databases.

Today most of these large medical databases can be accessed over the Internet. MEDLINE article abstracts and citations are now available free over the Internet. Professional full-text databases like Ovid, Lexis-Nexis, and Dialog still require a subscription fee, but a paid user can access them over the Internet by using a password as the key. The subscription cost for access to these databases by the individual user can be prohibitive so their use is primarily through universities, medical schools, and medical libraries. Free searches are restricted to professionals served by the facility with the subscription. Some of these facilities, however, will do a search for you for a fee.

New lower cost database subscription services like MD Consult, *http://www.mdconsult.com,* and E-Library, *http://www.elibrary.com*, offer full-text articles to individual researchers. MD Consult provides access to the full text of nearly 40 major medical textbooks and at least that many journals. It has a free trial period as do many of the other subscription databases. Many newspapers and magazines offer archive searches, but require registration and sometimes a monthly fee to view and save the full-text articles to your computer.

In summary, throughout this chapter we've mentioned many places to locate medical information, including libraries, bookstores, associations, and many, many more. We've also explained that many of these information centers have either a physical address or a virtual Internet address or both. Table 5-2 summarizes access information for the major resources mentioned throughout the chapter.

Table 5-2. Summary of Information Resources

Resource	Best Access	Way(s) to Locate	Additional Information
Public library	Direct visit	Telephone book	May have Internet catalog
Academic library	Direct visit or Internet web site	Telephone book or Directory	May have Internet catalog
Medical school library	Direct visit	*http://www.aamc.org/ meded* to find location	Over 125 medical schools nationwide
Hospital or consumer health library	Direct visit	Telephone book or *http://www.njc.org/ CAPHIS*	May have Internet catalog and online information
Bookstores	Direct visits or Internet web sites	Telephone book or web site (*http://www. amazon.com*), etc.	Online price comparisons can be useful
Government health agencies	Internet	Telephone Book for local agencies	*http://www.lii.org* under "Health" very helpful
Professional societies	Internet web sites	Use search engine	*http://www.dir.yahoo/ Health/organizations* very useful
Nonprofit organizations	Direct visit or Internet web sites	Use Directory or search engine	Libraries have directories
Medical product manufacturers	Internet web site or conference	Use Directory or search engine	Large libraries have directories
Internet	Computer/ modem or direct link	Internet Service Provider (ISP)	Adult education Internet classes offered in most places

CHAPTER 6

Effective Search Strategies

The ultimate goal of every librarian and information seeker is to find the highest quality, most up-to-date, relevant information, written at an appropriate level of complexity—and to find it as quickly as possible. In reality, librarians first determine exactly what they are looking for, find the most logical place to start, and then follow the trail where it leads. Sometimes they hit dead ends and have to start again. You seldom find a straight path to the answers.

In this chapter, we pose some specific research scenarios and consider the questions that a librarian or a professional researcher would ask in order to focus the question. We illustrate ways to begin the search, find a starting place, suggest things to look for as you search, and offer tips to make the search more efficient. If you don't have the time, resources, or inclination to do your own searching, we also describe how to find a qualified researcher to help answer your questions.

Things to consider before you begin

Here are questions to ask yourself each time you begin a new search:

- **What sources of information are readily accessible to me at this time?** Look at your situation. Do you have your own computer and Internet access or easy access to a computer? Is a medical library available to you? In the beginning you will be learning about the resources available to you as well as looking for answers to specific questions. As you become familiar with the resources available to you locally, you will gain an intuitive feeling for where best to go to find answers to a particular question.

- **What is my current level of technical understanding?** Are you looking for basic overview information, written at an average consumer level of understanding, or have you become familiar enough with the technical jargon to understand materials written for the professional? Note that even when the details of an article are difficult to follow, the conclusion of the article may be meaningful in your search, so don't be afraid to stretch the limits of your current understanding a little and note the terms that are unfamiliar to you. Some medical databases are general and consumer oriented and some will yield very specific information.

- **How much time do I have to learn about this?** The greater the urgency of your question, the more you will need to rely on easily accessible resources. If you have more time, you can be more creative in your search, tapping into resources that might require some waiting time before you get a response. You also might be willing to try some approaches that are less likely to yield helpful results.

- **Am I looking for standard treatment information or for clinical trials or complementary and alternative approaches to treatment?** You may be looking for a well-established explanation of your condition and standard medical approach to treatment. Or, you might be exploring other theories about the disease and new or experimental treatments.

- **Are there limits to what I want to know?** As we have said before, think about how much detail you feel ready to face and respect your own limits. A detailed description of a procedure you are about to have or unusual side effects from a drug that impacts some, but not all, patients may not be something you want to read at this point.

Research tools and scenarios

Listed in this chapter are generic questions that are representative of many types of health questions. In this list are a drug question, a treatment question, a question on finding a medical expert, a surgical question, a question on finding someone else with similar medical conditions, a prognosis question, and question about locating the best treatment centers. The suggestions for answering these questions will be specific, but you can use the answers as general guidelines for finding similar types of information. For example, finding information about one drug can help you find information about another drug or drugs in the same category of drugs.

If you have a computer with Internet access, you would be more effective if you look up information about your topic before you go to a library. By doing a preview search, you can more clearly define your terms and clarify your question. You might actually find your answers without leaving home!

A general research principle is to define your question and your terms and find general information first. Then, when you have an understanding of the larger question, you can narrow your topic to the specific areas of interest. There are many places to look for information. We could never present every resource that is available, but we have listed a few of the free and reliable research tools:

- A medical library. Call the National Library of Medicine at (800) 338-7657 for the location of a medical library in your area with public access.

- A medical textbook. One example of a free general medical book online is *The Merck Manual*, at *http://www.merck.com*.[1]

- Internet search engines. One subject-oriented search engine is Yahoo at *http://www.yahoo.com*, and one multiple search engine that searches 37 other search engines is 37.com at *http://www.37.com*. There are many excellent search engines. These are simply listed as examples of easy places to start. If you have your own favorite, by all means use it.

- MEDLINEplus from The National Library of Medicine (NLM). This is a good starting place because on the web site (*http://www.medlineplus. gov*), you can find medical dictionaries, atlases and visual models, and links to many useful consumer resources and organizations. MEDLINE-plus also has automatic links to preformatted searches in PubMed and the entire MEDLINE database.

  This is an excellent place to start any medical search. Note in Figure 6-1 the dictionary link in the upper left part of the screen, the topic choices by letter at the top of the screen and the pull down menu of topics by category. The medical encyclopedia contains excellent medical images.

- MEDLINE, accessed through PubMed. (See Figure 6-2.) An online database of more than 4,000 medical journals at *http://www.nlm.nih.gov/ pubmed*. PubMed is one of the most user-friendly formats for MED-LINE. Because it, too, is produced by the National Library of Medicine, the PubMed database is available free.

  Note in Figure 6-2 the links to "Limits," "Index," "History," and "Clip-board" under the box for the search statement. The "Limits" link allows you to limit your search to English, specific age groups, certain years,

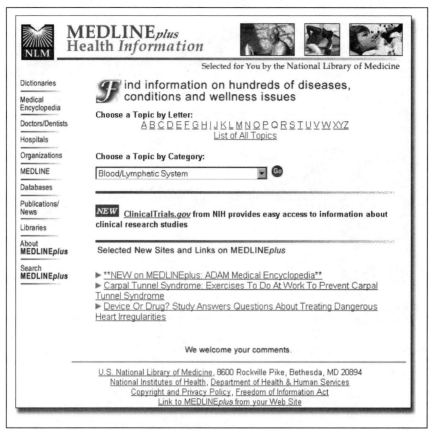

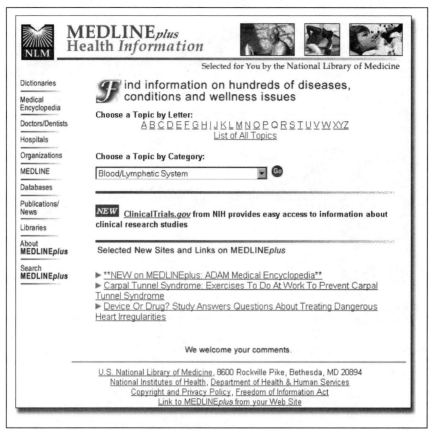
(contents of the figure image)

MEDLINE*plus*
Health *Information*
NLM

Selected for You by the National Library of Medicine

Dictionaries

Medical
Encyclopedia

Doctors/Dentists

Hospitals

Organizations

MEDLINE

Databases

Publications/
News

Libraries

About
MEDLINEplus

Search
MEDLINEplus

**ind information on hundreds of diseases,
conditions and wellness issues**

Choose a Topic by Letter:
A B C D E F G H I J K L M N O P Q R S T U V W X Y Z
List of All Topics

Choose a Topic by Category:

Blood/Lymphatic System   Go

NEW ClinicalTrials.gov from NIH provides easy access to information about
clinical research studies

Selected New Sites and Links on MEDLINE*plus*

▶ **NEW on MEDLINEplus: ADAM Medical Encyclopedia**
▶ Carpal Tunnel Syndrome: Exercises To Do At Work To Prevent Carpal
Tunnel Syndrome
▶ Device Or Drug? Study Answers Questions About Treating Dangerous
Heart Irregularities

We welcome your comments.

U.S. National Library of Medicine, 8600 Rockville Pike, Bethesda, MD 20894
National Institutes of Health, Department of Health & Human Services
Copyright and Privacy Policy, Freedom of Information Act
Link to MEDLINE*plus* from your Web Site

Figure 6-1. MEDLINEplus from the National Library of Medicine

and much more. The "History" feature allows you to track your questions and combine them to focus your search. The "Help" screens are also very useful.

For the sample research scenarios, we list the question, then give the questions a librarian might ask to help focus the search, suggest good places to look for information, particular things to look for, and search tips.

Question 1: What are the side effects of blood pressure medication?

This is a question you might ask about a specific drug. You can use the following search procedure to find information about other drugs as well.

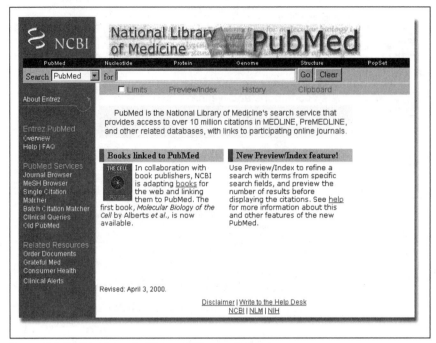

Figure 6-2. PubMed from the National Library of Medicine

Questions a librarian would ask to focus the search

- Is there a specific drug name that is of interest, or is this a generic question about all blood pressure medications? If it is a specific drug, is it over the counter or prescription?

- Is this medication to be prescribed for an adult, a child, or a geriatric patient?

- Does the patient have any coexisting diseases, conditions and/or medications that would complicate treatment for high blood pressure?

- Are there any other terms for high blood pressure that would help make a search more effective and complete?

Starting places to look for information

Start with MEDLINEplus, *http://www.medlineplus.gov.*

You can start with MEDLINEplus if you have computer access because it is easy to search. You can select "H" from the alphabetical list and scroll down to "High Blood Pressure" and click on that link. Then look for treatment or drug therapy. You may also want to search the dictionaries, especially Merriam-Webster, from the dictionary list at the top left of the screen for definitions.

By searching MEDLINEplus, you find out that high blood pressure is called hypertension and medications are called antihypertensive agents. If you want more information you can go to the MEDLINE box on the screen and click on the "Therapy" link. You'll immediately go into PubMed and a pre-formatted search of recent articles. If you know the name of a specific drug, you can type it in the search box at the top of the screen.

Some of the abstracts may actually have enough of an answer, and you need look no further. If you need assistance in searching, there are some very useful help screens for PubMed and other services on the main National Library of Medicine web site at *http://www.nlm.nih.gov*. You may also want to search a specific web site that has basic drug prescribing information such as Rxlist at *http://www.rxlist.com*.

Next, or if you don't have a computer, go to a library. They may have a computer you can use. The reference librarian can help you find a recent medical reference book and a *Physicians' Desk Reference (PDR)*, which is a well-known drug reference.[2] Other recently published drug references may also have the answers for you.

Armed with the information from your MEDLINEplus and PubMed searches and your drug references, you can compile a list of questions for your physician so that you can understand how antihypertensive agents will affect those who are taking the drugs.

Things to look for

When searching PubMed, look carefully at the numbers of people in each study mentioned in the abstract and where the studies are taking place. Find a review article if you can, or one in a general family physician journal such as *American Family Physician*. You want to look for large studies that are about people like you, not some group that may have other specific traits in common, such as diabetes, pregnancy, or obesity, etc.

Search tips

Keep a list of pros and cons for taking or not taking blood pressure medications as you go along. Keep copies of relevant information you find and note the sources of that information in case you want to find it again and so you can tell your physician where you found the information.

Question 2: Are there nonsurgical options for carpal tunnel syndrome?

This is an example of a question you might ask about various treatments for a specific condition. You can use the following procedure to locate information about treatments for other conditions as well.

Questions a librarian would ask to focus the search

- What treatments have already been tried?

- Is this for a man or woman? Is this for someone who needs to use their hands a great deal?

- How did the injury take place?

Places to look for information

With the advent of high computer use, carpal tunnel syndrome has become almost an epidemic. One good place to start in finding information about a well-known condition is a reliable consumer site such as the National Library of Medicine's MEDLINEplus web site: *http://www.medlineplus.gov.* Click on the letter "C" for carpal tunnel and click on the link to carpal tunnel syndrome. Pages of relevant information will come up.

If you need further information, go to a medical library and look through the section on orthopedics, hand surgery, and rehabilitation and look in the index of those books. Look up carpal tunnel syndrome in the library catalog for a specific book on the subject. You can also do a MEDLINE search in PubMed by just typing "carpal tunnel" in the search box. Check the titles and see if the library has some of the articles that look useful to you. Note that when doing a PubMed search the database goes all the way back to 1966. You need to be aware of the dates of the information since new treatments are constantly being discovered and what worked ten years ago may not be the best option today.

Things to look for

When you are reading medical articles, be aware that the writers will have a point of view just as with writers of any type of information. Therefore, if a surgeon is writing the article on carpal tunnel syndrome the article may favor surgical treatment since this is what the surgeon knows more thoroughly. An internist or a physical therapist might favor a nonsurgical approach.

Search tips

The articles will not often come to a clear conclusion. It is a good idea to read several to reach some sort of consensus when you are making a decision.

Question 3: What does an elevated PSA on my blood test mean?

This is an example of a question about a medical test for a specific condition. You can use the following procedure to find information about other medical conditions.

Questions a librarian would ask to focus the search

- What does "PSA" stand for?

- What is considered a "normal" PSA and what is the range of measurement, i.e., is the PSA slightly elevated or extremely elevated? This information will influence further research.

- Who is asking for the information, i.e., is it for a young person or an elderly person and have they had treatment for the condition PSA is used to diagnose?

Places to look for information

Find a medical dictionary to define PSA. If you don't have one, there are several available on Internet. One web address listing medical dictionaries is MEDLINEplus, *http://www.medlineplus.gov*, mentioned earlier. Of the online dictionaries listed, one of the easiest to use is *The Merriam Webster Medical Dictionary*.[3]

Finding out that PSA stands for prostate specific antigen, you would then either do a MEDLINE search or consult a medical textbook in the area of urology and look in the index of that book for PSA. Note that you will want to look for the most recent textbook and journal articles since this is an area of medicine that is still generating research and improved treatment options.

Things to look for

One of the most important things to look for is the date of the information you are reading as well as the credentials of the author. You also want to find good overall coverage of the prostate specific antigen tests and what they mean in different age groups.

Search tips

After you define your terms and check a textbook and/or MEDLINE you may have enough information to understand PSA. You may be able to find a great deal of information on the Internet for this topic but be extremely cautious regarding the author of the information. Always check with your doctor if you are making medical decisions based on information found on Internet. After you have your information, you can bring your test results and confer with a urologist if there are elevated numbers that indicate you should have additional screenings. In the current healthcare system, your tests will usually be recommended by your primary care physician who can make a referral to a urologist if you are worried about elevated PSA levels.

Question 4: What are the treatment options for acid reflux?

Here is an example of a question you might ask about treatments for a specific condition. You can use the same process to find information about treatments for other conditions as well.

Questions a librarian would ask to focus the search

- How long has the condition been a problem?
- Has there been an official diagnosis by your physician?
- Have you found other terms for the same condition such as gastroesophageal reflux or GERD?
- Are there other coexisting conditions or situations that would exacerbate the acid reflux such as dietary problems, other gastrointestinal problems?
- Is this question for an adult or child?

Places to look for information

Since this is a treatment question and you already know the diagnosis, you can start with a search in PubMed, *http://www.ncbi.nlm.nih.gov/PubMed*. Type the words "acid reflux treatment" in the opening search section. You want recent information and PubMed brings up the most recent medical journal references first. PubMed is the most current MEDLINE database you will find.

Things to look for

In the PubMed abstracts, look for summaries of outcomes of various types of treatment. The more recent these summaries are, the more relevant this information will be for your decision making. If you get too much information you can limit your search by date or by typing the word "review" at the end of your question so the string of terms will be "acid reflux treatment review." That should help you retrieve articles that give reviews of all of the treatments.

Search tips

If the abstracts of the articles you find in PubMed do not give enough information, you would want to obtain copies of the full text of the articles most relevant to your question. You can obtain these from a medical library or an information broker or through interlibrary loan at your public library.

Question 5: Historically, what is the treatment for tuberculosis?

This is an example of a question you might ask about the historic changes in the treatment for a specific condition. Sometimes earlier treatments are brought back because they have been most effective over time.

Questions a librarian would ask to focus the search

- Is this only an historical question or do you need to know how tuberculosis is best treated currently for yourself or a loved one?

- If it is for a current patient, has any treatment already been started? If so, what is it and what has been the outcome?

- What type of tuberculosis is this? There are several new strains that are resistant to many drugs.

Places to look for information

The best place to start if this is a current treatment question is PubMed, *http://www.ncbi.nlm.nih.gov/pubmed*. If this is only an historical question, there will be a great deal of information in public health history textbooks in large public libraries or colleges and universities, as well as in medical libraries. Tuberculosis has been with us for a long time and has been called consumption and other names.

Things to look for

Look for current outcome studies for tuberculosis treatment. Since tuberculosis is an infectious disease, look for studies that discuss control of this disease in high-risk populations such as homeless groups or others with little access to healthcare. For historical information and public health history, look for the place tuberculosis has played in the whole picture of the public health movement starting before 1900.

Search tips

As stated above, start with PubMed. Then go to the most current medical textbooks on pulmonary medicine and/or infectious diseases. Antibiotic resistant tuberculosis is a very real problem in recent years and you want to search for treatments that will discuss this recent problem.

Question 6: Are there any new drugs for asthma?

Here is an example of a question you might ask about drug treatment for a chronic or long-term condition. You could use the example to find information about other chronic conditions, as treatments may improve over time.

Questions a librarian would ask to focus the search

*   Is this for a new diagnosis or for someone with long-term chronic asthma?
*   Is this for an adult or child?
*   What treatments have been tried and are they still effective? Are there any allergic reactions to current treatment and/or drug therapies?

Places to look for information

For this question you can again start with PubMed and then look elsewhere on the Internet. You might try one of the consumer-focused search engines such as NetWellness at *http://www.netwellness.com*. NetWellness has an "ask an expert" feature with excellent information. Another starting place for this question would be to find an internet mail list of asthma sufferers at *http://www.liszt.com*. Since asthma is a chronic condition, there are probably many people discussing this same question. Some of their answers may be very useful. Always be cautious and a little skeptical when hearing about unusual cures or self-treating certain illnesses. Check the information out with a doctor if it involves taking any unknown drug or herbal remedy that may cause a reaction or serious side effects.

Things to look for

In the PubMed or NetWellness search look for the names of new drugs or new studies on effective treatments. If one drug or therapeutic regimen comes up several times in the most recent references, especially those involving a large group of people, look up the drug itself. You can continue in PubMed or check one of the pharmaceutical web sites such as *http://www.pharminfo.com* or *http://www.rxlist.com*. Evaluate the information about the treatment in terms of your own health history. Some of the studies are done only on children or only on newly diagnosed asthma cases, etc. Compare your situation to those of the people in the studies. If your situation is similar to those in several of the studies and you have no conditions that would contraindicate a new drug, bring the information to your physician to discuss trying this new therapy.

Search tips

When you're searching for new therapies, whether it is a drug therapy, a new surgical technique or some other therapy, be very cautious. Research into new therapies is usually announced as a promising and exciting breakthrough. Both the researcher and the agency or company funding the research will present results in most favorable terms, since they have a commercial agenda. New therapies have not been tested over a span of time that would allow for the discovery of any long term adverse effects. You should try to verify the results of any single study to see if researchers were able to duplicate the results as well as check any drugs mentioned. Often an older drug designed to treat one condition will be used for an entirely different condition. Dapsone, for example, was used to treat leprosy and is now being used to treat asthma. The drug itself may have a long history of side effects that have nothing to do with treatment of asthma, so if you can read up on the drug itself, you'll have a clearer understanding of its properties.

Question 7: Who specializes in treatment of narcolepsy?

This is an example of a question you might ask about finding a medical expert. You can use the following process to locate information about other medical experts as well.

Questions a librarian would ask to focus the search

- What is narcolepsy? Is it a nervous system disease or a psychiatric condition or both?

- Have you been treated for narcolepsy before and what was the outcome?

- Are you looking for a specialist for treating this disease or a general practitioner?

- If you are looking for a certain physician, do you have geographical or insurance limitations affecting your search?

Places to start looking for information

If you need to know more about narcolepsy, consult a medical dictionary or textbook such as *The Merck Manual* for basic information. MEDLINEplus directs you to "sleep disorders" when you look for information on narcolepsy. Another starting place might be the American Board of Medical Specialists (ABMS) web site, *http://www.abms.org*, or the AMA web site, *http://www.ama-assn.org*, to search for specialists, usually neurologists, in your area.

In looking for people who treat a given condition, another good starting place would be a search engine to see what is out on the Web about the condition. One of the multi-site search engines such as Dogpile, *http://www.dogpile.com*, or Inference, *http://www.infind.com*, might be more effective than the larger search engines such as AltaVista. Simply type "narcolepsy" or "sleep disorders" on the search line. There may also be a discussion list where individuals discuss their own experiences and may name certain therapists. You can note whether these are neurologists or psychiatrists or experts on sleep disorders, a new subspecialty. You could then search for a list of certified sleep disorder specialists or clinics.

Things to look for

Look for training and certification of any experts for treating narcolepsy. Who does the certification and what does it mean? It's good to learn the initials of certain respected certification programs, such as those for specialists certified for sleep disorders. The specialized web sites on sleep medicine and a current medical book on sleep medicine will both explain the credentials of specialists.

Search tips

As you collect information about narcolepsy, you will find that it is categorized as both a neurological disorder and a sleep disorder. You can probably receive excellent treatment from specialists in either area. Credentialing specialists in sleep disorders is quite recent. You would want to be certain, however, that whoever you consult has treated a number of people with this condition.

Question 8: What are the complications with hip replacement devices?

This is an example of a question you might ask about orthopedic surgeries. You can use the search process to find information about complications of other surgeries as well.

Questions a librarian would ask to focus the search

- Is this for someone contemplating hip replacement surgery, or is it for someone who has already had the surgery?

- If it is for someone who has already had hip replacement surgery, what type of prosthesis was used and how recent was the surgery?

- Are you looking for a specific complaint or complication or just considering all of the possibilities?

Places to look for information

The starting place would be with the orthopedic surgeon performing the surgery. The surgeons have followed many, many patients with hip replacement surgery and they would have a very good idea of complications that occur. You can also find information in orthopedic textbooks, especially *Campbell's Orthopedics*,[4] or a text specifically on the complications of orthopedic surgery such as *Epp's Complications in Orthopedic Surgery*.[5] To find discussions of complications, you can access PubMed and type in the phrase "hip replacement surgery complications" and read the abstracts from the orthopedic journals. Remember that journals often report unusual findings or unexpected results and that the generally expected course of treatment will be found in the medical texts.

Things to look for

Look for studies of large numbers of surgeries to determine complication rates and types of complications that may occur. Also note that the age of the patient is often a factor in complications for surgeries like this one. If you see discussions of some complication that you are experiencing or that you want more information on, you would consult your surgeon. Your own surgeon will know your particular situation and will know if you may be susceptible to specific complications.

Search tips

Surgical questions require a full range of answers including textbook information, information from recent journals, and the information from surgeons who have experience with this type of surgery. The surgeons can answer your specific questions and relate them to your specific case. It is a good idea to understand a full range of complications and how they are treated, since your own surgeon may not even mention those that he thinks may not affect you unless you ask.

Question 9: What are the current surgical procedures for gallbladder removal?

Here is an example of a question you might ask about different types of surgery for the same condition. You can use the search procedure for many types of surgery.

Questions a librarian would ask to focus the search

- Is this a question for someone who needs surgery immediately or is it for someone who's been told they may need gallbladder surgery at some time in the future?
- Has a physician and/or surgeon already recommended one type of surgery over another and what type was that?

Places to look for information

Start with the MEDLINEplus or the most recent surgical textbook available, no more than two years old. You'll find that the surgeons call gallbladder removal "cholecystectomy."

Gallstones do not usually cause trouble until one lodges in the bile duct, which can cause abdominal colic, identified by severe pain occurring in spasms. The term for this is "cholelithiasis." It is very useful to have a medical dictionary handy for quick consultation when the terms used by the medical community are so different from terms in popular use. A physician or other health professional may discuss "gallbladder surgery" with you, but then your chart and other medical records will have these strange terms such as cholecystectomy. So a medical dictionary is definitely a good idea.

The next place you would look would be either MEDLINE, through PubMed on the Internet, or a graphical web site for surgeries titled "Your Surgery," at *http://www.yoursurgery.com*. Both sites are free. In PubMed look for review articles, those articles that review current treatment, by limiting to review.

Things to look for

Look for the different procedures and also look for the effectiveness of each. A laparoscopic cholecystectomy is a less invasive surgery with a much shorter recovery time, but it is sometimes not effective, and the more standard operation must be done later. Your surgeon has a great deal of experience in selecting one operation or another. If you are leaning towards requesting the less invasive surgery, ask your surgeon how many of these laparoscopic surgeries he has performed. Experience can enhance the success rate of a procedure as well as your own recovery after the surgery.

Search tips

When you are searching MEDLINE, look for complication rates and the reasons for complications. Discuss these with your doctor. You may want to make a list with the pros and cons for each type of surgery. If you choose the less invasive laparoscopic procedure, the surgeon will usually only agree to try to honor your choices because he won't know until the actual surgery if laparoscopic surgery will work in your case.

Question 10: How do I find someone to talk with who has had a bone marrow transplant?

This is a question you might ask about finding others who have similar medical conditions.

Questions a librarian would ask to focus the search

- Are you personally considering bone marrow transplantation or is it for a family member or friend?

- Bone marrow transplantation or BMT may be autologous or ABMT, i.e., using one's own marrow, or the marrow may be from a donor. Which type do you want to know about?

- What condition is this bone marrow transplantation for? BMT is used as a therapy for some types of leukemia, cancers, and other diseases. It is used with varying degrees of success in both adults and children. To find someone with whom you can compare notes, you need to be very specific about the type of bone marrow transplant, the condition for which it is a treatment, and whether it is for an adult or child.

Places to look for information

The first place to start is with the physician who has recommended a bone marrow transplant procedure. This physician, or those in his group, will most likely have other patients who have undergone this therapy. If it is for a child, the physician will know parents who will be able to share information about the experience.

The next place you could go would be to find a support group in your community. Usually these groups are organized by hospitals, cancer centers, or health information agencies.

The third place to look is on the Internet for a discussion list on the topic of bone marrow transplantation. There is an Internet site for finding these discussion groups. The URL is *http://www.liszt.com*. To focus in on your interest you would be most effective looking for discussion groups that share information and support for the condition being treated, i.e., look for a group discussing leukemia, breast cancer, or parents with children undergoing bone marrow transplantation, etc. For example, you can submit a question to a leukemia list asking for people who have had the experience of bone marrow transplantation. There may not be a discussion group focused specifically on the topic of bone marrow transplantation since the experiences are more directly related to the specific disease being treated.

Things to look for

Whether you find contact through your physician, through a support group, or through an email discussion group, you want to find people whose experiences most closely resemble yours. You also want to be cautious about strong biases. Bone marrow transplantation is a serious and difficult therapy. Some people respond well and others have many complications. Listen to many sides of the discussion to get a full picture of the procedure and its impact on a patient and her family. You can find out the chances for success or failure of the treatment from your physician or in medical textbooks. The information that individuals can add is that they can suggest coping strategies, offer support, and give some hope that patients can recover after such a serious procedure. Since the online discussion groups are international, you may learn of a trial or new treatment showing success in another part of the country or the world.

Search tips

Find people like yourself as well as people who have had similar experiences. In other words, if you are a grandfather, find a grandfather. If you are the mother of a child with leukemia, find another mother who has helped her child and herself get through the experience. Advice and sharing can be very supportive and even more useful if you can locate someone from a similar situation and background.

Question 11: What is the prognosis for heart bypass surgery?

Here is an example of a question you might ask about the prognosis or long-term outcome of a medical procedure.

Questions a librarian would ask to focus the search

- Is the individual considering a coronary artery bypass graft (CABG) considered high-risk, i.e., advanced age, poor health, with concurrent diseases such as diabetes or kidney failure, previous heart surgeries, etc.?

- Have less invasive alternatives such as diet, drug therapies, and/or lifestyle change been tried? Is there time to try these alternatives?

- How much experience has the surgeon and the hospital had with this procedure? Several studies conclude that surgeons and hospitals with the most experience with this procedure have the best outcomes.

Places to look for information

There is a great deal of information on coronary artery bypass graft surgery because it has become a relatively common procedure in the last fifteen years. You would start by asking the surgeon or the cardiologist recommending the surgery. Another place to look is on the web site for the Society of Thoracic Surgeons, *http://www.sts.org*. It has outcome studies for heart bypass posted, as well as links to studies done by different state medical societies and other groups.

You might also want to consult a recent cardiac or thoracic surgery text for basic information on the procedure.

Things to look for

Look for information on outcomes that are comparable to your own situation. Try to find studies that refer to cases that are similar to your case in age, sex, previous surgeries, medical condition, etc.

Search tips

Often you will be in a situation where there is little time to decide whether or not bypass surgery is a good option. If you or a family member has been admitted to the emergency room because of a heart attack and the physician recommends bypass surgery, you could ask for a second opinion. If your condition mandates that you need help immediately, it would be foolish to ask for more information, but there may be a nearby medical center that performs many of these surgeries. It is always a good idea to check on the surgeon's experience. The prognosis is more positive in centers where many of these surgeries are performed.

Question 12: Where should I go for cancer treatment if I can afford to go anywhere in the US?

This is the type of question you might ask if you need to locate places that specialize in the treatment of certain conditions. Use the following search process to locate expert providers and treatment centers for any condition.

Questions a librarian would ask to focus the search

- What type of cancer is to be treated?
- What stage of cancer has been diagnosed?
- Have you consulted with your own oncologist for recommendations?
- Would you be willing to be a part of a clinical trial?
- Have you already had surgery, chemotherapy, radiation, or all three?

Places to look for information

You want to find out who the experts are and where they work. A good place to start is with major cancer textbooks. Two leading cancer texts are DeVita's *Textbook of Cancer Diagnosis and Treatment*[6] and Holland's *Cancer Medicine*.[7]

Consult the chapter(s) for the specific cancer or cancer treatment and note who wrote these chapters. Then turn to the list of contributors at the front of the book and note where these experts work. The next step would be to look up the cancer in MEDLINE through PubMed. In the full citation, the institution is listed. Narrow your search to review articles and note the institutions where the articles are being written. They will probably include many of the same institutions you found in the two cancer texts. After this, check Cancernet, *http://www.cancernet.nci.nih.gov*, for clinical trials for the type of cancer you are dealing with. Another place on the Internet to find clinical trials is *http://www.clinicaltrials.gov*. Note the institutions where these clinical trials are taking place. Finally, check the American College of Surgeons web site, *http://www.acs.org*, for accreditation information on cancer treatment centers. You will begin to get a picture that three or four centers seem to have the medical experts doing research on the type of cancer you are facing. The names of the experts who are writing and setting up the clinical trials may not be the actual treatment specialists, but they will often be the teaching experts at the centers that have strong programs.

Things to look for

Look for the same institutions showing up again and again in the research, the textbooks and the clinical trials. Some of the largest cancer centers such as Memorial Sloane-Kettering in New York, M.D. Anderson in Houston, or the Mayo Clinic in Rochester, Minnesota may have experts on all types of cancer, but other centers may have experts on certain types of cancer. You would look for experts who write on the traditional as well as experimental treatments.

Search tips

Don't get frustrated if you end up with a list of eight or nine cancer centers. You can narrow this list down in several ways:

- Look at the types of experimental treatments being performed at different centers and consider if these sound reasonable to you. The published research in your MEDLINE search may give you some idea about the outcomes of these treatments.

- You can also call the centers to ask if they are accepting patients and if there are any restrictions. The National Cancer Institute has a hotline that can help you with contact numbers. Their phone number is (800) 4-CANCER or (800) 422-6237. With those contact numbers, you will be able to reach different centers for information and you will also have some idea about how well they deal with questions.

- Share your list with your oncologist and ask for his opinion about which center may be the best for you.

After you collect your information and compile a list of several excellent cancer centers, your final decision will come from your intuition. Which place feels the best to you? You want to have confidence in the place you go and the people who will be treating you.

Ways a librarian can help

Librarians are trained information professionals who have a master's degree in Library and Information Science. This training and subsequent work experience has given them knowledge of basic important reference sources, both electronic and in print. Medical librarians have experience using the important medical reference tools and they have experience showing others how to use them effectively. They can help you in your research in several ways:

- A librarian can help you refine your question and focus on the real information that you need.

- A librarian can help you determine the level of answer you are seeking, whether you want a brief overview or complete in-depth study.

- A librarian, especially a medical librarian, can help you clarify your question and formulate a search strategy.

- A librarian can help you determine the quality of the medical information you have found.

- A librarian will direct you to the indexes, texts, directories, and web sites where authoritative medical information can be located.

- A librarian can refer you to other libraries and organizations which may have the exact information that you need.

Medical librarians can save you a great deal of time by directing you quickly to the best resource for your question. Also, through experience, a librarian may have heard questions similar to yours and may be familiar with the information you are seeking, including several follow-up questions.

You can find medical librarians in the same ways that you would find medical libraries. The National Network of Libraries of Medicine can give you the name and number of the nearest medical library open to the public and staffed by medical librarians by calling (800) 338-7657.

Hiring a professional researcher

Self-education takes time: time to concentrate, time to learn new terminology and concepts, and time to evaluate and filter information. Research expertise is learned with practice. An expert is a person who has already made all the beginner's mistakes. If you find yourself running into dead ends at a time when you need to make a decision quickly, you might find it is more efficient and cost-effective to seek the help of a professional researcher or research group.

Why you would use a professional researcher

A professional will be familiar with the tools and experienced in knowing where to go first to look for the information you are seeking. A professional researcher will know how to evaluate information and filter out irrelevant items and unreliable sources of information.

A professional researcher will have access to resources that you cannot access, such as a subscription to a large collection of medical databases like Ovid and Dialog. A researcher will probably also have collaborative relationships with a network of librarians and other specialized researchers at specialized medical libraries. An experienced researcher will know where to look first and will recognize more quickly when to proceed or when to begin again. This can significantly reduce the time it takes to gather the information you need.

Unusual treatments and rare diseases are much more difficult for a new researcher to find. A local professional contracted on an hourly basis can supplement or augment your own search efforts. Even medical experts rely on help from the professionals at their local medical libraries and institutions.

Finding a professional researcher

If you live near a medical library, ask the staff if they offer search services or can recommend an independent professional researcher. If you are not near a medical library, your public library is the next best place to ask for a local recommendation.

The yellow pages in your local phone book will not provide you with a recommendation, but you can look for professional researchers under "Information Retrieval." This listing will include researchers who specialize in business-oriented research such as trademarks, patents, and other marketing issues as well as those with experience in medical research.

The Association of Independent Information Professionals (AIIP) offers a free referral service, called the IP Access Program. They will give you the names and contact information for up to three AIIP members. Contact AIIP Headquarters at (888) 544-AIIP and ask for a Request for IP Services form.

You can also find companies that do medical research. Examples include The Health Resource, (800) 949-0090 or *http://www.thehealthresource.com*; and Schine On-Line Services, (800) 346-3287 or *http://www.findcure.com*. Both companies were founded by survivors of unusual diseases who found help through research.

Qualifications

There is currently no certification process for an independent information professional or an information broker. (These two terms can be used interchangeably.)

Information professionals come from a wide variety of fields. While many are freelance librarians with degrees in library and information science, others come from the professions of law, science, education, journalism, and medicine. Researchers specialize in a variety of services, including online research, document retrieval, analysis, and summary.

The two professional organizations for independent information researchers are the American Society for Information Science (ASIS) and the Association of Independent Information Professionals (AIIP). The web sites for these two organizations are *http://www.asis.org* and *http://www.aiip.org*, respectively. Members of AIIP must have a master's in Library Science (MLS) or equivalent degree in a professional or academic discipline.

How much will a search cost?

There is no standard fee. An individual researcher will probably charge you by the hour, while a research service is more likely to have a package price. The Health Resource currently offers a four to five working day turnaround at a cost ranging from $275 to $375.

Billing can be hourly or by the project. Hourly fees may be $50 to $75 per hour plus the cost of any fee-based database. You may be asked to pay up front, upon receipt, or given 30-day terms. Some researchers have a minimum charge. You might want to request an hourly search, not to exceed a certain amount.

What to look for when hiring a researcher

Here are some things to compare when you are interviewing professional researchers:

- **References.** Request references and talk with previous clients to find out if they were satisfied with the work of the researcher. Ask if they are planning to use this service again.

- **Experience.** Ask about the individual's research background. Does she have MEDLINE and Dialog training and experience? Does she have college training in information retrieval? How many years experience does she have? How much experience does she have in medical research? Does she continue to take classes in Library and Information Science and online database training?

- **Communication skills.** In preliminary discussion, do you feel you are able to communicate easily with this researcher? Does she ask questions that help you to focus in on what type of information you would like to receive?

- **Resources.** Does the researcher have access to major fee-based medical database collections such as Ovid or Dialog? What other resources does she use? Will she search print resources and make phone calls as well as accessing online resources?

- **Full text.** Find out if you will receive the full text of documents, chapters of medical texts, abstracts, or just bibliographical information.

- **Range of information.** Does the researcher have access to information on complementary and experimental treatments, names of experts, and information on support groups and associations?

- **Form of delivery.** Will you receive the information by fax, email, overnight express, or standard mail delivery?

- **Follow-up.** Ask what sort of follow-up the individual or service does to insure that you are satisfied. Will they redirect the search if the material is not focused enough? Do they offer a money-back or a satisfaction guarantee?

Information to give the researcher

The development of a satisfying research relationship depends on the success of your communication with the person or service. If you have a clear idea of what questions you are trying to answer and what technical level of information you expect and can communicate that to the researcher, you have a much better chance of getting a report that meets your expectations. Prepare to provide the following information:

- **Diagnosis.** Specific details of your diagnosis

- **History.** Background of previous treatment for this or any related condition

- **Depth and range of information.** Types of information you are seeking, i.e., introductory, overview, or detailed medical research; mainstream or experimental options; names and addresses of experts in diagnosis and treatment; support groups and associations

- **Previous research.** Areas of information that you have already covered

- **Purpose.** How you plan to use this information; what types of decisions you will be making

- **Time frame.** The level of urgency you are experiencing

- **Specific questions.** Any pivotal questions that will affect your decision-making process

- **What information to avoid.** A clear statement of approaches you are not willing to consider and also details you would prefer not be covered

CHAPTER 7

Understanding Standard Treatment Options

STANDARD TREATMENT OPTIONS are traditionally defined as therapies in current use by physicians that have proved to be effective based on past studies and physician experience. "Proven effectiveness" is the key concept in defining and understanding standard treatment.

In this chapter, we go over standard treatment options—what they are and where you find them. We cover the various forms that standard treatment can take and how to look critically at each. You will find some guidelines and questions you can ask so that you can determine for yourself whether the standard treatments seem appropriate to you.

Defining standard treatments

Standard treatment options have several names. They are published in medical textbooks simply as treatment or as clinical practice guidelines or association guidelines. Another growing movement is evidence-based medicine, which is defined as "the explicit and judicious use of current best evidence in decisions about care of individual patients."[1] Standard treatment options are also increasingly published as clinical pathways by hospitals, HMOs, and clinics.

Those publishing the standard treatment options maintain the concept of "proven effectiveness" in producing those treatment options. By gaining an understanding of what is or is not considered effective standard treatment, you have a basis for your own medical choices. You also gain a foundation for research into various alternative therapies and/or clinical trials.

There is no single standard used for developing treatment options other than generally acknowledged proven effectiveness or best evidence of a positive outcome. The treatment recommendations that are based on large, long-term studies are stronger. Those that have incorporated important follow-up of the patients receiving the treatment are stronger still. One such study is the Framingham Heart Study that has spanned the past 50 years.[2] The Framingham study identified risk factors for heart disease such as high cholesterol, high blood pressure, and smoking that have all become standard guidelines today. Because the study has gone on so long, it has been able to include offspring of the initial subjects and even addresses the genetic component in heart disease. Smaller studies, not subject to review or subsequent tests of the conclusions, will rarely evolve as standard treatment. Standard treatments also vary from one country to another as well. It may be beneficial for you to compare treatments of other countries in order to determine the optimum treatment for yourself.

A woman who has been struggling with a cancer recurrence has been comparing cancer treatments in the United Kingdom to other countries:

> *Our cancer survival rates in the UK are appalling—equivalent to Estonia and Poland! We find that some drugs and treatment regimens that are available elsewhere are not always available to us here. Or they are available but in a very patchy fashion. It depends on your zip code and whether you are lucky enough to live in an area where the health authority is "generous." This has been the case with Taxol—women in some areas can't get it as it's deemed too expensive!*

How doctors select and recommend treatments

The best doctors keep up with research in their area of expertise and continue to follow up on patients. When you are in treatment, a physician will usually give you several options for your situation and explain the risks and benefits of each option. Medicine is not an exact science because each patient has unique physical and psychological profiles, and the effectiveness of a given treatment varies widely from patient to patient. There is a great deal of art in the practice of medicine.

Doctors select among treatment guidelines, critical pathways, and "best evidence" of successful outcomes for their patients, based on proven effectiveness. However, there are always limitations. For example, guidelines are always evolving and a better treatment might not yet be considered the standard. Other factors, aside from effectiveness, also come in to play.

Additional criteria are used in determining standard treatment options. Cost-effectiveness is one consideration, local norms are another, and limitations imposed by insurers and HMOs now all enter into the equation. Factors such as the patient's condition, the physician's particular medical expertise, and external limitations can all impact or restrict what is called "standard treatment."

Physicians want to choose the best option for each patient. If there are cost-restraints imposed by insurance guidelines or HMOs, you would want to know this. Sometimes the outcomes and risks of more experimental treatment options are not very favorable and used only as a last resort. Some minor conditions, such as a sprained ankle may be painful, but the standard treatment is usually a verbal recommendation for nonprescription pain medication and an ankle wrap, but no formal treatment.

If your doctor recommends a certain therapy, you can ask if this is the standard treatment for your condition and what other treatment options exist. If your physician is recommending a nonstandard treatment option, you will want to know why that treatment has been recommended.

A doctor explains why he doesn't always prescribe balloon angioplasty, even when it may be the standard treatment:

> Occasionally patients with severe atherosclerosis or an elderly
> patient will develop new-onset hypertension. In these cases we might sus-
> pect reduced blood flow to one or both kidneys as a cause of the hyperten-
> sion. Although the standard treatment might be balloon angiography or
> even surgical revascularization, the treatment that is recommended may
> vary with the expertise of the physicians and the sophistication of the
> medical center. Also, a variety of less invasive intermediate tests can be
> used initially to establish the diagnosis, since there is small but real risk to
> angioplasty. Finally, we need to weigh the risks of the disease itself against
> the potential benefit of treating each individual with that disease.

An expanded list of factors used to determine standard treatment appears in the following sections.

Patient's condition

A number of factors about the patient will impact a doctor's recommendations, including:

- Severity of illness

- Age and physical condition

- Early versus late diagnosis (i.e., if immediate treatment is needed)

Severity of illness, your age, and your physical condition are critical factors in selecting a treatment option. Some treatments are more effective for younger patients and some more effective for older patients. Some treatments may be tried only after milder therapies have proved ineffective for a particular patient. Other treatments may be selected because of a coexisting condition such as diabetes or heart trouble. Finally, in an emergency there may be not be time to consider options, as would be the case if you arrived in the emergency room with a burst appendix.

One woman who found herself in the emergency room explains the need to act quickly:

> All day I had been feeling kind of "punk"—I thought maybe I was getting the flu. At 3 a.m. the next morning, I knew it wasn't the flu. I had such severe pain in my abdomen I thought surely I would die. I couldn't even think—I hurt so badly I could only cry. Somehow my husband and my daughter got me to the emergency room. All I wanted was to get the pain to stop. I was doubled up, could barely walk, and didn't even want to think.

> At the hospital, there was a swirl of activity—people asking questions, blood drawn, x-rays taken, papers signed. I could overhear snatches of conversation between my family and the staff. I didn't know most of the people who poked and prodded. They told me it was severe appendicitis and I needed surgery right then. A doctor I had never seen before was to be my surgeon. All I could say was "okay – do it now!"

> I always thought if I got sick I would investigate all the options and choose the best one and then choose the best doctor. Well at 3 a.m. that morning I was just very happy to be in a good local hospital with a licensed physician readily available. Research on appendicitis was not on

my mind. Later I discovered I could have had a severe infection or even died if treatment had been delayed even a short while.

A cancer survivor was surprised that age of the patient could make a difference in treatment choices:

> *When I was diagnosed with cancer, my oncologist told me I was young and that we'd treat aggressively. I guess in the world of cancer patients, I was still young at 45. I was glad I was otherwise healthy and able to handle the more aggressive treatment he recommended.*

Medical expertise

The doctor's medical experience and training impacts his recommendations. For example, a doctor will take into account:

- Known outcomes and risks of a given treatment
- Preferences for and experience with certain therapies

Physicians follow the medical research and adapt their treatment recommendations when a convincing body of evidence shows one therapy more effective over time. When there are several treatment options known to be effective, your physician will probably recommend those he has used before with success.

Having seen many "miracle" cures abandoned because of unforeseen side effects, a physician offers this explanation:

> *A time-tested doctor's adage advises, "Be not the first nor the last to prescribe a given treatment." We've all seen the latest heralded "cures" become yesterday's has-been disasters due to unexpected or dangerous side effects.*

> *It is all right not to immediately prescribe the latest treatment unless there are compelling reasons to do so. It's safer to await the "track record," especially since newer treatments are typically more expensive in dollars and potential risk than time-tested ones.*

> *One malpractice lawsuit has more influence on medical practice than ten papers in prestigious journals.*

New drugs, surgical techniques, and diagnostic tools are constantly being developed. You can act as a partner with your physician by following developments as they pertain to any treatment you may want to try or are already receiving. There is so much medical information and so many new discoveries that you may be able to bring new or additional information on your condition and/or course of therapy to your doctor. You may also want to be very alert to adverse effects of some of the newer medications as they are reported.

Limitations

Limitations that may affect recommended standard treatment include:

- Limitations of the local facilities
- Insurance coverage and limitations
- Your own preferences

If the treatment being recommended differs from the standard treatment options for your condition, you would want to actively investigate any limitations that exclude the widely accepted standard of care. These include limitations placed because of local preferences, insurance, HMO, and facility constraints. If your hospital does not have the capability of supporting open heart surgery, this may not be recommended.

One man graphically pointed out the difference between a small hospital and a large medical center in the level of expertise and experience available:

> They hit us with real bad news right away...that I had about a year to live. It was mesothelioma, which is a very aggressive cancer and it was a rare case since it was caused by exposure to asbestos. They said they would do as much as they could at the hospital....
>
> They said the malignancy was on the pleura of my lung and that they couldn't remove the pleura. They would have to take the whole lung. They said the mortality rate of that was about 35 percent in the operation and another 35 percent mortality in recovery. That didn't give us a lot of confidence. That's when my wife got on the Internet and started calling around. We had made an appointment at UCLA.
>
> Anyway, we got into UCLA and right away they said, "We have to take the pleura out," like it's no big deal. So in a couple of weeks we were down there and they took the pleura. At the smaller hospital they'd told

me it was impossible. I'm glad I didn't listen. They took a rib out to get to the pleura. It took the pathologist a week to find the malignancy.

So I had the operation and then had five weeks of radiation.

We did a CT scan a month or so afterwards and there was no evidence of the cancer. It was real clear. I had gained most of my strength back. No fluid. Everything was fine. I felt really good, back busy again.

Many people have had success in overcoming limitations and obtaining treatment at larger medical centers and in obtaining referrals to highly trained specialists when the research shows these referrals will lead to the best outcome.

One librarian reported helping several women when the policies of a local HMO changed:

The new policy of one of the large HMOs in our town was that women would be given a pap test for cervical cancer every other year, instead of annually. Several women came in to check this policy since it did not seem to be safe. We found that this might be acceptable for young healthy women, but not for any woman considered "at risk" such as cancer survivors or those with a family history of cervical cancer, etc.

They were still refused an annual pap test until they came to the medical library and found an OB/GYN textbook stating that annual pap tests are the standard, especially for women at risk. I photocopied that section out of the book for them and they brought it back to the HMO and got the policy amended. It seems like it took too much work just to get people to do what they are supposed to do in the first place.

While you may insist on receiving standard treatment, never forget that you also have the right to impose your own limitations on a given treatment. You may feel that the adverse effects outweigh the benefits, or you may simply want to stop treatment. Your physician or a counselor can explain the effects of limiting treatment. It is always your choice, because it is your body.

One man who had a seriously infected foot sought medical help but insisted taking the risks involved with having the standard treatment of intravenous antibiotics delivered his own way:

I was diagnosed with a serious streptococcal infection of my foot from a cut I got on a coral reef when I was in Hawaii. My foot was so swollen, I couldn't even stand on it. Red streaks were coming up my leg. He (the doctor) tried to lance it, but nothing came out—the infection was too deep. That's when they wanted to put me in the hospital and I refused.

The doctor almost denied care because I wouldn't come to the hospital. The doctor said if I wasn't under direct care I risked losing my foot. In my mind I was risking a lot more by the possibility of getting another infection. I've spent enough time in hospitals and I don't like them. It's so infectious in there and I already had an infection I couldn't fight.

We came to a compromise. He said it was unorthodox. But I asked him "Are you going to be with me every minute I'm in the hospital?" He said, "No, the nurses will take care of you."

I said, "How about if I get my own nurse and she can teach my housemate how to change the antibiotics without killing me? We'll call the minute my condition worsens." I even had to promise to come to the hospital immediately if my condition didn't improve. So I took over my own care.

I had a nurse from Visiting Nurses come in on a periodic basis and she taught my housemate how to change the IV line and take care of me when the nurse wasn't there. I had to take the antibiotics ten days intravenously and I had to take them for another two weeks thereafter in pill form. I never did go to the hospital and I survived—I think even better.

Your own research

Your own research can help you make a decision based on reliable medical information. You can ask your own doctor about treatment options. You can also ask for a second (or third) opinion and look up expert guidelines for your situation. Many people reach out to friends or through the Internet to see what others have decided in a similar situation. Through contacting others around the country and even the world, you can find out what types of treatments are proposed in other places. You can pull together all of this information and then ask yourself what you want.

One patient used Internet, word-of-mouth, and physician recommendations to track down treatment for a rare and aggressive cancer:

Finding out about the San Antonio drug trials was a real adventure. I had found it on the Internet. I got on and just started looking for anything with mesothelioma, anybody that I could find that ever had mesothelioma. A lot of times the information was sponsored by an attorney because of lawsuits connected with asbestos exposure. That was good because those attorneys had done a lot of research. Trying to entice me to come to them, they would put out lots of information. I followed through with all that information. It was helpful and I didn't feel like I owed them anything. That's how I found out about San Antonio. It turned out my nephew had the same thing and was also directed toward San Antonio where they had this drug.

Questions to ask your doctors

When considering treatment there are some key questions you would want to ask whether this is the standard treatment or some variation of that treatment.

Some of these key questions are:

- What are the side effects, both short- and long-term, of the proposed procedure?

- What are the known survival rates with and without treatment?

- Is this treatment covered by my insurance or HMO?

- What treatment or specialists would you recommend if there were no restrictions or insurance guidelines?

- What life changes will be necessary during treatment? Will I need to quit my job? Will I need to travel to a medical center for some period of time? Will I need help in my home during the recovery period?

- What will be my expected quality of life during and after treatment? Will I be bedridden for a long period of time or permanently? Will I be in a great deal of pain or rendered nearly unconscious from the effects of drugs? Will I regain energy and control over my life soon after treatment? How soon?

- Does the HMO or insurer compensate you for selecting this course of treatment over others?

- What medical assistance will I need during recovery? Will I need and have access to physical therapists, home nursing, etc.?

Getting second or third opinions

Most medical treatments and tests would not warrant getting a second opinion. But there are situations when getting a second opinion or a second reading of a diagnostic test is the most prudent option. The following guidelines can help you determine when to request a second or third opinion.

- Will the results of the laboratory tests or pathology results be used to initiate irreversible or highly invasive procedures?

- Is the recommended procedure or surgery invasive, i.e., does it involve entry into the body such as a surgical incision? Are there less invasive options to this procedure such as physical therapy or laparoscopic surgery?

- Is the proposed drug therapy or series of drug treatments potentially toxic?

- Is the recommended procedure extremely painful, and is there a less painful alternative?

- Is there any uncertainty in either the diagnosis or course of recommended treatment?

- Is the recommended procedure much less costly than one that is considered a standard treatment option?

If your whole course of treatment is based on laboratory tests and/or pathology results, it would make sense to have a second reading of those results. One man was relieved to learn that the interpretation of his first test was inaccurate. A second test resulted in a different diagnosis:

> I was visiting friends who lived in a rural area. I'd been having some stomach and back pains, but all of a sudden the pain was nearly unbearable. I went to the small clinic they had in the area. At the clinic they tested my blood and when they saw the numbers for the liver function test, they told me I might have liver failure or liver cancer. I thought "This is it—I'll be dead in a few months."

> They told me to fly home immediately and talk to my own doctor. As soon as I got back I called my doctor and he told me to go to the emergency room at the large medical center in our town. I had more blood tests and then an ultrasound. It turned out that gallstones were causing bile to back up into my liver. All I needed was gallbladder surgery. I was so relieved!

If the physician recommending surgery is not a specialist in that area, it would be prudent to request a second opinion from a specialist. For example, if a general surgeon recommended a complex gastrointestinal procedure that he had only performed a few times, you would benefit from the opinion of a colon and rectal surgeon who specializes in those procedures.

One patient was glad she had gotten a second opinion because it reassured her that she had made the right choices:

> The second opinion I got was mostly to relieve my own mind. I hadn't had time or energy to research a full range of treatments, with all that was going on with my family. My gut instinct was to trust my doctor: he'd had good training and experience. However, the outcome (the length of my life) felt too important to leave to instinct.
>
> I was relieved when the specialist I went to confirmed that my doctor's treatment recommendation was sound and that he even knew of my doctor's background and work. With that second opinion, I could put to rest my uncertainties and get on with treatment and healing.

Getting a second opinion is now even mandated by many of the major insurance plans because they have found that some surgeries and diagnostic tests are unnecessary. Even Medicare, and in many states, Medicaid, pays for the cost of second opinions. If your insurer will not pay for a second opinion or a second evaluation of laboratory and pathology findings, you may want to personally pay for these consultations. When you are about to undergo treatment that will have a great impact on your life, it's in your own best interests to make certain the recommended therapy is appropriate and necessary.

One man got second and third opinions before making a treatment choice:

> I got a PSA test—prostate specific antigens, a marker in the blood. The PSA test results came back at 9.8, several points above the minimum safe zone and bordering on a dangerous number. My doctor sent me off to a urologist.
>
> The urologist then did a biopsy and ultrasound examination and discovered that I, indeed, had a tumor. From the biopsy he was able to determine a code, which they call a Gleason scale for prostate cancer, for the relative aggressiveness of the tumor. That was in the moderate range. So then he recommended what he considered to be the "gold standard" of

treatment for prostate cancer which was surgery, a radical prostatectomy.
But he invited me to get a second opinion.

He gave me the name and phone number of a radiological oncologist
whose opinion was that I should get external beam radiation. So now I
had two opinions. I had a surgeon tell me I should do surgery and I had a
radiologist tell me I should do radiation. I wanted a third opinion.

I saw a small display ad in a magazine with an 800 number for
another prostate cancer treatment. I called that number. Within a matter
of days, they sent me a booklet on their approach, which is the implanta-
tion of radioactive seeds directly into the prostate gland. They also gave
me some information about the closest place to have that procedure,
which is in Seattle, and then I began making my decision.

I decided to go with the radium seed implant. The reason I chose that
is that it seemed to be the least invasive of all of the modalities, the one
with the least side effects. Some of the side effects of the other therapies
seemed to be more frightening than the disease itself. I choose the one that
let me be in the most control of my own body and what has been happen-
ing to it.

Another reason for getting a second opinion is for your own emotional and
psychological acceptance of a given course of therapy. Surgery and invasive
diagnostic procedures can cause anxiety and fear in any normal person. For
your own well-being, you should understand a recommended procedure
and feel confident that you are getting an accurate diagnosis and appropriate treatment. Facing a course of therapy with confidence can only enhance
the healing process. While the mind-body connection is still being discussed in traditional medicine, it is well known that our emotional and psychological status affects our health.

One man used every kind of healing he could find to help him cope with a
serious diagnosis:

I didn't report this to all of my doctors, but along the way I also
talked to a homeopath, an acupuncturist, and a Chinese medicine per-
son. I talked to an astrologer, and I've had a couple shamanic healing ses-
sions. I have had all kinds of prayers spoken for me. I have had candles
lighted all across the country. So I think I have done what I can. I feel
good about it. I am not sure of the outcome, but it has felt good to be in
charge of this process.

Locating and contacting experts

Getting a second opinion or a second evaluation of test results may involve some effort on your part. Usually your own physician can recommend an expert for consultation. You should probably look to the larger medical centers and medical schools outside your own physician's office or HMO for second opinions. The local physicians may be more likely to agree on recommendations and may have already discussed your case. You can find outside sources in many ways such as consulting the county medical societies, through recommendations of friends, family, and other medical professionals.

One way to locate experts is to consult medical textbooks and/or do a MEDLINE search to get the names of physicians and institutions that specialize in state-of-the-art treatment for your condition. You can also get a list of specialists in your area from the American Board of Medical Specialists. They publish an annual directory that is in large public libraries and most medical libraries. The American Board of Medical Specialists oversees the evaluation and certification of the 24 medical specialist boards in the United States. The toll-free number is (800) 776-2378; the web site is *http://www.abms.org*.

A librarian tells about one patient who was especially creative in locating an expert:

> *I showed a new book on lung cancer to one man who said he had just received that diagnosis. He made a lot of copies and he said he would call the medical school where the lung cancer expert who wrote the book was teaching. The next day he told me he just asked for the secretary of the oncology program. He then asked the names of all the specialists near him who had trained with the expert who wrote the book. He's active in his own alumni organization and he knows know they keep track of all their graduates, if only to ask for alumni donations. He got the names of three doctors within 200 miles of his own house. That way he got the benefit of the expert's knowledge and experience, without traveling thousands of miles.*

You can pay for your own outside second opinion(s) if your insurer is reluctant to assist you. You can also appeal your case to the manager of your health plan and demand to know why your request for an outside opinion has been denied. Physicians are accustomed to requests for second opinions and most of them actually welcome the opportunity for verification of their diagnosis and plan for treatment or the recommendation of a different course of treatment.

By getting a second opinion, one man avoided an unnecessary and even, for him, a dangerous surgery:

> I was told that I would have to have my prostate gland removed to stop the progression of recently diagnosed prostate cancer. Since removal of the prostate is delicate and major surgery, irreversible, and subject to complications, I naturally wanted a second opinion. I also read everything I could find on the subject on the Internet and in the medical library and learned that there were several other non-surgical approaches. To compound my fears and uncertainties, I found that the surgeon recommended by my HMO for this procedure performed only about fifteen to eighteen prostate surgeries per year.
>
> I arranged for a second opinion from a well-known urologic surgeon at a large medical center not too far away and he emphatically stated that surgery was not the optimum treatment for my condition. This was because of potential serious postoperative consequences related to the fact that I had had several major abdominal surgeries years ago. He recommended a non-surgical approach of placing radioactive pellets in the prostate. I will always be grateful I insisted on that second opinion.

Reading guidelines that doctors use

When you have been diagnosed with a serious medical condition, you quickly become familiar with medical vocabulary. By asking questions and referring to a medical dictionary, you can learn to understand the medical terms appropriate to your situation. With so much access to information today, you can read most of the medical literature that the doctors consult. A great deal of the information about standard treatment options is readily available on the Internet or in nearby medical libraries. Physicians consult a mixture of textbook recommendations, clinical practice guidelines, clinical pathways, and evidence-based medicine. You, too, can locate and read these recommendations and guidelines.

Textbook guidelines

Medical textbooks list the standard treatments for given conditions. Since the textbooks often take a year or more to publish, standard treatment options found in textbooks may be older than treatments discussed in medical journals. Newer and more effective therapies may have been developed since the publication of even a very current medical textbook. Several excellent textbooks are updated each year and these would be a good place to start:

- *Conn's Current Therapy: Latest Approved Methods of Treatment for the Practicing Physician.*[3] Published annually, this book has been an authority for over 50 years. *Conn's* includes contributions from over 300 authorities providing the expert therapies for over 870 conditions.

- *Griffith's 5 Minute Clinical Consult.*[4] Published annually, *Griffith's* covers over a thousand medical topics set up in a user-friendly two-page format that covers the diagnosis, treatment, follow-up, prognosis, and additional references for each condition.

- *Current Medical Diagnosis and Treatment.*[5] Published annually, this text covers the currently accepted medical treatment for all major conditions, arranged by body system. The *Current Medical Diagnosis and Treatment* is part of the Appleton & Lange series that includes current recommendations for more specific medical therapies as well. These specialized books are updated every two to four years. For example, *Current Surgical Diagnosis and Treatment* is updated every two years and *Current Diagnosis and Treatment in Gastroenterology* is updated every three years.

Doctors regularly check the textbooks and journal articles to update their own information in a given area and to provide reassurance to a patient. One doctor describes gathering information for a very cautious patient:

> One of our most popular surgeons was in the medical library early one morning. He was doing a routine hernia repair and wanted to find the most recent textbook on that subject. He also asked if we could do a quick MEDLINE search on surgical approaches for this type of hernia. He then asked if the textbook he was reading was considered the latest and the best textbook on the topic. We said, "Yes, it is."
>
> The surgeon requested two copies of the textbook section and two copies of the journal article we'd identified in MEDLINE that confirmed the textbook recommendations.
>
> When we asked the surgeon why he was spending so much time researching such a routine surgery, he laughed and said, "This time I'm

operating on an attorney. Attorneys just won't sign a consent form until they know they're getting "gold standard" treatment. They have to be certain they're getting the latest and the best—those extra copies are for him!"

Who publishes textbook guidelines?

The general medical textbooks listed previously and other, more disease-specific textbooks, are published by several different medical publishers to assist physicians in maintaining current information. These textbooks reflect the consensus of standard treatment options. Annual textbooks provide you with a good starting point for determining what the standard treatment for your condition may be. You can also use basic textbooks in each specialty as a place to start a discussion with your physician. Usually there are several options given for each condition. These options will most likely be listed in the order of the least invasive to the most invasive recommended therapy.

One woman was quite pleased that she found a much more acceptable treatment option for her situation:

> *I was helping a friend of mine get some information. She's a mother of six and a grandmother of eleven. When she visited the doctor last week, he said her stress incontinence is being caused by prolapsed pelvic floor muscles. They have an operation where they would insert a Teflon mesh sling for support. That sounded pretty extreme to both of us.*

> *We went to the medical library and looked in a current OB/GYN textbook they had. The book did mention the Teflon surgery, but one of the other recommendations for that condition was the use of estrogen cream. We made a copy and she showed it to her doctor and although he was skeptical he wrote a prescription for the cream.*

> *After two weeks her symptoms disappeared. Her doctor was impressed and we were both relieved. At her age, there are always extra risks with surgery and she wants to avoid it whenever she can.*

Evaluating textbook guidelines

Because the textbook guidelines have evolved over a long period of time and are generally conservative, the main criteria for evaluating their relevance would be the currency of the information and the relevance to your particular situation. You should always check the date the textbook was published. The information is usually a year or more old at the time of publication.

In addition to the currency of information in the medical textbooks, you would want to know if the information was accurate and well reviewed. Besides the reviews in the medical journals, there are three major reviewing sources for medical textbook, CD-ROM, and database information:

- *Brandon/Hill Selected List of Books and Journals for the Small Medical Library.* Published every other year in the *Bulletin of the Medical Library Association.*[6] It lists recommended titles for each medical specialty and notes a select group of the very best in each area.

- *Library for Internists.* Published every third year by the American College of Physicians. This recommended list is published in the *Annals of Internal Medicine.*[7]

- *Doody's Rating Service.* Contains reviews by experts in each medical and scientific field. It is published monthly with an annual list of "A Buyer's Guide to the 250 Best Health Sciences Books." Each inclusion is given one to five stars, with five being the highest recommendation.[8]

Thanks to some excellent web sites put together by the medical and trade book dealers, it is relatively easy to determine which books have been well reviewed. One of the web sites is from Login Brothers Book Company, a medical book distributor, *http://www.lb.com*. Each book in the Login Brothers list contains a notation if it has appeared in the Brandon-Hill list, and if (and how many) the Doody's reviewers awarded the title stars. At least two web sites in the trade books arena also list medical books with readers' reviews. They are *http://www.amazon.com* and *http://www.bn.com*. Both web sites list reviews by readers and give publishers information. Amazon.com lists medical best sellers while Barnes and Noble gives the table of contents for selected medical titles. Both sites are extremely useful.

The textbook guidelines are usually excellent treatment guidelines, but there may have been medical breakthroughs concerning your condition since their publication. Sometimes textbook treatment guidelines are very general in nature and don't give enough detailed information for you to make a final decision about your care. So, you would usually consider the textbooks a first step in medical research.

Clinical practice guidelines

Medical associations and government research organizations have enlisted their expert members in publishing guidelines for treatment in a response to the growing demand for basic standards of clinical practice. Clinical practice guidelines have been defined as "systematically developed statements to assist practitioner and patient decisions about appropriate healthcare for specific clinical circumstances."[9] The professional associations' practice guidelines also serve to protect physicians and patient choices in the face of budget cuts, shorter hospital stays, and possible HMO restrictions.

The clinical practice guidelines vary a great deal. Some are very specific, well-researched and well-presented. Others are more general and even philosophic in scope.

Many of the medical associations such as the American College of Surgeons have published "statements" on treatment for specific conditions. These statements are less comprehensive than the longer guidelines, but they can still assist you in determining what is considered the best treatment for your condition. The more elaborate and specific guidelines will, of course, be most useful.

Who publishes clinical practice guidelines?

Clinical practice guidelines are published by the Canadian and American government health services and by professional medical associations such as the American Heart Association, the American College of Physicians, the American College of Surgeons, the American Diabetes Association, etc. These are published as guides for association members and to set a standard of treatment endorsed by the association. You can search for association guidelines on any association's web sites and locate those association web sites through the use of almost any search engine.

For example, to find an association's clinical practice guidelines, you might go to a search engine such as *http://www.37.com,* which searches 37 different search engines. You would type in the name of the medical association that would reflect your interest. It's always best to type the name in quotation marks so that the entire phrase is searched for, such as "American Heart Association." When you find a link to that association, click on it and look for practice guidelines, standards, or recommended best practices listed on their home page. Find those that interest you on the list. These guidelines are also published in the medical journals published by each organization.

A clearinghouse for clinical practice guidelines has been created by the Agency for Health Care Policy and Research (AHCPR). The web site for that clearinghouse is *http://www.guideline.gov*. Practice guidelines are constantly updated on this web site. Another source is a fee-based Internet research service, MD Consult, which lists over 600 clinical practice guidelines on its web site, *http://www.mdconsult.com*. MD Consult charges monthly fees but has a short free trial period for potential users.

Evaluating clinical practice guidelines

If you find an association guideline or a clinical practice guideline appropriate to your situation, there are a few questions you can ask to determine if you would feel comfortable following that particular guideline's recommendations.

- Do the recommendations in the guidelines include recent medical discoveries and innovations? In other words, are they current?

- Are guideline recommendations based on large reliable studies? Were large enough groups sampled and could the results be duplicated? Were variables in the outcomes of these large studies mentioned? If the conclusions were based on a study of 100 people in one area of the country, they may not be relevant to your situation.

- Do the guideline recommendations mention several possible therapies and explain why one practice is recommended over others? For example, one ACP guideline recommends hormone replacement therapy, or HRT, for the treatment of symptoms of menopause, but it specifies this may not be appropriate for every woman. That study does not include women at high risk for cancer, and it does not mention natural hormone therapies as an alternative.

- Finally, are the guideline recommendations applicable to you? If the recommendations are for treating an elderly male for stroke, and you are a younger female who has recently had a minor stroke, treatment guidelines may have no clinical relevance.

There is an excellent series of articles in *JAMA, the Journal of the American Medical Association,* entitled "User's Guides to the Medical Literature," which gives further insights into the creation, evaluation, and use of clinical practice guidelines. These articles have been published over the last six years and can be located through a MEDLINE search or the AMA (American Medical Association) web site: *http://www.ama-assn.org.*

Clinical pathways

The clinical pathway (sometimes called critical pathway) is an attempt to put forth an actual flow chart and sequential steps in therapy and recovery practices for the most frequent medical conditions treated in the hospital or clinic.

The pathways are utilized in hospitals and HMOs as a way to maintain a high quality of treatment and keep treatment costs down. The clinical pathways are created through consensus of groups of physicians, nurses, physical therapists, pharmacists, and other allied health professionals. In implementing clinical pathways, hospitals and HMOs can become much more efficient in handling preoperative and postoperative patient care, since this care will be similar for most patients and does not need to vary widely with each physician's preferences.

The clinical pathways are an evolving set of recommended practices for given conditions that include surgery, drug therapy, length of stay, recommended tests, physical therapy, drug interventions, and type of nursing care. The orthopedic procedures such as total hip replacement have been some of the first pathways to be published because these have many similarities from patient to patient. Hip replacement candidates can be asked to lose weight, change diet, etc., prior to surgery in order to optimize the results of the surgery. Since this surgery is elective and not usually life-threatening, the patients can be put on programs to make them surgery-ready.

One patient noted that they had sequential steps and policies when he had his hip replacement surgery:

> Even though I needed the hip surgery, the doctor told me I would
> have to lose 20 pounds before they would do the surgery. I'm a big
> guy—6'7" and 250 pounds. By the time I got to surgery I only weighed
> 220 and was in good shape. The guidelines say I'll do better if I carry less
> weight, which makes sense.
>
> Then they determined that since I was still young and active, they
> wanted to put in a titanium hip. This is known in medical circles as the

"Bo Jackson hip," since he played two seasons of professional football on his new hip. That sounded good to me—we even joked about a new career.

We had to go to a different hospital for that operation because the hip itself is more expensive and recovery takes a longer hospital stay. With that titanium hip, parts of the prosthesis are porous and your bone has to start growing again into the hip before they let you go home. With the other types of hips, they just use cement. I guess the change of hospitals was a managed care thing.

Even though I stayed in the hospital a whole week, they got me walking in the first 24 hours after surgery. That was in their recovery plan, but it was the hardest 18 feet I've ever walked!

I feel great now—in fact, my new hip is the good one.

Clinical pathways are a work in progress because a study of the outcomes is supposed to be built into each pathway. If the outcomes are seen as ineffective, the pathway will be altered to include treatment seen as more beneficial.

The long-range plan for clinical pathways is that results can be followed and monitored for outcomes and they will evolve over time to truly reflect optimum treatment(s). Differences in patients' conditions also impact the way the pathways are applied. For example, in a total hip replacement pathway, it may state: "the patient will be walking with assistance on the first day after the surgery." However, a patient may have a secondary knee problem that would delay his progress towards walking.

The risks and benefits of each procedure are determined before implementing or making changes in a pathway. Not only are the potential risks weighed against benefits, there is also consideration of the cost-to-benefit ratio. If the addition of a certain procedure such as additional physical therapy is included in a pathway, the added costs would have to be justified in terms of greatly improved outcomes for the majority of patients. Cost containment is one of the objectives for clinical pathways.

Who publishes clinical pathways?

Clinical pathways are produced by many different entities, including the US and Canadian governments, hospitals, HMOs, and clinics. Initially they were part of the Quality Improvement process. Quality Improvement programs in hospitals are geared towards improvement of performance and medical procedures to achieve the best patient outcomes. Pathways create a method of comparing patients who have similar procedures so that the best outcomes can be duplicated whenever possible. Clinical pathways have also become a way to predict or control costs of given procedures by standardizing care and limiting some of the options available to physicians and hospital staff.

How to evaluate clinical pathways

If you are to be admitted to a hospital for a given procedure, ask if there is a clinical pathway for that procedure. You can benefit by seeing it in advance and by being able to ask about any aspect of the recommended treatment that you do not understand. The pathways reassure many patients, allowing them to see each step of their progress including the day they will be able to leave the hospital. Some of the doctors and other caregivers worry that these clinical pathways may become cookbook medicine and not allow for individual patient requirements.

You can use many of the same questions for evaluating clinical pathways as for evaluating the practice guidelines discussed earlier. In addition to those earlier questions about guidelines, you may want to ask some of the following:

- How was this clinical pathway developed? Was the entire patient care staff involved in creating this procedure? Did nurses, therapists, pharmacists as well as physicians all have an opportunity to contribute to the pathway?

- Is the pathway based on sound medical research and outcome studies?

- Does the pathway take into account individual differences and reactions or complications that may arise? For example, some women and infants may do very well with a 24-hour hospital stay for childbirth, but some mothers and infants may develop serious complications and end up back in the hospital if they are sent home that quickly. Which therapeutic options were dropped from the pathway because the benefits were not high enough to justify increased costs? Who decided?

- Does my physician have the authority to alter the clinical pathway if my condition warrants a change, or must a hospital utilization team or clinic committee approve any changes?

Evidence-based medicine

Evidence-based medicine (EBM) is a relatively recent movement created to assist physicians in identifying best clinical practices as determined by the most reliable studies in most fields of medicine including internal medicine, surgery, psychiatry, pediatrics, and obstetrics and gynecology. The field of evidence-based medicine was developed in the late 1980s and early 1990s at McMaster University in Canada, the University of Oxford in the UK, and the University of Rochester in the United States. Now nearly every medical school in the western hemisphere is participating in identifying the best practices.

EBM is a concerted effort to sift through the quantities of medical research to identify those studies whose results are most likely to be useful and true. EBM has some important inclusion criteria. One of these criteria is that real—not hypothetical—patients must determine a recommended course of treatment. Evidence-based medicine recommendations must be clearly stated and include a clear description of how the evidence for that recommendation was tracked down. Each recommendation may include an abstract of several studies and review articles. Experts in that field also review each recommendation.

Similar to clinical pathways, evidence-based medicine includes references to the costs as well as effectiveness of a given therapy. Unlike clinical pathways, the focus of evidence-based medicine is directed towards individual patients and may actually raise rather than lower costs. Quality of life and patients' preferences and situations are considered along with clinical expertise in making medical decisions in the evidence-based medicine model.

Evidence based medicine is not cookbook medicine because it places all treatment decisions on the clinical expertise of individual physicians and the choices of their patients, based on the evidence of best practice. It may be seen as a way to take the extensive body of medical literature and select those studies that clearly show evidence of improved patient outcomes. Medical care decisions for each patient will differ due to their individual situations and preferences. Sometimes the best evidence will include references to basic sciences such as genetics or immunology. Scientific facts combined with review of randomized trials help physicians and their patients select the "best practice."

Who publishes evidence-based medicine guidelines?

There are several journals and at least two medical databases that publish evidence-based medicine recommendations. One journal is appropriately called *Evidence-Based Medicine*. Another journal covering evidence-based medicine is the *ACP Journal Club*, published by the American College of Physicians.

There are at least two databases that disseminate evidence-based medicine guidelines. One is *Evidence Based Medicine Reviews: Cochrane Database of Systematic Reviews*, which summarizes articles from over 800 journals in several languages. The second database is *Evidence Based Medicine Reviews: Best Evidence*, from the American College of Physicians. Both are available on the Web or in CD-ROM format. Both are, however, fee-based, and so the user must pay for access to these resources. Both are available in university medical libraries and many larger hospital libraries.

How to evaluate evidence-based medicine recommendations

Studies published as "evidence-based medicine" or "best practice" have already been painstakingly scrutinized by practicing medical experts. Each recommendation should contain a list of references and experts consulted in producing that recommendation. If the references are solid, the only question in evaluating the recommendation would be the date of the study. There may be some more recent medical research that changes a recommendation. Also, some of the evidence-based medicine recommendations will apply to a very narrow and specific patient diagnosis. You can read the whole study to be sure that it applies directly to your own situation.

Standard treatments change constantly

In preceding sections, you may have noticed terms like "updated annually," "changing," and "evolving." In fact, there is probably no standard treatment that will remain static for long, except possibly "take two aspirins and call me in the morning." Treatments change through medical discoveries, outcome studies that determine certain treatments are more effective than others, clinical trials, and observation. What is standard treatment one day may be considered poor medicine the next.

Medical history is full of examples of treatments that have gained acceptance, been discarded, and then gained acceptance again. One of the most fascinating is the use of maggots to clean wounds. The Mayans used maggots for this purpose. In recent history, one surgeon on the battlefields of World War I noticed that the soldiers whose wounds had been infested by maggots had less infection and gangrene than those wounded soldiers whose wounds contained no maggots. The maggot-infested soldiers had better outcomes and fewer amputations. When World War I was over in 1918, doctors returned to begin research into the beneficial wound cleaning talents of the otherwise disgusting maggots. By the 1930s over 200 hospitals and medical centers were using maggots for gangrenous wounds. Then sulfa drugs and finally penicillin were discovered, so maggots were abandoned. Recently, laboratory raised maggots have been reintroduced to assist in the healing of some very deep wounds which have been resistant to even the most sophisticated antibiotics.

Another constantly changing scenario is the standard treatment options for HIV and AIDS. As each new drug has been discovered, treatment options have changed. Researchers have the opportunity to evaluate the failures and success of each successive treatment modality from AZT to the protease inhibitor "cocktail" that is one current standard treatment option. As research continues and new drugs are developed, a cure for AIDS and a protective vaccine may be developed. You can watch this standard treatment evolve constantly. Similarly, researchers are expanding modes of treating every type of cancer. Each discovery brings a new "standard."

Vaccines, such as the Salk vaccine for polio, changed the standard treatment option for that crippling disease. In fact, the most dramatic changes in standard medical treatment options throughout history have been to substitute prevention of the disease for treating it. Thanks to continuing efforts of our healers and researchers, most of us no longer have to contend with smallpox, diphtheria, or even measles. When we travel we are protected by cholera, typhoid, and hepatitis vaccines.

Standard treatment options for surgery have also changed dramatically over the years. The discovery of antiseptics in the nineteenth century elevated surgery to a true medical occupation. More recently, biomedical technologies—such as the introduction of laser surgery and laparoscopic procedures—have made surgical procedures less invasive and therefore less dangerous and less expensive. Surgeries such as gallbladder removal (cholecystectomy) have been streamlined through the use of laparoscopic techniques. A patient who may have faced a week's hospital stay and four weeks of recovery with traditional gallbladder surgery now faces a one-day hospital stay and a one-week recovery period.

One patient had been told about both procedures and wanted the laparoscopic surgery. The doctors couldn't guarantee which surgery would be most appropriate until they started the surgery:

> The first thing I asked when I woke up in the recovery room was "which surgery did I get?" I was thrilled that they had been able to do the laparoscopic surgery, since that meant I could go home sooner and could fully recover faster. No surgery is a piece of cake—even this less invasive surgery was tough. I hate to think what people endure with the full gallbladder surgery.

Another example of how medicine can change with technology is brought out by the Dean Ornish, MD study, published in the *Lancet* in 1993. The study found that major lifestyle and diet changes could control serious atherosclerosis, or blockage of the arteries to the heart.[10] That study was considered a radical treatment recommendation. "Conservative" treatment for atherosclerosis had evolved to the use of heavy doses of drugs to lower cholesterol and coronary artery bypass graft surgery or CABG. Drugs and surgery were the current standard treatment.

As one healthcare worker commented:

> I couldn't believe that putting a person on an operating table and cutting him from navel to Adam's apple to work on the arteries leading to his heart is considered conservative or standard treatment...not when it is compared to the radical therapy of diet and exercise!

When a change in lifestyle—your activities, your diet, or even your occupation—has the potential to restore or preserve your health, it certainly needs to be considered as a standard treatment option.

However, if you are researching treatment options for a loved one, resist the urge to preach or to present only that option. Although lifestyle changes may be inexpensive, noninvasive, safe, and effective, they do need to be fully embraced by the person involved in order to work. Present all options dispassionately, and let the person with the problem make the choice.

As you are told of standard treatment options and you research alternate options, keep in mind that these options are constantly changing. You would always want to find the most current treatment option that has proven effective. It may be useful to you to understand what the earlier treatments for the same condition may be and why those options have been replaced. As in the case of the maggots, sometimes the oldest options may prove to be the most effective.

Identifying your own comfort level

After all of your research, your own instincts and comfort level will help you determine which treatments you can accept and which you reject. As you read through the medical textbooks, practice guidelines, clinical pathways, and evidence-based medicine to determine the most effective treatment for a given condition, you always will be considering how any specific treatment would impact your life. If you are dealing with a chronic or recurring condition, you have already experienced some choices for treatment and you have a clearer idea of what is in store for you.

Some recommended invasive therapies may not have much better outcomes than less invasive or alternative treatments. You are the final decision-maker. You know your own limits and constraints. You know about the demands from the other areas of your life: family, work, commitments, etc. Basically, *you* know yourself. You know how much risk and how much pain you can tolerate. You know your physicians and caregivers. Is there a bond of trust that you can rely on? Do you have a large network of family and friends to help you recuperate or are you on your own? Are there friends you can recruit or support groups you can find to help you in your decision making?

Finally, how do you feel? Your own feelings can have profound effect on your outcome. When you combine all of the available medical information with your own situation and feelings, you make the best decisions for your own care.

In later chapters you'll find more in-depth discussion of some of these concepts. Chapter 10, *Support: Learning from Others*, discusses ways to find and use support when facing illness. Chapter 12, *Reviewing Information with Your Doctor*, includes guidelines for discussing options with your doctor, and in Chapter 13, *Making Your Decision*, we go over techniques for making medical choices and decisions.

CHAPTER 8

Researching Clinical Trials

"I'VE EXHAUSTED MY STANDARD TREATMENT OPTIONS. Are there any experimental treatments being studied that might be effective for my condition?" This is one question that brings patients to clinical trials, but there are other valid reasons to take a look at clinical trials as well as pros and cons to consider before entering a clinical trial.

In this chapter, we first briefly describe clinical trials. Next, we discuss at some length why you might consider participating in or at least gathering information about the trials relevant to your condition. We describe the safeguards designed to protect your interests and explain the structure of a clinical trial. We take a look at the issues you will need to consider, such as the location of the trial and the possibility that you might end up in the control group receiving standard therapy, rather than the group receiving the experimental therapy. We end this chapter with a discussion of how to find clinical trials.

What is a clinical trial?

Medical research is done in a variety of ways. Clinical trials study human volunteers for their physical or psychological responses to specific biomedical or behavioral interventions.

The US Food and Drug Administration (FDA) regulates and monitors the medical marketplace. A clinical trial is considered the most reliable way to evaluate the effectiveness and safety of a new treatment. The FDA requires clinical trial testing before giving approval for a new medical drug, biologic, or medical device to be marketed in the United States. Some trials evaluate the effectiveness of completely new forms of treatment. Others compare the current standard treatment with newer experimental treatments or new delivery methods in the hopes of expanding treatment options. In this chapter, we focus on trials of medical treatments involving drugs and biologics (such as vaccines and anti-toxins).

Who designs a clinical trial and why?

Drug companies, medical device manufacturers, and other biotechnology companies sponsor clinical trials to verify the safety and effectiveness of a new product prior to application for marketing approval and to provide support for a company's marketing claims. There is a clear economic incentive for medical product manufacturers to support clinical trials, but other groups also sponsor and design trials.

Government agencies sponsor clinical trials as part of their directive to work toward the advancement of medicine. The National Institutes of Health (NIH) is the largest sponsor of clinical trials in the United States.

Professional cooperative groups of researchers, such as the Southwest Oncology Group (SWOG) or the Pediatric Oncology Group (POG) sponsor trials designed and conducted by their members to find new treatment options. Academic medical researchers depend on clinical trials to validate their research hypotheses.

Insurance companies, managed care groups, and professional associations rely on clinical trial data to develop treatment guidelines that define the normal course of treatment. Clinical trial results identify newer treatments that offer better outcomes or verify that an older treatment is still the safest and most effective choice.

Why research clinical trials?

There are many reasons to participate in a clinical trial. Even if you do not expect to enter a trial, it is still worthwhile to take a look at what is being offered. The information you gather now could help you in the future if your standard treatment options become more limited. You might also learn about research on a new treatment that would not be available to you any other way.

The following sections explain the advantages you might gain from reviewing clinical trials at this point in your treatment, or later if needed.

Benefits of participation

This section describes some of the advantages to participation in a clinical trial. Always bear in mind, however, that clinical trials are experimental. A treatment that looks promising today might, when the results are in, turn out to be less effective or more toxic than your current standard treatment options. You might also be assigned to the control group that receives "standard treatment," rather than the experimental group. If there is currently no standard treatment available for your condition, you could receive a placebo (a substance that looks like the experimental drug, but has no active ingredients), or no treatment at all.

Leading-edge treatment

It can take eight to ten years to develop and qualify a new drug for FDA approval. For a treatment that is not yet approved for marketing to the general public, your only access to it may be through participation in a clinical trial.

If you have exhausted the list of standard treatment options available to you, a new treatment under study in a clinical trial might offer you hope for effective treatment. A man with mesothelioma recounts how his wife tracked down a trial to treat his recurrence:

> When I had another CT scan in August, they found new growths. When I went back to the treatment center, they said they really couldn't do any more. The x-ray treatments wouldn't help any more and they couldn't operate. They'd done all they could.
>
> They mentioned a drug that is having good results in clinical trials. They had planned to offer it, but had not been able to put together a trial for it. So my wife got on the Internet and found trials on this drug being offered in three other places. We called for information and visited two of the trial sites. I will be starting the treatment next week.
>
> I think people get frustrated running into so many dead ends. What's scary to me is that we might have just gone home and thought this was all we could do.

Regardless of the stage of your disease, clinical trials provide additional options when no standard treatments are currently available for you. Hope for cure is not the only reason to look at ongoing clinical studies. New treatments can also offer the hope of longer life or improved quality of life through symptom management. A woman with early stage Parkinson's talks about joining a trial:

I went to see my doctor when I noticed a tremor in my left thumb. My father had Parkinson's so I knew a little about it. She wanted to do some tests but we were getting ready to leave for Arizona. I asked if I could have the tests at the Mayo Clinic branch there.

Two doctors at the Mayo Clinic examined me and both came to the conclusion that I had Parkinson's. They told me about a trial that was being offered at their clinic. My diagnosis was early, so there is no medication available for me at this point.

The medications that are available now are used to control the symptoms of the disease. They don't stop the progression. They have to keep increasing the dosage. At some point it becomes toxic. This medication is being used to stop the progress of the disease, not just the symptoms. I knew right away that I was interested.

I have been in the trial for two years. I feel lucky that we were going to Arizona. If I'd stayed in Indiana, I probably would have gone to a neurologist there and not heard about this trial.

Quality of care

Clinical trial participants are closely monitored for their response to treatment and possible side effects. Patients often feel that they get better care and follow-up when they participate in a clinical trial. A woman from Britain says:

My family physician is married to a hospital consultant. She told me that her husband recommends joining a clinical trial because he feels participants get far superior monitoring of their condition and progress. Monitoring is an area where our services are lamentable. The idea of prevention or early diagnosis seems strangely absent here.

In addition, some of the brightest medical and scientific minds are brought together in the design and implementation of a clinical trial. Participation in a trial gives you access to this network of forward-thinking professionals.

Advancement of science

Some people enter trials to make a contribution to medical research. Taking a chance on an experimental treatment is a gamble, but even if you do not respond to the treatment, the information gathered from the trial will help researchers refine future treatments. One woman in a clinical trial expressed her feelings this way:

I just feel like I'm doing something positive that will help others like me in the future.

Benefits of researching current trials

In addition to learning about experimental treatments you might qualify for now, through trial participation you will also learn about the latest research on treatments that may be available to you in the future and about new uses for previously approved drugs that are being studied for possible expanded use.

New approaches

When you look at clinical trial protocols, you will find:

- Information about new treatment approaches before they are published in the medical literature

- Explanations of the most current scientific thinking about the disease process along with background on why the proposed experimental treatment shows promise

- Pointers to the scientists, clinicians, and centers who are at the forefront of innovative thinking and treatment for your condition

Off-label prescriptions

Sometimes drugs that are being used experimentally for one condition have already been approved for use for another condition. Once a drug is FDA-approved, a physician can prescribe it, at her discretion, for any condition where preliminary studies show promising results. This is called an off-label use. Research into clinical studies can help you to identify an off-label use long before the drug is publicly marketed for that use. Off-label use does not require participation in a clinical trial, since the drug is already FDA-approved.

Be aware, however, that while preliminary evidence is hopeful, that does not mean the effectiveness is proven. It is important to separate good marketing from good medicine. In a preliminary report on raloxifene, investigators noted a reduction in breast cancer incidence among the participants. The study showing this association, however, was not designed to evaluate breast cancer incidence. The subjects were chosen for risk of osteoporosis, not breast cancer risk, and the preliminary report was made only two and a half years into the study. A future study of women at high risk for breast cancer may or may not have the same results. In considering an off-label use of a drug, look at the study data carefully with your doctor to determine if the promise of benefit outweighs the potential risks for you as an individual.

If you and your doctor are considering the off-label use of a product, it is worth looking for a clinical trial to participate in so that your use of the drug can help to qualify its effectiveness for future users in your situation.

Emergency treatment options

A treatment that has not yet been approved by the FDA for general use can sometimes be given outside of a clinical trial to a patient in a desperate situation. This is referred to as "compassionate use." If you or a loved one is desperately ill, your research into clinical trials might bring to light a drug, combination of drugs, or treatment process when all other avenues are closed.

In March 1998 a 9-year-old boy fell from a rope ladder in his backyard and broke his neck. He was rushed to Children's Hospital in San Diego where the doctors told his parents that he would probably face a lifetime of paralysis as a result of the accident. The boy's father found a high school English paper on the Internet that mentioned an experimental drug, GM-1 ganglioside, for spinal cord injury. With the help of his son's pediatric neurologist, the father contacted the drug manufacturer and the FDA to get emergency approval for the use of the experimental drug in the hopes that it would reduce the extent of paralysis. The hospital reviewed the case and approved the use of the drug as well. The drug is most effective if used within 72 hours of injury. The boy's recovery may or may not have been the result of compassionate access to this drug.[1]

The FDA refers to an Investigational New Drug as an IND. When a drug shows sufficient hope for patients with serious to life-threatening disease, a drug company can submit a Treatment IND protocol to the FDA along with the standard IND application. If the Treatment IND application is approved, special case patients can be treated without participating in a multiple-patient trial.

Treatment INDs are available for treating two categories of patients:

- Seriously ill patients can be given individual access to drugs, usually during Phase III testing or in the time between the application for New Drug Approval (NDA) and the actual approval. The sponsor must be able to present data offering sufficient proof of safety and effectiveness.

- Patients with immediately life-threatening disease can be treated with drugs that have been identified as potentially effective and not likely to expose the patient to unreasonable or significant risk of additional illness or injury and for whom all other avenues of treatment have been exhausted.

There are several reasons a physician might request an unapproved product for single-patient use:

- A new treatment for a rare disease might not generate enough participants for a full multiple-patient trial.

- Single-patient use allows for more flexible interaction with a seriously ill patient. Dosage levels can be adjusted according to the patient's response.

- A drug in short supply can be tested without the production demands of a larger clinical trial. Sometimes, if the supply is limited, access to a drug through a Treatment IND may be by lottery.

- A patient can be treated who does not meet trial criteria.

- A patient can be treated who lives too far from the trial sites to participate in a trial.

Are clinical trials safe?

Some people hesitate to participate in a clinical trial out of fear that they will be treated like guinea pigs—that their personal needs would be secondary to the pursuit of science. This section will give you background on the safety measures in place today to protect the rights of individual patients.

While clinical trials are highly regarded for the evaluation of the safety and effectiveness of a new treatment, the practice of medical experimentation on humans has had some bleak moments. World War II brought the most notable abuses of human research ethics when the Nazis developed a eugenics program, calling it "racial hygiene," and conducted medical experiments on the prisoners in their concentration camps without the prisoners' consent and with the expectation that many would die during these experiments. This is the reflection of human experimentation at its worst.

Universal guidelines in the Nuremberg Code

As a result of the war, the scientific world addressed the need for universal guidelines. A statement of research ethics was drafted as a result of the Nuremberg Trials in 1946, when the scientists and medical doctors who directed the Nazi experiments were tried and convicted for their actions.

The following is a summary of the ten points outlined in the code:[2]

1. Any person involved as an experimental subject should have the capacity to give consent, be given the free power of choice, and should be informed about and understand the purpose, method and means, duration, nature, risks, and benefits of the proposed experimental treatment.

2. The anticipated results should benefit society and it must be determined that the information could not be gathered in any other way than by the use of human subjects.

3. Experiments should be based on previous animal experimentation and knowledge of the disease. The anticipated results must justify the performance of the experiment.

4. Unnecessary physical and mental suffering should be avoided.

5. No experiments should be performed with reason to believe that death or disabling injury will be the result.

6. The degree of risk should not exceed the importance of the problem to be solved by the experiment.

7. Precautions should be taken to protect the subject from injury, disability, or death.

8. Only scientifically qualified persons should conduct experiments.

9. The subject should be at liberty to withdraw from participation at any time during the experiment.

10. The scientist in charge must be prepared to end the experiment if he finds that the continuation is likely to cause injury, disability, or death.

Informed consent

All clinical trials in the United States require some level of informed consent.

The US federal requirements for informed consent[3]—which includes the following basic elements for any research involving human subjects conducted, supported, or sponsored by any federal department or agency—are summarized as follows:

1. Procedures and purposes of an experiment must be clearly identified.

2. Discomforts and risks must be explained.

3. Benefits must be reasonably stated.

4. Disclosure of alternative procedures must be made.

5. Extent to which confidentiality of subject's records will be maintained must be explained.

6. If more than minimal risk is involved, any compensation offered or medical treatments available if injury occurs must be explained.

7. Contact information for questions about the research, subject's rights, and whom to contact in the event of a research-related injury must be provided.

8. Statement that any participant can withdraw from the study at any time without prejudice, penalty, or loss of benefits must be given.

One clinical trial participant describes the informed consent process:

> *They told me about the drug and possible side effects. This drug is already in the last phase of research, so they already know a lot about the side effects. They gave me about five pages of written information to read about the trial and the drug. They gave me some time to read it and then they came back and I signed it and they signed it.*

Trials that do not receive federal funding or direction are not required to follow these guidelines, but reputable trials will observe them whether or not they are federally funded.

In the United States, some states have laws governing informed consent for trials within that state. Where there is a conflict between federal and state law, the stricter law applies. You can check with the department of health in the state where a trial is being conducted for rules that apply in that state. A woman who serves on an institutional review board in California says:

> California law requires all subjects in a study to read and sign the Experimental Subject's Bill of Rights before they sign the specific consent form. Even if you don't live in California, you should know what is in it. It says you have the right to know what the study is about, what the risks are, and that you can drop out of the study at any time without your doctor saying, "Then I can't see you anymore." If you are on a drug that can't be stopped suddenly, there must be an appropriate transition provided to subjects who drop out of the study.

Institutional review board

Clinical trials at respected institutions are highly structured and well monitored. An institution's reputation depends on careful, ethical management of its trials, often by establishing its own ethics committee or Institutional Review Board (IRB) to approve, monitor, and review all trials at that site. Other institutions rely on external IRBs to review and monitor trials conducted at their site and others throughout the area or country.

An IRB usually includes scientists, doctors, clergy, and members of the community. An IRB member describes her role this way:

> We review the study design, looking particularly at the potential benefits of the study versus any additional risks that are involved and make sure that the consent form is accurate, honest, and written in language that a typical patient can understand.

The IRB evaluates the scientific merit of the trial. The treatment must potentially be as effective or more effective than the current standard treatment.

The IRB monitors the trial and reviews any serious adverse event reports submitted by the principal investigator or study coordinator. The IRB makes sure that participants are informed of any new information that might affect their willingness to remain in the trial.

An IRB may add to the list of safeguards to address special concerns about a treatment, but here are some standard IRB patient safeguards:

- The control group will receive the best available standard therapy unless there is no treatment proven effective for the condition at the time of the trial. In that case, the experimental therapy would be compared to a placebo or no treatment.

- A patient may reconsider his consent to participate at any time during the trial and may withdraw from the trial without repercussions.

- The patient will be informed of any unexpected risks discovered during the trial.

- The patient's doctor will be informed of the patient's progress. If the treatment becomes detrimental to a patient, the doctor may withdraw the patient from the trial.

- In a double-blind study (neither the research staff nor the patient knows which treatment the patient is receiving), a code will be assigned to each patient so his treatment can be revealed in an emergency situation.

- If one arm of a trial is showing significant side effects, that arm will be terminated. (The whole trial will be terminated if the design only includes one experimental arm.)

- If, during the trial, the results in one arm are significantly better than in the other arms, the trial will be terminated to allow all participants to receive the superior treatment.

How is a clinical trial structured?

In this section, we discuss the things you should know about clinical trials in general. We cover trial design, phases, criteria for acceptance, and financial sponsorship.

Trial design

To minimize variations that might affect outcome, every possible effort is made to eliminate bias and insure that the population of each group has the same basic characteristics.

Group size and composition

The final size and distribution of the patient groups within a trial will affect the reliability of the trial results. The trial designer structures the treatment groups with as much attention as possible to the following considerations:

- Control group. A control group provides the baseline for comparison and evaluation of effectiveness of the treatment. Volunteers in this group do not receive the experimental treatment. The treatment for the control group is usually the most effective standard treatment available at the time. When no standard treatment is available, this group receives no treatment. When studying a new drug, "no treatment" might be in the form of a *placebo*, an inactive pill or substance that looks exactly like the drug being tested.

- **Blinding.** Whenever possible, patients are assigned randomly to the control or the experimental groups. In a single-blind study, the medical caregivers know the patient's group assignment, but the patient does not. This prevents a patient's expectations from affecting his response to the treatment. In a double-blind study, neither the patient nor the medical personnel know which treatment the patient is receiving. Group identification is not revealed until the trial ends.

- **Randomization.** Patients are usually distributed to the treatment groups by computer. This insures that the trial population will be distributed evenly into all groups, without bias.

- **Multiple arms.** Sometimes several different treatment options will be compared in the same trial. Each treatment group is referred to as an "arm" of the trial.

- **Sample size.** A minimum size for each group must be calculated to offset the placebo effect. About one-third of the patients in a trial will respond whether or not they are actually receiving the intervention, even on a placebo. Group size is calculated to allow for a statistically significant response rate, large enough to offset the placebo effect. If the groups are too small, the significance of the response can be questioned.

The protocol document

The trial protocol is described in an overall design document. The principal investigator or study chairperson submits the protocol document to the sponsoring agency, monitoring agencies, and to participating physicians. It identifies the following:

- Purpose of the study
- Length of time the trial is expected to last and number of people expected to participate
- An explanation of how this study will further research and what previous studies led the researcher to develop the hypothesis being tested
- Details on the planned treatment procedures

- Information on the testing methods that will be used to measure the effectiveness of the treatment

- Identification of the participant profile, including restrictions that will be placed on who can enter the trial

- A list of potential side effects, along with a description of how they will be monitored, and an explanation of how they will be treated

- A record-keeping and reporting plan

- Any plans for follow-up after the trial testing period has ended

The protocol document is a guideline. If new information becomes available as the trial proceeds, the protocol may change.

A copy of the full protocol may or may not be readily available for patients to read. In trials sponsored by drug or biotech companies, the document may contain proprietary business information. Open disclosure of the information on a drug that is not yet patented can prevent the drug from meeting the requirements for patent.

The protocol document may also provide detailed descriptions of common side effects or specific treatment procedures that indicate to a patient which treatment group she has been assigned to in a blinded study. Access to the full document is sometimes limited for this reason.

Patient-oriented information on risks, benefits, safeguards, and patient rights is available as part of the informed consent process. Some patients want to know more than others. One woman describes her reaction to the informed consent process:

> I entered a clinical trial to test a new diagnostic procedure. By the time they finished the informed consent process, I'd almost changed my mind. They gave me papers to read describing what they were going to do. Then they came in and told me exactly what they were going to do, to be sure I understood. I was better informed than I really wanted to be.

If, however, you feel you need more detail or background information, check with the trial coordinator to see if you can read the full protocol or parts of it that might help you decide whether or not to participate. If the information is proprietary, you can offer to sign a non-disclosure agreement.

Phases of clinical trials

Drugs and biologics (such as vaccines) progress through three phases prior to application for FDA approval for marketing. A fourth phase sometimes follows FDA approval. A pilot study may be done prior to an official Phase I trial.

Pilot study

This is a small study, usually privately financed, conducted with the expectation that the experimental treatment will generate enough positive data to justify and solicit support for a Phase I study.

Phase I trial: Maximum safe dosage

The Phase I trial focuses on product safety. The goal is to observe how the human body processes the drug, establish a safe dose range, and look for initial signs of its effectiveness. A Phase I trial enrolls a small group, in the range of 20 to 80 participants, and typically lasts several months.

Participant groups are given increasing doses of a drug or drug combination until signs of toxicity are noted. Researchers monitor how the drug is absorbed, metabolized, and excreted. They look for and record side effects. Phase I information is used to design a Phase II trial. About 70 out of 100 products move successfully from Phase I trials to Phase II trials.

If you have advanced disease that has not been successfully treated with standard therapies, a Phase I trial might interest you. An oncologist describes working with a patient whose soft tissue sarcoma wasn't responding to chemotherapy. Knowing that his particular tumor was unlikely to respond to any standard chemotherapy or radiation, she suggested that a clinical trial with a new agent might be a good option to consider. Here is how she explained a Phase I study to him:

> In this Phase I study, we are studying the side effects and toxicity of a new drug that hasn't been used very much in humans, but has been shown to be effective against some cancers in animals. We don't know if your cancer will respond to the drug. We are starting at a low dose, and then working up, so the drug may not work at all at the lower doses, and in the higher doses it may be very toxic. There is a small chance that your cancer will respond to the drug, which is why I am offering it as one of your treatment options.

However, the brief duration of this type of trial and the lack of information on effective dosage may be too much uncertainty for your particular situation. A woman looking for more treatment options describes talking with her doctor about a Phase I trial:

> I asked my physician if we should begin fighting to get me into the antiangiogenesis trial now. He said chances are I wouldn't get in because of the small number of patients, but even so, he said that Phase I has too many risks—I might get in the placebo group, or the very high dose most toxic group, or get a very low dose ineffective group. He felt we shouldn't bother until (and if) Phase II begins.

Phase II trial: Effectiveness

A Phase II trial continues to look at safety and side effects. However, the primary objective in this phase is to study effectiveness in the case of a treatment or immune response in the case of a vaccine or antitoxin, or to determine if the treatment is sufficiently robust as a preventive measure. This type of trial will enroll up to several hundred participants and may last from several months to two years.

Researchers record treatment response during a Phase II trial, which often requires measurable disease (such as a measurable tumor). The need for measurable disease in Phase II trials tends to select for patients with advanced disease.

If the treatment shows significant clinical response rates, the trial will be repeated to confirm the original findings. About one-third of the trials complete the first two phases and move on to Phase III trials.

Phase III trial: Comparison to standard treatment

Phase III trials are large-scale multi-center trials, which include 1,000 to 3,000 people at sites throughout North America. They typically last several years. An experimental treatment is compared to the most effective proven treatment, unless there is no proven standard treatment, in which case it will be compared to a placebo or no treatment.

The goal of the Phase III trial is to confirm a drug's safety, effectiveness, and proper dosage for future labeling and marketing. The increased trial period and large number of participants in a Phase III trial offers researchers more opportunity to observe longer-term side effects, note variations within the larger population of participants, and further define the benefits and risk of the treatment.

Of every 100 drugs that complete Phase III testing, 70 to 90 finish the trial successfully and are sent to the FDA for approval for marketing.

Phase IV trials: Follow-up

Phase IV trials are not required for FDA approval, but they are sometimes specified in the approval. These trials provide added information about long-term risks, benefits, and most appropriate use. They can be used to compare a drug to other drugs on the market, evaluate different dose levels or dose schedules, and study long-term effects.

Financial sponsorship

Trials funded by government agencies are supported by government tax money. Private donors, private institutions, pharmaceutical and other medical companies also fund research. Trials may have more than one source of funding.

A trial sponsor typically contracts with a physician to act as the principal investigator and may offer reimbursement on a per patient basis to cover administrative costs, or a physician may solicit private or government sponsorship for a trial she designs herself.

Criteria for acceptance

Eligibility criteria are designed to eliminate as many conflicting variables as possible and to protect any group of people that might be at increased risk for harmful side effects. Each trial protocol outlines specific requirements for acceptance in these areas:

- **Stage of disease.** Many trials, particularly Phase I and II trials, require participants to have advanced disease.

- **Type of disease.** Most trials limit the study to one type of disease such as breast cancer or colon cancer, but some trials study the effect of the treatment on more than one type of disease.

- **Measurable disease.** A trial may require participants to have measurable disease, such as a measurable tumor, which may decrease in size in response to effective treatment.

- **Previous treatment.** Some trials require patients who have had no previous treatment or no prior treatment of a particular kind. Others simply require a specific period of elapsed time since a particular treatment.

- **Age and gender.** Some trials put restrictions on the age or gender of eligible participants.

- **Health.** Many trials require participant performance or disability status to fall within a certain range. Two commonly used methods of evaluation are the Eastern Cooperative Oncology Group (ECOG) performance status and the Karnofsky scale. Both systems are used to rate a person's level of functional activity.

Issues to consider

Cancer studies are responsible for a substantial number of clinical trials, yet it is estimated that less than 3 percent of the adult cancer patients in the United States are treated in clinical trials. While in many cases this is because patients are not aware of trials that are available to them, there are also other considerations that come into play that might limit a person's ability or willingness to participate.

Take a close look at the flexibility of your situation and weigh your willingness to be treated in a less familiar environment. Recognizing your limitations will help direct and filter your search.

Travel and lodging

Are you willing and able to travel to seek experimental treatment at a distant location or would you prefer treatment nearby? Do you have job or family responsibilities that keep you close to home?

What are your time constraints? Do you have time to travel to visit an out-of-town treatment facility? How long can you stay away from home? How often will you need to be at the treatment site? What if you experience unexpected complications? Can you afford to take unplanned time away from your family or your job? One couple explains their travel considerations:

> We have to fly to Texas every 21 days from California and we will be staying 2 to 6 days, depending on which tests they do. We have decided not to take planes that change in Denver during the winter because we don't want to get stuck in the airport and miss the treatment appointments.

Are you willing to pay out-of-pocket for the added expense of participating in a clinical trial? The medication, extra tests, and doctor visits are sometimes provided as part of the trial, but you also need to consider the cost of travel and lodging. Some insurance companies will pay your medical costs for an approved trial, but travel and lodging expenses will be your responsibility. Some trial sponsors pay participants a small reimbursement for trial participation, but there is no standard rule.

In his book, *Cancer Clinical Trials*, Robert Finn provides some information on this issue:[4]

> *Because cancer trials can sometimes be quite onerous for the patient, some cancer patients are actually compensated for their participation and that adds to the cost of a clinical trial. Often the compensation is limited to reimbursement of out-of-pocket travel expenses.*

> *Cash payments tend to be rare in NCI-sponsored trials, but are more common in trials sponsored by pharmaceutical companies. Payment tends to be higher in early-phase trials, which are more risky.*

Here is how the one couple has solved their lodging problem:

> *We stayed in a hospitality house associated with a large medical center. It was like a resort across the street from the treatment center. We kept trying to convince ourselves that we were on vacation in a beautiful hotel. After a couple of days it began to feel like a big prison—you couldn't get out of there. We talked to people in the elevator who had been at this hotel for six months. We were there for almost a week and it cost us over $800. It was convenient but it wasn't cheap.*

> *Someone told us about extended stay facilities for business travelers. I called and sure enough we found one ten minutes away from the treatment center we are going to. It's a little apartment with a full kitchen and living room. It's $74 a night, which isn't bad compared to hotel prices.*

Organizations such as Mercy Medical Airlift's National Patient Air Transport Helpline at (800) 296-1217, the Corporate Angel Network at (914) 328-1313, and the Air Care Alliance at (888) 662-6794 may be able to provide some travel assistance. Low-cost lodging and ground transportation can often be arranged through the treatment facility.

Treatment costs

Often a pharmaceutical company will provide the drugs being tested, but generally will not cover the cost of treatment delivery or testing. Monitoring and follow-up require extra tests. Insurance coverage for these services varies. Treatment costs can include hospitalization, diagnostic tests, physician fees, supplies, and medication.

Institutions vary in how much financial support they offer their trial participants. Some of the testing and treatment expenses may be provided at no cost. More often, however, the participant must pay at least some of the costs.

One trial participant says:

> I don't pay for anything. The medication, the visits to the clinic and blood tests are free.

Another says:

> My treatment is covered but not the extra CT scans, x-rays, blood tests. Yes, our insurance covers clinical trials. But since going out of state, we don't know if it's going to be touchy to get reimbursed. We'll do as much of the follow-up testing as we can at home.

The National Institutes of Health (NIH) offers free treatment for those who can go to the NIH facility in Bethesda, Maryland to participate in the clinical trials conducted there.

If you are considering trial participation, get notification in writing of what your insurance plan will cover. If you are denied coverage, you can contest that decision, but you must be prepared to show that the treatment has scientific merit for the treatment of your condition.

If your insurance does not cover these expenses, you can check with the social services office at the clinic or hospital that is offering the trial to find out about their financial assistance programs. Patient support organizations like the American Cancer Society or the NIH Cancer Information Service (CIS) offer help finding financial aid for those who need treatment they cannot afford on their own.

Congress is expanding insurance assistance programs like Medicare to cover more trial costs. The state of Maryland has a law that insurance companies in their state must pay for all trials for patients with life-threatening disease. Rhode Island requires insurance companies to cover all Phase II and III clinical trials. Check with your local, state, and federal legislators' offices to find out the status of current legislation on insurance coverage of clinical trials.

Compliance

Be clear with yourself about how motivated you are to stick to the trial protocol. Consider carefully whether or not it will fit easily into your lifestyle or whether you can accommodate the changes. One woman talks about how she schedules her visits to the clinic in another state where her treatment is being monitored:

> I have been in the trial for two years. At first I went in once a month for monitoring. Now I go every three months. It takes us about eight hours to drive there. We have friends in Arizona, so we visit while we're there. I see the nurse who is assigned to the trial first. She runs me through some exercises and then I talk to the doctor. Sometimes they do a blood test.

Risk taking

The side effects of standard treatment vary from person to person. Even less is known about the short-term and long-term effects of an experimental treatment. As an IRB member warns:

> The worry is that someone who is really hoping for a cure or dramatic improvement will have the expectation that the new type of treatment or drug is going to be better. If the trial sponsors knew the treatment was better, they would not be allowed to do the study. In fact, the experimental treatment may turn out to be worse than the standard treatment, in terms of efficacy and/or toxicity.

Phase I studies help to determine safe, yet effective, dosage levels. Some patients will receive ineffective dosages while others may receive dosages that border on toxicity. If you are in a low-dose group, the treatment may not offer you any benefit. While Phase I and II are gathering dosage and side effect data, by Phase III, the investigators have developed a better understanding of the risks. Some Phase III trials are repeated to substantiate the results of a previous Phase III trial.

Phase III trial documents will have the most complete listing of known side effects. In any phase trial, if continued treatment with the protocol therapy is determined to be dangerous to you, the treatment will be stopped and you will continue to be followed by your doctor for response duration and long term survival.

Long-term effects will be harder to predict unless you are looking at a treatment that has already been approved and in use for another condition. Even standard treatments carry some risk of long term side effects, but the risks are better known. A woman in Europe describes her initial response to being offered a stem cell rescue trial and how further research tempered that response:

> My first reaction on being offered entry into the stem cell rescue trial was that I wanted it—desperately! I felt that if I believed in chemo at all, then more must be better. I'd been told it was really tough, so I felt I really should do it—more pain, more gain. This is warped thinking.
>
> I soon got more rational (it took about a week) and started looking at whatever real evidence I could find. I came across a recent study comparing stem cell rescue to FEC [fluorouracil-epirubicin-cyclophosphamide] chemo that showed no difference in outcomes. I read a lot about FEC and found it was the gold standard in Europe for women with my stage disease. That made me feel a lot more comfortable about opting for the FEC and ditching thoughts of stem cell rescue.

Consider the level of risk that you are willing to take. All treatment involves unknowns. Experimental treatment may offer you more hope than your standard treatment options, but the experimental treatment might not be as effective for you.

When less is known about a treatment, expectations are greater. Weigh what you have to gain against what you have to lose. Take as much or as little risk as you personally feel comfortable taking. As a woman with advanced cancer points out, your willingness to take a risk might depend on your situation:

> When I was first diagnosed with cancer, I looked at the large number of women cured and expected to be one of them. Now that my cancer is metastatic, I look at the small numbers that a treatment has helped and think that I could be one of them.

Changed relationship with your physician

Unless your physician is participating in the trial, you may be treated and monitored at the trial site. Most trial investigators will periodically report to your primary physician on treatment and tests given at their facilities.

A woman explains extra precautions her physician takes:

> My doctor here doesn't get any reports on my progress because the trial is blinded. She is very careful when she prescribes a new medication for me. She has me call the clinic to find out if there is any concern about interaction with the trial drug.

As your treatment team expands to include a more distant circle of participants, it may slow your primary physician's access to the most current information on the progress of your treatment. Here is how the wife of one trial participant is keeping her husband's doctors updated:

> We've made a point of keeping all our doctors totally involved. Everything that we do, whether it's related to them or not, we write up a letter and fax it to all three doctors. We want everyone to stay in the loop. When my husband is at home we want his doctor at home to be up-to-date on what has been done at the trial site. Whenever we have a test, we say, "Make sure you send the results to the other doctors."

Discuss the trial with your primary physician. If complications arise when you are home, will your primary physician have enough information to treat you? Are you comfortable with this? Determine the level of communication between trial investigators and your physician that you require to feel confident that your individual needs can be addressed during your participation in the trial.

Blinding and randomization

A clinical trial will have at least two groups of participants—one or more experimental treatment groups and a control group. The control group will receive the most effective standard treatment available at the time or a placebo if there is no proven standard treatment for the condition being treated. In a randomized trial, you have no control over which group you are assigned to. Consider how you feel about this. One woman who has not participated in a trial says:

> I guess clinical trials scare me a bit. They're designed with statistical correctness, rather than my odd case of cancer in mind. Treatments for this disease are unpredictable at best, so being in a blinded group isn't very appealing to me. I keep reading and looking though.

If you prefer a particular treatment, a clinical trial will not insure that you get it. If the trial is blinded, you will not know which group you are in until the trial ends. The only guarantee is that you will have a chance at a treatment that might not be available in any other way. No guarantee may be better than no chance, as one woman points out:

> In Britain, joining a trial is sometimes the only way to get a treatment that has already shown promising results elsewhere in the world.

Sometimes you can find trials that use the experimental drug in both control and study groups but add another drug to it in the study group or vary the dosages as in the following case:

> There are two groups in the trial I'm in. Both groups get the experimental drug. This study is comparing it with and without the addition of a pain medication. I joined the trial for the experimental drug. To me the pain medication would just be an added bonus.

List of questions to ask about the trial

As you read through the informed consent document or if you are able to get a copy of the protocol design document, look for answers to the following questions. Some questions will not have clear-cut answers, but look for a willingness on the part of the trial investigators to answer questions and address potential problems.

Purpose

Questions to ask about the trial goals include:

1. What is the purpose of study? Is the trial studying dosage levels, safety, effectiveness, or making comparisons to other forms of treatment? Is the trial being conducted to collect data to support an FDA application for marketing approval or is the goal to gather marketing data?

2. Who is the sponsor? Does a government agency, national organization, medical institution, medical product manufacturer, or private individual sponsor the trial?

3. Who is the investigator? Who is conducting the trial? Are there multiple investigators? Does the investigator have a financial interest in the treatment being studied? Does the investigator receive compensation for recruiting enrollees?

4. Has this treatment been studied in previous trials for this condition? Has it already been approved for other conditions?

5. Why do researchers feel this treatment will be effective? What advantages do they expect to see over treatments that are already in use? What previous studies or experiences have led them to this conclusion?

Trial design

Detailed design questions to ask include:

1. Are all qualified applicants accepted or is there a further selection process?

2. What extra tests, treatments, medications, hospitalization, and follow-up exams will this trial involve?

3. How will the trial investigator keep my physician updated on my treatment and progress?

4. Will there be long-term follow-up care? Who will treat me if I experience long-term complications?

Location and cost

Questions to ask about logistics include:

1. Is the trial being held at multiple centers? What is the closest center to my home? Can my physician manage my treatment?

2. What expenses will I be responsible for? Is my insurer likely to pay these expenses?

3. Will the trial investigators negotiate with my insurer for coverage? Is this my responsibility?

4. Are there any provisions made for travel and lodging if I have to travel a long distance to participate?

Safeguards

Questions about patient protections include:

1. Who is in charge of evaluating trial design, patient safety, and ongoing reports? Will I be informed of unexpected side effects that occur during the trial? Who will inform me?

2. Who will have access to my records? How will my privacy be protected?

3. What will be done to treat expected and unexpected side effects?

4. If I experience a serious complication in a blinded study, what is the process for finding out what treatment I have received? What are the criteria for revealing this information? Who would make the decision? How long would it take?

5. If the treatment causes me unanticipated long-term harm, will my treatment expenses be compensated?

6. If I have concerns during the trial, whom do I speak with? What if I have more questions during the trial? What if I am unhappy with the way I am treated?

Treatment expectations

Questions about expected treatment benefits and risks include:

1. Is this treatment available outside a trial setting? What are the advantages of participating in the trial?

2. Does this treatment offer me the expectation of significant advantage over standard treatment options?

3. What is a realistic expectation for type of response? Is it realistic to expect total cure or prevention, slower progression, or easing of symptoms?

4. What is the anticipated response rate and duration of response? How effective do they expect this form of treatment to be in a situation like yours? How does that compare to standard treatment response rates? How will they measure response?

5. What are the potential side effects? Which ones are likely and which ones are possible, but less likely? What other organs could be affected? Could the damage be permanent?

Personal concerns

Questions to ask about how the trial will affect your daily life include:

1. Who will be in charge of my care? When should I contact trial personnel and when should I contact my primary doctor?

2. Can I take my regular medications?

3. Will the treatment affect my daily life? Will I be temporarily disabled? Will I be sick? For how long? Do I need to schedule extra time off from my job?

How to find clinical trials

Up until recently, there has been no central clearinghouse of information for all clinical trials. However, a new government web site now available at *http:/ /www.clinicaltrials.gov* will become a clearinghouse for clinical trials that are both federally and privately funded. The site is being developed by the National Library of Medicine as a service of the National Institutes of Health. As of this writing, however, not all trials in the US are listed in this database.

When looking for trial information, seek out respected, reliable resources. A pamphlet describing a trial is one starting place, but you will want to gather information about the trial from other sources as well. A woman explains how the source of the information affected her confidence in the trial she was considering:

> *I almost went into a trial at Columbia, but for reasons of timing, I didn't. The things that made me consider it were: 1) the trial had been reviewed by oncologists I respect, 2) they had a very competent research nurse in charge who answered or got an answer to every question I asked, 3) I have a friend who works at the company making the drug who gave me information on what had been found up until then and the ability to get in touch with the person in charge at the company.*

Ask your doctor

The first place to ask about trials is your own doctor's office, particularly if you are seeing a specialist. Your doctor is likely to know about the most prominent trials being conducted in your region for your condition. If you let your doctor know that you are interested in clinical trials, he can help you identify specific things to look for as you widen your search and he may be able to help you find trials that you can participate in without traveling to another area.

Your doctor's office should not be your only stop if you are searching for trial options. Relying on your doctor alone is sometimes hit-and-miss. As one trial participant found:

> I met a man who is participating in the same trial. He lives 40 miles from the trial site. The doctors in his town told him there was nothing they could do. His wife found the trial on the Internet. No one had told them that there was a trial just 40 miles away.

Clinics, hospitals, and academic research centers

Since most clinical trials are conducted in medical treatment centers, you can contact your nearest clinic, hospital, or medical school to find out if they are conducting any trials that might interest you. Most medical school web sites have a listing with the screening criteria for open ongoing trials. If you ask about trials at a larger local medical clinic, you will probably be directed to the clinic's trial coordinator who will be a helpful source of information.

Nationwide, look for respected treatment centers that specialize in research and treatment of your condition. Even if you do not find a trial that fits your needs, you may be able to identify a research specialist in your disease who can direct you to an appropriate trial at another major center. Scientists and clinicians focused on a particular specialty can be valuable allies in the search for information on current advances in treatment and promising upcoming studies.

Be aware, however, that an expert who is conducting his own clinical trials might not be a well-balanced source of information on the risks and benefits of that program. It is important to do further research to gather other viewpoints. After declining a clinical trial, one woman found that her doctor had withheld his opinion because of his association with the trial he was offering as one of her options:

> The oncologist I was then seeing wouldn't give his opinion on the relative merits of stem cell rescue or the alternative he was offering. I guess he felt he shouldn't influence patients. Later after I had decided against the trial, he confessed that he didn't think stem cell rescue would turn out to be superior in his study.

If you find a center offering a trial that interests you, get verification that the trial is still open before you travel to the trial site. Sometimes you will be encouraged to come for evaluation without being told the trial is closed, with the idea that you might be willing to participate in some other trial. One man recounts such an experience:

> At the very beginning we told them we were interested in a particular drug and asked if they had a trial open. They said yes, sent us the literature, and made an appointment. We spent four days at the trial site being tested.

> On the fifth day, we met with the doctor to be told that the program had been closed. They wanted to start us on another program. I said, "What's the track record of that drug? I have confidence in the other stuff." They said they didn't know. We packed our bags and left.

Funding or sponsoring agencies

The National Institutes of Health (NIH) outside Washington, D.C. is the best-known and most complete source of information on clinical trials in the United States. You can contact the NIH by phone at (301) 496-4000 or through the Internet at *http://www.nih.gov.*

For information on cancer trials, the NIH offers a searchable database of all types of NIH-sponsored cancer trials. The database can be accessed at their CancerNet web site at *http://www.icic.nci.nih.gov,* or you can phone the Cancer Information Service (CIS) at (800) 4-CANCER for information about ongoing trials. Trial information changes rapidly—new trials are offered and older trials fill up. Be sure to check back regularly.

Other national agencies such as the FDA, the Centers for Disease Control and Prevention, and the Department of Defense also sponsor trials, but the most complete listing of federally-sponsored trials will be on the NIH web site at *http://www.clinicaltrials.gov.*

Some state agencies fund medical research. Contact your state's department of health for help finding listings of state-funded trials.

Manufacturers

Most clinical trials are designed to support the approval process for new medical products and techniques. If you hear about an interesting new treatment for your condition, call the company to find out about their ongoing and upcoming trials.

If you hear something about a new drug under study, but cannot remember the name, you can check EurekAlert at *http://www.eurekalert.com* for recent medical press releases. You can also find product development information for US publicly traded companies at the Edgar web site *http://www. FreeEDGAR.com*.

The Pharmaceutical Research and Manufacturers of America (PhRMA) publishes a brochure called "New Medicines in Development." You can request a copy by calling them at (202) 835-3450. They also offer a searchable version of the database on their web site *http://www.phrma.org*.

For patent protection reasons, commercial companies are careful about how much information they release about their un-patented products to the non-professional. You can expect to find out where their trials are being conducted and by whom, then you can contact the clinical investigator. Access to treatment details and rationale may be limited to medical professionals. In that case, you will need help from your doctor in gathering the information you need to evaluate the trial for your situation.

Patient organizations and support groups

National organizations that specialize in patient support for a specific type of disease, like the American Foundation for AIDS Research, are an excellent resource for finding ongoing research information. Their newsletters often refer to new studies or the latest research that shows enough promise to go to clinical trial.

Local support groups are another way to learn about ongoing and upcoming trials. You may even meet people who are already participating. This woman heard about a trial from several patient resources:

> Once I got involved in the patient community, I heard about the trial
> I'm in from several sources. I read about it on an Internet mailing list, I
> read it in a patient newsletter I get, and I heard about it from someone at
> my support group.

Patient advocacy organizations are especially valuable sources of information on trials. Advocacy organizations monitor the more commercial aspects of medical research to keep their members informed about potential problems.

They can direct you to current research, alert you to the questions that you need to ask, and make you aware of the risks that you need to consider.

Patient groups are becoming important lobbying forces for changes such as access to information, more timely publication of results, or increased government funding for research. Patient groups sometimes promote clinical trial participation among their members for research directions they consider promising.

Professional organizations

If your doctor is a member of a professional organization such as the Southwest Oncology Group (SWOG) or the Eastern Cooperative Oncology Group (ECOG), he will receive regular updates on clinical trials being conducted by other members and non-members. Details of these trials are usually restricted to member physicians, but you, as a consumer, can look on the Internet for a listing of the trials they sponsor. With that information, you can discuss the trial with your doctor to decide if it warrants his request for further information or you can contact the institution conducting the trial for more details.

Learn which professional organizations include your disease in their field of focus. Find out what organizations your physicians belong to. Conferences for groups like the American Society of Clinical Oncology (ASCO) are held to keep physicians in that specialty up-to-date on the latest research. While membership is limited, some conferences are open to patients and other non-professionals. You can also look for the association journals at your nearest medical library or look the association up on the Internet. The association often publishes its conference agendas and session summaries. This information may help you find a specific trial or direct you to a center doing research in that specialty.

Nationally known specialists often serve on the board of directors for these organizations. A look at who is on the board will help you find experts in the field. You can look for articles written by those experts and contact them about research studies that they are conducting.

Media reports

Newspapers, popular magazines, radio, and television all carry reports on the latest breakthroughs in medical research. Follow-up on a news report is sometimes disappointing. The media often selects stories more for their headline potential than their likelihood of increasing your current treatment options. Although only 1 in 5,000 animal studies ever makes it into human trials, newscasts are filled with references to the latest "breakthroughs" in the treatment of mice.

If a report has even a glimmer of value to you, follow it up. Look for the institution and the name of the researcher in the report. Also find out what, if any, written information the report is based upon. You may not find what you thought you were looking for (i.e., a simple painless treatment that will cure any disease), but you may find a research center or an expert who can help you identify your next step.

Trials on the Internet

More and more individual institutions are posting information about their trials on the Internet.

Internet trial databases

The two most comprehensive sites for trial information are the government's ClinicalTrials web site and CenterWatch:

- ClinicalTrials.gov. This new database at *http://www.clinicaltrials.gov* will eventually include public and privately funded US trials as well as some international trials. It can be searched by disease or condition, treatment, or phase, as well as by location or sponsor. You will need to check back regularly for updates.

- CenterWatch. The CenterWatch web site at *http://www.centerwatch.com* provides information on clinical trials of all kinds. Their listing includes both private and corporately funded trials. You can search by disease categories or by keyword. CenterWatch will send you email updates on the latest new trials in the areas you specify.

- HSTAT. The National Library of Medicine provides access to an NIH clinical study database in the Health Services/Technology Assessment Text section of their web site at *http://text.nlm.nih.gov/ftrs/gateway*. To get to the search form, choose "NIH Clinical Studies" in the pull-down menu.

- CRISP. Another resource for finding federally-funded biomedical research studies is the Computer Retrieval of Information of Scientific

Projects (CRISP) database at *http://www.crisp.cit.nih.gov*. This database lets you use keywords to select projects and investigators working on a particular condition.

- **CancerNet.** For cancer-specific trials funded by the federal government, look at the CancerNet web site at *http://www.icic.nci.nih.gov*. This database is searchable by cancer type or by keyword.

- **CancerGuide.** Steve Dunn's CancerGuide web site has a section on clinical trials. Start with his article "Finding Clinical Trials on the Net," *http://www.cancerguide.org/clinical_trials.html*. He not only provides a list of places to look for trials, but he also gives a clear explanation of how the trial process works and offers some excellent suggestions on what to look for and what to avoid. This site is useful to anyone looking into clinical trials, not just those looking for cancer trials.

- **European Organization for Research and Treatment of Cancer (EORTC).** This searchable database of cancer protocols in Europe is found on the Web at *http://www.eortc.be/protoc/default.htm*.

Some web sites require you to fill out a patient profile so they can notify you if you qualify for a trial. Be cautious when you fill out medical profiles. Make sure that you understand how the information will be used and protected. Read the privacy statement carefully and do not provide any personal information that you do not feel comfortable sharing.

Trial sponsors, clinics, and research group web sites

Professional organizations have web sites with information on clinical trials they sponsor and those being conducted by their members.

Most institutions conducting clinical trials have trial listings on their web sites. First, however, you must identify clinics, hospitals, and medical schools doing research in the disease area that you are researching. One way to identify these institutions and individual investigators is to do a MEDLINE search in PubMed *http://www.ncbi.nlm.nih.gov/PubMed* to bring up published research articles about that condition. You can use the keyword phrase "clinical trials" along with the name of the disease.

Note, however, that the time between the evaluations of a study to the article publication may be about three years, so unless the article is describing an ongoing trial, most articles will not help you to find current trials. A search of the literature will, however, help you identify institutions and researchers working in your area of interest. Then, you can look for an institution's web site to see if they have a listing of ongoing clinical trials. If not, contact the researcher (look in the institution's phone or email directory) or contact the institution by phone.

Be sure to check the web sites of hospitals, medical schools, and clinics in your region. You might find an appropriate trial nearby.

Check the web sites of groups that fund medical research. They have information on the grants that they have awarded which will direct you to the place where the research is taking place. Government agencies such as the FDA, CDC, and the US Public Heath Service are all trial sponsors. Some disease-specific organizations also raise money for research.

Internet discussion groups

Internet mailing lists provide access to discussion groups on most diseases. In large gatherings of people with the same disease, you are likely to find some are participating in or familiar with current clinical trials. You can search for a newsgroup or mailing list discussion along with information on how to participate at the Liszt.com web site *http://www.liszt.com*.

Some medical web sites have live chats and bulletin board type discussions where people also share experience and research tips with others dealing with a particular disease.

Search engines

As a last resort, you can try a keyword search in your favorite engine. Be aware that unless you are researching a rare condition or use a highly specific search phrase, you are likely to be overwhelmed by the number of references the search will display, and many of them will not yield much useful information.

Drugs and trials overseas

Occasionally in your research you will come across a promising trial being done overseas or a drug that has been approved overseas that is not available in the United States.

Here a woman describes her unexpected discovery of a more effective delivery method available in Singapore for a drug sold here in the US in a different form:

> While on a vacation with a friend who lives in Singapore, I got a case of intestinal flu. My friend gave me some Voltaren suppositories she had with her. Back in the United States, I was having a bout of intense bone pain, so I decided to try one of the Voltaren suppositories. The suppository worked like magic in 20 to 30 minutes. The oral form does nothing for me. I routinely use Voltaren suppositories to control the bone pain that I have from my cancer.
>
> I can only get the medication in suppository form from Asia or Canada. I've inquired at Novartis/CIBA about distribution of the suppositories in the US. I was told that they'd looked into this market, and the market simply wasn't large enough to justify the expense of producing that form in the US. I have recently had a compounding pharmacy (Liberty Drug, 195 Main Street, Chatham, New Jersey 07928), formulate Voltaren in suppository form for me in 50, 75, and 100 milligram doses.

Some patients are willing to go across national borders for access to a treatment or substance not available in the US. One woman talks about how she has been able to gain access, with the help of doctors in both countries, to a drug approved for use in Canada, but not in the US:

> I read about a promising new drug in the New England Journal of Medicine. The company apparently has no intention of doing the testing necessary to have the drug approved in the US. I have a friend who works for the drug company that makes it. I was given my first three-month supply by the drug company via my friend.
>
> This same friend found me a doctor in Canada. My doctor in the US sent him a prescription for long-term use. Every three months, I send the Canadian doctor a check and he pays his hospital pharmacy to send it to me. We had some FDA import problems at first, but things are going more smoothly now.

A drug used in a foreign country, but not approved for use in the US, can sometimes be imported for personal use. This is called "personal importation" and may be permitted for compassionate use when domestic drugs are not meeting the needs of a seriously ill patient or when a course of treatment begun outside the US must be completed in the US.

It is, of course, wise to evaluate such a drug with the same care as you would a domestic treatment and give additional attention to patient safety regulations in that country, the quality of the manufacturing process, and studies done on its effectiveness. Even if the FDA allows you to import the product, that does not assure you of its safety, quality, or effectiveness.

The decision to allow the importation of an unapproved drug for personal use is up to the discretion of the FDA enforcement agent in the district where the product passes through US Customs. Documentation accompanying the product that can be helpful to the FDA enforcement agent includes:

• A letter stating in writing that the product is for your own personal use

• The name and address of the US physician who will be overseeing your use of the medication

• A letter from your doctor stating the expected benefits of this treatment over an approved domestic treatment for your condition or a letter from a foreign doctor providing evidence that the drug is a continuation of treatment started under his care in a foreign country

If you are interested in importing an unapproved drug for personal use, contact the FDA Center for Drug Evaluation and Research (CDER) at (888) 463-6332 for additional information. You can also find a document called "Information on the Importation of Drugs," prepared by the Division of Import Operations and Policy, on the FDA web site at *http://www.fda.gov/ora/import/pipinfo.htm.*

CHAPTER 9

Complementary and Alternative Therapies

COMPLEMENTARY AND ALTERNATIVE MEDICINE (CAM) includes a range of approaches for preventing and treating illness, such as diet and exercise programs, herbs, chiropractic treatment, and the healing power of the mind, among others.

We will not attempt to cover or even list all the individual modalities. Instead, we focus on defining complementary and alternative therapies, taking a new look at these therapies, concerns about the risk of using unproven treatments, evaluating nonstandard therapies, talking with your doctor, expenses and insurance coverage, and where to look for reliable information.

Defining CAM therapies

Complementary and alternative therapies are defined and grouped in a somewhat confusing variety of ways. This confusion can lead to misunderstandings about what exactly is being discussed or compared.

In his landmark study on the frequency and distribution of alternative therapy use in the United States,[1] Dr. David Eisenberg defined alternative therapies as "medical interventions not taught widely at United States medical schools or generally available at United States hospitals." But therapies that qualified in his 1993 study may not qualify under that definition today, as more medical schools and hospitals add some of these therapies to their programs.

The National Library of Medicine Medical Subject Heading (MESH) defines Alternative Medicine as "An unrelated group of unorthodox practices, often with explanatory systems that do not follow conventional biomedical explanations."

In a 1993 article on alternative AIDS therapies, Carola Burroughs defines "alternative" as a "catch-all phrase" used for "various treatments which simply have not been accepted by the medical establishment."[2]

Terms like "unconventional" or "unorthodox" make a political distinction. Distinctions like "modern" medicine, versus "traditional" or "folk medicine" denote cultural variations and imply a superior level of advancement.

"Unproven" is another often-used distinction. However, there are standard medical treatments used today that have gained their acceptance through history of use, rather than formal clinical testing. Drugs tested and approved for one use can be prescribed off-label for a new use when preliminary outcomes look hopeful and the physician feels the situation warrants the risk. Although not yet thoroughly tested and proven for that use, off-label uses are common in clinical practice.

In this book, when we refer to *alternative or complementary therapies*, we will mean *nonstandard* forms of treatment—those therapies not formally accepted as standard clinical practice. Experimental therapies currently in clinical trials are not included in this category. They are in the process of crossing over into acceptance as standard treatments. They are viewed here as pre-standard therapies. (See Chapter 8, *Researching Clinical Trials*.)

Classification of complementary and alternative therapies

The National Center for Complementary and Alternative Medicine (NCCAM) at the National Institutes of Health divides alternative and complementary therapies into seven major classifications of practices.

An NCCAM listing has identified over 340 terms related to CAM practices and modalities. A disclaimer states that this classification and listing of therapies is neither complete nor authoritative and will continue to be refined.

Table 9-1 shows the seven major categories and descriptions from the National Center for Complementary and Alternative Medicine.[3]

Table 9-1. Classification of CAM Practices

Classifications	Subcategories	Description
Mind-body medicine	Mind-body systems Mind-body methods Religion and spirituality Social and contextual areas	Behavioral, psychological, social, and spiritual approaches to health.
Alternative medical systems	Acupuncture and oriental medicine Traditional, indigenous systems Unconventional Western systems Naturopathy	Complete systems of theory and practice that have been developed outside of the Western biomedical approach.
Lifestyle and disease prevention	Clinical preventative practices Lifestyle therapies Health promotion	Theories and practices designed to prevent the development of illness, identify and treat risk factors, or support the healing and recovery process. Lifestyle and disease prevention is concerned with integrated approaches for the prevention and management of chronic disease in general or the common determinants of chronic disease.
Biologically-based therapies	This category is divided into four subcategories: Phytotherapy or herbalism; special diet therapies; orthomolecular medicine; pharmacological, biological and instrumental interventions.	This category includes natural and biologically-based practices, interventions, and products. Many overlap with conventional medicine's use of dietary supplements.
Manipulative and body-based systems	Chiropractic medicine Massage and body work Unconventional physical therapies	Systems that are based on manipulation and/or movement of the body.
Biofield	No subcategories	Systems that use subtle energy fields in and around the body for medical purposes.
Bioelectromagnetics	No subcategories	The unconventional use of electromagnetic fields for medical purposes.

Distinguishing complementary from alternative therapies

Complementary therapies are used in addition to standard therapy with the hope of reducing side effects, enhancing the outcome of the standard treatment, or improving your quality of life. For example, acupuncture can be used to reduce nausea during chemotherapy, guided imagery can be used to enhance the action of the chemotherapy and reduce the physical and emotional stress of treatment, or yoga can be used to increase flexibility after surgery.

While nutrition and exercise may not be listed as standard treatment for a particular condition, most physicians encourage complementary lifestyle changes that will improve the patient's general health and quality of life.

A therapy is technically only truly alternative if the patient chooses to use it in place of the standard recommended treatment. It is a complementary therapy when used in combination with a standard treatment, but most often the term "alternative" is used to indicate both complementary and alternative practices.

Taking a new look at complementary and alternative therapies

Contemporary fads often color what we see as progressive and modern treatment. We can look back at the popularity of the healing water spas in the early 1800s or the patent medicine cure-alls of the 1880s and 1890s. The words "scientific" and "modern" were commonly used to market these forms of treatment and many treatments looked on as useless or even dangerous today were endorsed by respected physicians of those periods.

On the other hand, some popular therapies dismissed by the medical community as unsubstantiated in the past, upon closer examination have been shown to be effective. Dr. William Fair, former head of urology at Memorial Sloan-Kettering says:

> When I was in medical school, acupuncture was thought to be really hocus-pocus. We now know (especially in the area of oncology) that nausea and vomiting can be very effectively controlled by acupuncture.[4]

Since Dr. Eisenberg's 1993 study showing the widespread use of alternative therapies was published in the *New England Journal of Medicine*, medical professionals have begun to take a closer look at nonstandard therapies. Dr. Eisenberg found that 34 percent of the people he surveyed had used at least one unconventional therapy to treat a serious or bothersome condition in the past year. In fact, their visits to unconventional care practitioners exceeded visits to primary care physicians that year.[5] A 1997 follow-up study showed the use of non-conventional therapies had increased to 42.1 percent and total out-of-pocket expenditures had more than doubled.[6]

By 1998 a survey of US medical schools showed that 64 percent offered some coursework in complementary and alternative medicine.[7] Another group of surveys conducted between 1982 and 1995 showed that 43 percent of the physicians interviewed made referrals for acupuncture, 40 percent for chiropractic, and 21 percent for massage therapy. The authors concluded:

> This review suggests that large numbers of physicians are either
> referring to or practicing some of the more prominent and well-known
> forms of CAM [complementary and alternative medicine] and that many
> physicians believe that these therapies are useful or efficacious.[8]

Clinics offering the combination of standard and complementary medicine, sometimes referred to as integrative medicine, are opening up in association with major medical centers.

Chronic incurable conditions and deadly diseases have been, and still are, an area where hope for a cure drives our willingness to look beyond the range of proven standard therapies. Non-standard therapies of today may become some of tomorrow's standard treatments.

Traditional medicine: The foundation of modern medicine

The World Health Organization (WHO) estimates that 80 percent of the people in most developing countries rely on traditional medicine for their basic healthcare. The World Health Organization defines traditional medicine as healing traditions that existed before the arrival of modern medicine—traditions handed down from generation to generation.

The use of traditional medicine remains high even among people in developed countries. Herbal preparations account for 30 percent to 50 percent of the medicinal consumption in China. Japan is estimated to have the highest per capita use of herbal medicine in the world. Interest in the use of traditional medicine is on the increase in European countries and in the United States.

Some medical traditions are very old. According to the National Center for Complementary and Alternative Medicine's Unconventional Timeline[9]

(Figure 9-1), herbalism can be traced back 200,000 years, as the oldest known form of medical treatment. Spiritual healing and shamanism date back 20,000 years, acupuncture 2,000 years, and homeopathy 200 years.

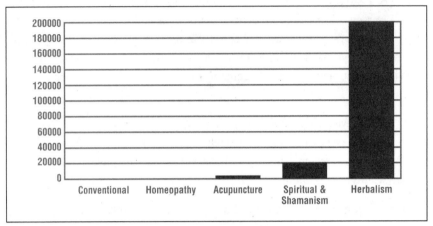

Figure 9-1. The unconventional timeline

Some drug companies send ethnobotanist plant hunters to interview traditional healers and search the rain forests for sources of new commercial medicines. Pharmacognocists study plant samples and microbes to isolate active ingredients that hold promise as future pharmaceuticals. Medical chemists study the relationship of chemical structure to biological activity in the hope of synthesizing drugs from these natural products and to learn how they work to protect us from or treat our diseases.

Traditional use of plants by indigenous people has provided the source of some of our most valued and respected modern medicines. African folklore led researchers at Eli Lilly to the discovery of the Madagascar periwinkle, which was developed into vinblastine and vincristine for the treatment of childhood leukemia and Hodgkin's disease. The taxanes, used to treat advanced breast cancer, come from the bark and needles of the Pacific yew tree. Curare, a deadly herb applied to blowgun darts, relaxes the muscles during anesthesia. Aspirin comes from white willow bark and morphine from the opium poppy, both used by the ancient Greeks. Even the smallpox vaccine has its roots in medical folk belief. Edward Jenner developed the vaccine after a milkmaid told him that local farmers believed that a mild case of cowpox made them immune to smallpox.

The limits of scientific proof

As mentioned earlier, not all accepted standard methods of treatment have been subjected to the rigorous scientific scrutiny required for the initial marketing of a new drug. Estrogen, for example, is approved for eliminating symptoms of menopause and reducing risk of osteoporosis. Estrogen has also been studied and promoted for lowering the risks of heart disease and Alzheimer's, but these are not uses for which estrogen is officially approved. Various studies showing associations with reductions in risk have lead to the promotion of these potential benefits as reasons for using estrogen replacement therapy. They are not listed as proven uses in FDA-approved insert information, yet the use of estrogen is often recommended by doctors to reduce those risks.

Even proven standard treatments have a risk of unexpected side effects, drug interactions, and long-term complications. Drugs such as diethylstilbestrol (DES), thalidomide, and fen-phen were approved as standard treatment options, and then later withdrawn from the market for re-evaluation after significant complications developed as the result of their use.

A former biologist who is being treated for cancer explains how she evaluates both standard and nonstandard treatments:

> I know how to read scientific literature, but the most important thing
> for me when deciding on a treatment, traditional or alternative, is the
> simple notion that "you can never know for sure." If someone recommends something to me as a sure thing, I immediately become suspicious.
> Even with treatments that have been thoroughly studied, there is always
> at least one question that the researchers have forgotten to ask.

The economics of product development

The research process is slow and expensive. According to the Pharmaceutical Research and Manufacturers of America (PhRMA), the cost of moving a new drug through the development process in the United States averages $500 million. While a drug patent gives a company exclusive rights for twenty years to develop and market a new drug, development and approval take up about twelve to fifteen of those years. That leaves a short period of exclusivity for a drug manufacturer to recoup the cost of development. Only about 1 out of every 5,000 drugs tested in US pharmaceutical labs survives the development process to reach the marketplace.

If a remedy is already in use, or has been described in the scientific litera-ture, it cannot be patented. Many CAM treatments, derived from age-old remedies cannot be patented, so they are not cost-effective products for drug companies to pursue. In response to this dilemma, the National Center for Complementary and Alternative Medicine has begun to provide funding for the study of promising CAM treatments that don't offer the promise of high monetary profit that patent exclusivity provides.

Drug companies also hesitate to undertake the development of treatments for rare diseases because the number of potential users is small. However, the Orphan Drug Act of 1983 provides clinical research grants, tax credits, and exclusivity for seven years for those companies willing to develop these less profitable drugs.

Cultural variations in standard treatment

Some standard practices in the healing systems of China or India are consid-ered alternative practices in the US. Standard therapy varies from country to country.

In her book, *Medicine and Culture: Varieties of Treatment in the United States, England, West Germany, and France*, Lynn Payer observes that the French pre-fer gentler forms of medical therapies. Their standard treatments use lower drug doses and less invasive techniques than those recommended in the United States. West German doctors are more likely to prescribe mud baths, walks in the forest, or herbal medicine. The British emphasize relieving dis-comfort and are more skeptical about the expectation of cure. Payer says:

> American doctors perform more diagnostic tests than doctors in
> France, West Germany, or England. They often eschew drug treatment in
> favor of aggressive surgery, but if they do use drugs they are likely to use
> higher doses and more aggressive drugs....[10]

The line drawn between standard and nonstandard treatments is sometimes affected by cultural attitudes and traditions, rather than proven effective-ness. In some cases, this rigidity is being examined and reevaluated.

Considering an alternative
or complementary therapy

The question often raised in response to Dr. Eisenberg's studies is: why are patients going outside mainstream medicine for treatment and prevention? In a response to Dr. Eisenberg's first survey, Dr. Edward W. Campion wrote in a letter to the *New England Journal of Medicine*:

> *The public's expensive romance with unconventional medicine is a cause for our profession to worry. We need to demonstrate more effectively our dedication to caring for the whole patient—worries, quirks, and all.[11]*

In a 1998 Journal of the American Medical Association article, John Astin, PhD, reported on a survey at the Stanford Center for Research in Disease which asked that same question.[12] He concludes:

> *Dissatisfaction did not predict the use of alternative medicine. Only 4.4 percent of those surveyed reported relying primarily on alternative therapies.*

His results showed that those who use alternatives do so "largely because they find these healthcare alternatives to be more congruent with their own values, beliefs, and philosophical orientations toward health and life."

Astin found the level of an individual's education to be the top predictor. Of those respondents with a high school education or less, 31 percent used alternatives in comparison to 50 percent of the respondents with a graduate degree. Astin also found that as a person's health status declined, his alternative usage went up. Specific health issues like back problems, chronic pain, anxiety, and urinary tract problems also increased the likelihood of usage.

A physician offers her perspective on why more patients are visiting alternative and complementary care providers:

> *One big reason I believe interest in alternative treatments has increased is because these practitioners have and/or take the time to listen to the patient, something that is being taken away in normal clinical practice where managed care has reduced the amount of time allotted per patient.*

One might consider nonstandard treatments for a range of reasons:

- Physical and emotional comfort
- Empowerment
- Ease of access
- Simpler, less invasive approach
- Quality of life
- Treatment of chronic conditions
- Prevention
- Hope of survival

Physical and emotional comfort

Complementary and alternative practitioners tend to pay more attention to a patient's physical comfort. Soft music, lowered lights, and warm blankets provide a soothing atmosphere. Patients generally feel that alternative care practitioners spend more time with them. Treatments are more likely to involve touch and feel more nurturing. Even if the process is not as efficient or effective, the experience is more appealing.

Modern medicine relies on test results. When medical tests are used to evaluate your health or progress in treatment, your sense of well-being becomes dependent on the results of the test. Being sent home with a negative test result feels like a personal failure.

Sometimes in the face of a lot of bad news, you need to take a break from the responsibility of evaluation and decision-making especially when there are no obvious answers or clear-cut treatment choices. One woman explains:

> I find that when I'm overwhelmed with medical decision-making and frightening possibilities, I need to indulge in things that soothe my mind and emotions—that get me centered again.

A relaxing massage or an herbal tea designed to strengthen your body's healing forces goes a long way toward restoring your sense of well-being.

Empowerment

Your doctor does not cure you. Your body does the healing, with some skilled assistance from your doctor. After being diagnosed with an acute disease, you may feel your life revolves around doctor visits and treatment schedules with little time to pause and reflect about how you feel and what you want to do. Taking time out to consider and/or use nonstandard complementary or alternative treatments gives you the feeling that you are a more active participant in the development of your treatment plan.

Ease of access

Complementary and alternative therapies are explained in simple terms and you can purchase or practice them without a prescription. Access is easy. Initial costs are generally lower, particularly compared to the costs of medications and treatments for acute diseases.

Note that ease of access does not insure effectiveness or safety. You should inform your doctor of all other approaches you are using if you are under treatment for an acute or chronic condition.

Simpler, less invasive approaches

Standard therapy may be aggressive and have damaging side effects. The long-term safety of newer treatments is not known. Positive outcomes are not guaranteed.

You may want to try simpler approaches first, as did this woman who was concerned about becoming dependent on a prescription medication:

> *After being exposed to a concentrated dose of a pesticide that affects the nervous system, I was given antidepressants. I did not want to start taking these drugs without a clear understanding of how they would alleviate the symptoms or resolve the cause of the problem.*
>
> *I was concerned about becoming dependent on the antidepressants. I felt they should be my last-ditch choice, not a first-line response. After a series of tests that ruled out more serious complications, I decided to try acupuncture treatments. I experienced a noticeable reduction in the symptoms within a short time. My symptoms gradually disappeared. The acupuncture was expensive and most of it wasn't covered by my insurance, but I felt it offered me a less invasive approach with fewer potential problems than the antidepressants.*

In this example a man tries an alternative approach to relieve his back pain and avoid the need for back surgery:

> I have painful deteriorating disks in my back. In lieu of an operation, I decided to try proliferative therapy. It is a therapy developed in New Zealand where glucose is injected into the ligaments parallel to the disks to strengthen the tissue around the disks and give lateral support to my back. It doesn't do anything to the disks but the tissue around it is healed and strengthened so it gives support to the disks.

> It worked. I've had similar injections on a shoulder injury and in my knee. Using these treatments I was able to avoid rotator cuff surgery on my shoulder and arthroscopic surgery for my knee.

Quality of life

You may think of CAM therapies as a way to boost your immune system during and after harsh treatments like chemotherapy or to help alleviate the side effects. Acupuncture, for example, has been shown to significantly reduce the amount of drugs needed for pain and to reduce the duration of stays in treatment facilities.[13] As William Fair, MD, explains:

> The role of the physician should be to provide healing even if we can't cure, and to provide an expansion of life, even if we cannot extend life.[14]

CAM therapies sometimes offer healing even when they don't offer cure. One woman uses meditation techniques during treatment:

> My husband and I learned transcendental meditation about 25 years ago. It's a big help in learning to focus as well as for relaxing when the nurse is trying to find that elusive vein for the fifth time in ten minutes.

She also tells how walking, nature, and music help her cope with the effects of the disease:

> Walking in the woods, bird watching, and canoeing, these things that I love are hard for me to do now, but I work at them. For me, being in a fairly primitive natural setting is absolutely the most healing thing I can do. Using a music tape as I walk helps a lot with my breathing problems.

Treatment of chronic conditions

Both Eisenberg's and Astin's surveys showed that alternative therapies are most often used for chronic conditions. Eisenberg found that 36 percent of the people in his study sought treatments for back pain, 28 percent for anxiety, 27 percent for headaches, and 26 percent for chronic pain. These were the three top reasons for using alternative therapies. (Cancer accounted for less than 3 percent.) If you suffer from a condition that standard medicine has not been able to treat successfully, you may be more willing to look at nonstandard options as a woman with chronic pain recounts:

> Because I went through three years of intractable pain, I tried a number of things, hoping that something would work. I took a lot of different medications that would work partially or would work for a while and then fade away and not work anymore. I tried acupuncture, hypnosis, homeopathy, and hypnotherapy—I was pretty desperate—I was willing to do anything.

In her case none of these solved the problem, but she was willing to try anything that might possibly work before she found a medication that helped her control the pain.

Prevention

Both alternative and prescription treatments advertise protection as a hedge on genetic susceptibilities to the diseases that killed our parents and grandparents. Healthy women are given hormone replacement therapy to reduce risk of heart disease and osteoporosis even when they have no current symptoms of either. Blood pressure and cholesterol medications are given to reduce the risk of strokes and heart attacks.

For those who would prefer not to take prescription drugs for prevention, lifestyle changes and other nonprescription approaches such as vitamins, herbs, and food supplements may present an appealing alternative.

Hope of survival

Survival is a strong motivating force. When scientific medicine runs short of tools to stem the progress of the disease, patients feel like they are on their own.

In a 1998 article in *Health on the Internet*, Charles Wessel talks about helping HIV/AIDS patients find complementary and alternative treatments:

> During the first decade of the AIDS epidemic, with so few viable options available, many affected individuals began to seriously examine and pursue the possibilities of nontraditional regimens.[15]

Many cancer patients know this scenario well, as this woman relates:

> My 25-year marriage to a scientist has certainly had an influence on my critical thinking tendencies (which were pretty strong to begin with). But in January, something very different happened when an MRI showed indisputable metastases in my bones. The quest for the right treatment takes on a new personality, a new urgency, when the goal is saving my life (and our life together). Now this PhD scientist, who makes his living being a skeptic, an analyst, an experimenter, is willing to look into anything on the continuum from far-out to tried-and-true approaches.
>
> But notice that I said "look into," not "try." We still want some evidence, beyond the anecdotal, that there might be some efficacy in a particular therapy or practice.

The value of hope should not be underestimated. Sometimes all a treatment really has to offer is hope, but that's a lot as this woman explains:

> I've looked at all my medical options and none of them hold much promise. My oncologist agrees. I heard about a Qi Gong healer. Since I started going to her, it's the first time I have felt hopeful.

Concerns about complementary and alternative treatments

You may have valid concerns about the use of untested treatments, particularly when you are in active treatment for acute disease. It's challenging enough for your physician to control the known variables in your treatment—a job that requires careful observation, knowledge, and experience—without having to control for the unknown variables from non-standard treatments. The addition of complementary and alternative treatments to your treatment plan can increase the difficulty of foreseeing and preventing negative interactions and may interfere with treatment response.

Concerns about complementary and alternative therapies include:

- Lack of scientific studies
- Treatment delays
- Practitioner licensing
- Potential toxicity
- Unexpected drug, herb, and dietary interactions
- Dependence on testimonials
- Questioning effectiveness

Lack of scientific studies

HMOs often request scientific proof of effectiveness before they will cover an alternative or complementary treatment. This forces medical organizations to limit their range of treatment recommendations to those that are standardized or evidence-based.

The demand for written proof puts CAM therapies at an even greater disadvantage. Many of them are based on observation, but have not yet been formally studied in clinical trials. As previously mentioned, clinical trials can be extremely expensive and difficult to finance unless a chance of profit on a disease with millions of patients can be predicted.

The need for studies to evaluate the effectiveness of these therapeutic approaches is as important to you as a consumer as it is to your medical care provider. Dr. Yashar Hirshaut, author of *Breast Cancer: The Complete Guide*, writes the following about the importance of evaluating alternative treatments and standard treatments using the same measuring stick:

> It is more than a question of whether farmers and cowhands can be friends. Every medicine or treatment used for breast cancer must meet the same test. It must be shown to work. Testimonials or anecdotes are just not enough to bet your life on. There are too many shysters out there trying to sell you snake oil for whom dollars and not lives are the focus.
>
> We must respect each other as people but before jumping off tall buildings on someone else's say-so we have to have real, solid, unquestionable proof that we will have a safe landing.[16]

We also need reliable information on expected outcomes and side effects of nonstandard therapies as well as an honest evaluation of what aspects need further study–the same quality of information as we expect to be given for standard treatment regimens.

Studies show that most people look first to standard treatment options when diagnosed with a treatable condition or illness. They are more likely to add in complementary therapies to supplement the healing process or look for alternative forms of treatment when, all of the standard options are exhausted, as this woman explains:

> One of my friends wanted me to try an alternative therapy instead of chemotherapy. I considered it, but decided it was something I could try later if the chemotherapy didn't work. I didn't want to take the chance on an alternative as long as I had proven medical treatments available to me.

Other people choose to forego standard treatment when they feel the risks outweigh the benefits of the standard therapy or their belief systems are in conflict with the standard approach.

Treatment delays

Doctors who work with life-threatening disease often talk about working with patients who refuse standard treatment in favor of alternative therapy. Then, when the patient returns for help, it is sometimes after their disease has progressed to a point where standard therapy can no longer provide hope for a cure or even disease management. At the same time, doctors are keenly aware of the limitations they face. They currently do not have enough tools available to treat or to save some of their patients.

You always have the right to refuse standard treatment in favor of an alternative therapy when you feel the potential advantages outweigh the risks, but it is important to have a clear understanding of and acceptance of the risk you are taking. A woman with colitis recounts her experience using herbal therapy in place of the prescribed drugs:

> One of the hardest things for a colitis patient is that there is this never-ending cycle. You're healthy for a while and then you go through the whole nightmare again. During one of my recurrences, my doctor told me that not much had changed in the past seven years since I was last treated. A friend recommended I talk with her brother, an herbal

therapist. I talked to him on the phone, then went out and bought about $100 worth of all this stuff. Within three days, I was in total remission. I didn't tell my doctor about the herbs when I went back six weeks later. I wanted him to verify, without any prejudice, that I was in remission. Sure enough, I was.

I had another recurrence a year later. I told my new doctor about the herbal therapy. He said since he didn't have anything new to offer and the herbs had worked, I should go ahead and take them. But I had to promise that if they stopped working, I would come right in. Very shortly after, I had a catastrophic event. It was too late. Even the homeopathic therapist said, "You know, it's just too far gone."

My only option was surgery. I never wanted surgery. That was my last resort. But by the time I did it, I knew I'd tried everything else. Then I was ready and I was ready to deal with whatever happened afterward.

Practitioner licensing

Efforts are being made to standardize licensing within the various practices. Acupuncturists, Chinese medicine practitioners, and chiropractors, for example, all have some form of licensing. Chiropractors are the best organized with licensure in every state. Acupuncturists are licensed in two-thirds of the states and in Washington, DC. Some therapeutic practices may have association guidelines but no formal licensing requirements. There may be more than one type of license within a specific therapeutic community. Licensing requirements also vary from state to state.

Just as you rely on your physician for medical expertise and experience, look for nutritionists, Chinese herbalists, and chiropractors who are licensed and experienced in the therapies you are considering. If you are considering a nutritional supplement or dietary approach for example, talk with respected nutritionists about the rationale behind the approach.

An analysis of alternative practitioners appeared in the *Journal of the American Medical Association.* Looking at medical malpractice suits from 1990 to 1996, Studdart, et al., found that claims against chiropractors, massage therapists, and acupuncturists were less frequent and involved less serious injury than claims against doctors during that period.[17] This, however, does not minimize the need to look for experienced reputable practitioners.

Potential toxicity

There is a popular perception that natural substances are safer than synthetic. The word "natural" is used often in marketing CAM therapies. Many plants, however, are toxic at concentrated levels. Ironically, it is sometimes the toxic nature of a plant or animal substance that makes small amounts of it effective in the treatment of medical conditions and disease. Often the active ingredient is effective primarily because at lower dosages it is poisonous to undesirable organisms (in the plant world, natural toxins inhibit pests). At higher doses it may also be toxic to humans. The arsenal of nature includes snake venom, poisonous mushrooms, and deadly nightshade. Natural remedies require the same caution as synthetic drugs. And in nature, the concentration of the active ingredient may not be consistent from one plant to another.

Prescription drugs, on the other hand, are reported to be the fourth-leading cause of death in the United States. About three times the number of people killed in automobile accidents die each year from adverse reactions to properly administered drugs (the number reported did not include suicide or mistakes in dosage).[18]

Just as overdoses of prescription medications can be dangerous, so can overdoses of herbs and vitamins. For example, vitamin D, vitamin A, and iron have all been shown to have toxic levels. Look for documentation on potential side effects and symptoms of overdose with any medication you take.

The FDA has less control over vitamins, herbal remedies, dietary supplements, and nutraceuticals than they do over over-the-counter drugs and prescription medications. It is only when a nutritional supplement claims to diagnose, mitigate, treat, cure, or prevent a disease that the product is required to meet FDA premarket testing and approval. Nutritional supplement claims on how the product affects the structure or function of the body are not subject to FDA premarketing approval. Products with claims such as "maintains a healthy circulatory system" or "for common symptoms of PMS" do not need FDA pre-approval.

Countries like Germany, which are more supportive of the role herbs play in health maintenance and treatment of disease, have rigid standards for quality of ingredients, truth in labeling, and quality manufacturing.

It is critical when you consider using these products, to look for studies of dosage levels for effectiveness and for toxicity. It is also important to remember that individuals vary in their dosage needs and responses to medications and supplements. One patient comments that she finds this frustrating in standard as well as alternative approaches.

> *Traditional practitioners are only beginning to use their vast knowledge to design the best treatment for an individual. I found customtailored alternative treatments even more rare—the one-size-fits-all principle prevailed.*

Quality in manufacturing among non-pharmaceutical products can also vary. Studies have raised concerns about the variation in the actual amount and strength of the active ingredients advertised on the labels and the potential for contamination in the unregulated manufacturing process. Therefore, it is important to buy from reputable sources. Look for the U.S.P. notation on the label, which denotes that the manufacturer voluntarily adheres to the US Pharmacopoeia standards.

Unexpected drug, herb, and nutritional interactions

A 1997 survey of nonprescription supplement users showed that 18.4 percent of prescription users used herbal remedies and/or high-dose vitamins concurrently with their prescription medications.[19]

Be aware of the possibility of drug interactions. An herbal remedy or nutritional supplement might increase or decrease the action of a prescription drug you are taking. For example, the effectiveness of digoxin is decreased when ingested with products containing guar gum. Even foods can interact—grapefruit juice, for example, increases the effects of calcium channel blockers. If you are taking more than one therapeutic agent at a time, you may have difficulty figuring out which one caused the problem if you experience adverse effects. It's important to inform your physician and your alternative practitioners of all medications you are taking so they can alert you to possible problems.

Dependence on testimonials

Case studies appear frequently in conventional medical literature. Case studies include accounts of unexpected treatment failure as well as stories of unusual success. In a published case study, the diagnosis, treatment, and outcome are all carefully documented. A case study or a series of cases helps to identify areas that deserve further study.

Anecdotal stories are often used to promote complementary and alternative therapies. They may resemble case studies, but the details and documentation are vague and negative stories are left untold. You will have to look further than the product literature to find accounts from disgruntled patients. Dead people do not send in their stories.

When you see a testimonial that looks intriguing, ask for documentation and try to contact the satisfied customer yourself. Ralph Moss, PhD, founder of the Ralph Moss on Cancer web site at *http://www.ralphmoss.com* explains his approach when researching a complementary or alternative therapy:

> *If patients claim to have benefited from a treatment, I will generally try to track them down. I definitely would suggest that if you are considering a treatment based upon an anecdote, that you do your best to track down that anecdote and think logically whether or not, aside from the wishful thinking, there's really any objective basis to believe that that person was "cured" by that treatment. Sad to say, most of these things evaporate, fall apart in your hands as you look at them.[20]*

He further explains:

> *It's very common for people to mistake a secondary prevention effect for a curative effect. In other words, they had an operation for their tumor. They may have been told by somebody that they had a great chance of it recurring. They did x, y, or z, and now the cancer hasn't returned.[21]*

Questionable effectiveness

Controversy rages over whether or not healthcare money is being wasted on unproven treatments that are really just expensive placebos. A placebo is a biologically inert compound (usually a sugar pill) that produces a healing response because the patient expects it to.

Some herbal preparations actually contain very little of the ingredient promoted on the label. No US agency currently monitors this. According to a 1998 *Time* magazine article, premium-priced nutraceutical drinks sometimes have little more than a trace of mentioned herbal ingredients.[22]

In clinical trials, about one-third of the patients in the placebo group experience a clinically measurable response. The placebo appears to act as a catalyst to stimulate the body's own powerful healing capabilities. Perhaps this effect should be viewed as a non-toxic, low-risk form of healing, but it is unpredictable and should be presented honestly.

Evaluating complementary and alternative therapies

Often you hear about a complementary or alternative treatment by word-of-mouth or through advertising. As with conventional medicine, it is important to separate marketing information from primary research information. Whenever possible, read the source information referred to in the marketing documents.

Questions to ask about a complementary or alternative therapy

In Michael Lerner's book *Choices in Healing*,[23] he identifies three areas to evaluate when considering alternative options: the therapy, the practitioner, and the delivery of service.

Here is a list of questions to ask the practitioner or product sales person when considering a nonstandard treatment:

- Why do you expect this treatment to help me?

- How does it work?

- What will be required of me? How often will I need to have treatment, how long will the treatments take, and how many treatments does the standard course of therapy require?

- How much will this cost me? What are the cost per treatment and the total cost for the expected course of treatments. Are there extra costs like medications, equipment, or clothing that I will need?

- Will my insurance cover any or all of this treatment? If not, why not?

- How long should I expect it to take before I see results? How will the results be measured? At what points should we re-evaluate whether or not the treatment is working?

- How often has this treatment been successful in a case like mine? How many patients like me have you treated?

- How long do you expect the effects of the treatment to last? Will I need to come back after the initial treatment is finished?

- Does the effect vary according to variations in the way the treatment is given or the level of the dosage? Can this treatment be dangerous or toxic?

- What are the potential side effects or complications? What are the warning signs I should be aware of?

- Are there published studies to support this use? Are the expected outcomes based on clinical observation or lab studies on animals or human cells? Have there been any clinical trials done on people like me? Where are the studies published and how do I get copies?

- Do you have names and phone numbers of patients I can speak with about their experience with this therapy?

- What is your background and training? How long have you been working with patients? Are you licensed?

- What sort of licensing is required in this state?

- Are you willing to talk to and work with my primary care provider?

Red flags

Here are some of the red flags to watch for when looking for reliable information:

- **Cure-alls.** Long lists of unrelated conditions cured by one product.

- **Unreferenced studies.** Vague references to study results with no explanation of who did the study, where it was published, or other information on how to obtain a complete copy of the report.

- **Ambivalent wording.** Words and phrases like "should," "may," "probably," or "has been associated with," rather than "has been proven."

- **Medical experts listed as "Dr."** Don't assume that the expert is a medical doctor. Look for a qualifying degree after the expert's name, such as MD or DO.

- **Testimonials as primary evidence of effectiveness.** Be especially wary if the testimonials are not credited to a specific individual.

- **Sure-cures.** If it sounds too good to be true, it probably is.

- **Exposure of a conspiracy to suppress information on a miracle product.** The product should be able to stand alone on its credentials.

- **Secret remedies.** The remedies are so secret, an outside laboratory cannot test them.

- **"Distributorships available."** Recruiting you as a sales associate may be more important than treating your illness.

- **"The truth about."** It is unlikely that there is one truth about anything.

- **Exclamation points, and grandiose adjectives like "miracle," "world's best," or "amazing."** The number of exclamation points is usually inversely proportional to the validity of the claims being made.

- **Misspellings.** A professional company will not release literature with misspellings.

Cautious optimism

Sort your complementary and alternative treatment options by level of risk. Low-risk options are those where you think, "It can't hurt...it might help." Sometimes a lifestyle change can reduce your reliance on medical intervention as happened to this woman:

> *The doctor put me on medications for high cholesterol and for high blood pressure. Recently, I went on a diet to lose weight. I've changed my eating habits so much that both my cholesterol and blood pressure are back in the normal range so I have been able to stop taking the medications.*

Treatments with more potential for harm need to be monitored more closely. Examine your expectations and define markers for success. Some patients establish evaluation criteria with their doctor and alternative practitioners as this woman does:

> *Most of the alternative therapies I've tried have not been very successful for me. On the other hand, neither have the conventional ones!*
>
> *I never know in advance whether or not the treatment will work for me. If I trust the doctor or friend or article that recommends the treatment, and I've assured myself that the dangers are minimal (this is often the hardest thing to find out), I just try it and see if it works for me. For*

example, I took Essiac tea, a concoction of fresh herbs. I took it for three months, but my disease progressed during that time.

I consider several factors in deciding whether to stop or continue a therapy. I rely on my doctor's interpretation of blood tests and scans for traditional therapies, and on my own gut feelings for both traditional and alternative therapies.

I ask myself if I can stand feeling like this for x more months, or for the rest of my life. If the treatment makes me feel too bad and the doctor feels I should continue we discuss lowering the dose or having the treatment less often.

If I'm dissatisfied with an herbal therapy or dubious about its efficacy, I consult the practitioner or experiment myself with lowering the dose, taking the drug at a different time of day, or stopping it altogether and seeing how I feel, or if the disease is progressing. I also watch my body for good or bad results as I go about my daily life.

Talking with your doctor

A 1998 Journal of the American Medical Association article about the integration of alternative therapies into the curriculum of medical schools concluded:

Patients are increasingly seeking to identify a physician who is solidly grounded in conventional, orthodox medicine and is also knowledgeable about the value and limitations of alternative treatments.[24]

The boundary between "conventional, orthodox" medicine and an alternative approach, however, is not as sharply defined as health consumers are encouraged to believe. Polarization sells products and extremists on each side argue that their approach is more reasonable, logical, and safe. The bottom line is whether or not there is enough evidence to support the treatment's safety and effectiveness for treating your condition.

How much to tell your doctor

Your feedback and honesty are important to the quality of your care. Eisenberg's first survey showed that 89 percent of the people surveyed saw providers of unconventional therapy without recommendations from their medical doctors. Of those who used unconventional therapies, 72 percent did not inform their doctors. His 1997 follow-up survey showed no significant change in the rate of disclosure.[25]

Your doctor is responsible for recommending and monitoring your medical care. You are responsible for presenting a complete picture of your situation. Use of complementary or alternative therapy is as important a part of your health risks assessment as the use of drugs and alcohol or levels of diet and exercise. The picture you give your physician needs to be as complete as possible. In a time of emergency, it could be a matter of life or death.

A woman describes her hesitation to share her less acute symptoms with her physician:

> I think that I get better treatment from my Chinese herbalist because I give him more information. I imagine that if I tell my doctor about some of the aches and pains worrying me, he will send me upstairs for an MRI or some painful diagnostic test.

High doses of vitamins, ongoing use of herbal supplements, medications, creams, and visits to alternative practitioners should all be described when discussing a problem with your doctor. Some people may assume that unregulated remedies are safer because they are not controlled. They believe herbs and supplements are like over-the-counter drugs. However, over-the-counter drugs are more closely monitored and regulated to insure safe use and identify potential adverse effects. The lack of regulation in the case of herbal or dietary products is not a measure of safety as much as a reflection of the complex ongoing legal issue of whether these products should be regulated as food or as drugs.

Resistance

Remember that doctors have not been trained in how to include most complementary or alternative therapies. Be compassionate. When patients combine treatments and modalities, the outcomes become more uncertain. Doctors are in uncharted territory.

If your doctor is hesitant about a complementary or alternative treatment, ask for information to help you evaluate his concerns. Most treatments, conventional or unconventional, have some controversy associated with their acceptance. It's important to separate the unknown from known as you evaluate risks and benefits to make your decisions.

Keep a treatment diary

While a treatment diary would be useful to record standard treatment responses, it's even more important if you are adding complementary or alternative therapies into your treatment plan. Ask your doctor and your practitioner to help you identify potential side effects and warning signs to look for.

When a treatment goes on for a long time, it's not always easy to pinpoint changes. A diary provides a valuable record and helps you keep an eye out for the onset of possible complications. Record new symptoms along with treatment dates and dosages. You can also rate your level of improvement as the treatment progresses.

Working as a team and taking responsibility

In the best of all worlds your primary physician, nutritionist, herbalist, acupuncturist, and chiropractor would all work together to help find the most effective treatment for your situation. However, since time constraints and differences in value systems sometimes make this sort of collaboration difficult, you will usually take on the role of coordination yourself. (This may contribute to the sense of empowerment that a patient feels when bringing nonstandard therapies into the treatment process.)

It is your job, with the combined expertise of all of the members of your extended team, to put your complete treatment plan into a perspective that meets the criteria of your value system and gives you the most confidence in a successful outcome.

Expenses and insurance coverage

American consumers spent $21.2 billion in 1997 for alternative professional services. Less than half was reimbursed by insurance.[26] As a result of the surge in spending on alternative therapies, most major US health plans now include some form of alternative therapy.

Research by Kenneth Pelletier at the Stanford Center for Research in Disease Prevention (SCRDP) shows that decisions by insurance companies as to which alternative therapies to cover are based primarily on consumer demand for those services, not an evaluation of the medical effectiveness of these services. Pelletier hopes that insurance codes for these treatments will permit more extensive tracking and documentation, thus helping to determine which treatments are effective for which conditions.[27]

Landmark Healthcare, Inc., an alternative managed care company based in California, sells insurance coverage services for alternatives like chiropractic and acupuncture to other insurance providers. As they point out, some of these therapies are more cost-effective for the insurance company. Here are some examples:

- A 1996 report in *Medical Care* compared the costs of healthcare for back and neck pain in a managed care setting. The study showed that chiropractic patients paid $539 for treatment compared to $774 for standard treatment.[28]

- Other studies have shown that acupuncture can significantly reduce the need for drugs and the duration of stays in costly treatment facilities.[29]

- A study on acupuncture for osteoarthritis in the elderly at the University of Maryland found that 7 of 29 patients were able to avoid surgeries that would have cost approximately $63,000 per patient.[30]

Landmark Healthcare conducted a nationwide survey of health plans in 1996. They found that 58 percent of the companies they surveyed planned to offer alternative coverage within the next two years.[31] In 1999 Landmark conducted another nationwide survey. They found that 67 percent of the HMOs surveyed offered at least one form of therapy defined by the HMOs as alternative, such as chiropractic, acupuncture, or massage therapies.[32]

In addition to health plans that offer alternatives as part of their treatment coverage, some companies offer riders that supplement their basic health plan to include visits to alternative practitioners. These supplemental plans are available for add-on premium cost.

Other alternative coverage approaches include discount programs where members who visit a practitioner in an established network receive a discounted rate for services. The discount ranges from 20 percent to 35 percent off the usual and customary rates. It is paid at the time of treatment.

Ask your insurer if the company provides coverage for complementary and alternative therapies and which types of treatment they cover.

Where to look for reliable information

If others know about your condition, you will not have to look for people proposing CAM therapies: they will find you. Well-meaning family and friends scour popular literature for solutions to your problem. Many of the tips and clippings that you will receive will highlight experimental and CAM therapies.

If you find one that interests you, find out where the work on it is being done. Call the company or the practitioner. Ask for written information.

The resources listed here and further detailed in Appendix B, *Resources,* are simply starting points. Always look beyond the marketing literature and verify, verify, verify.

The Internet

The Internet is a good starting place because of the sheer amount and diversity of information you will find there. An AltaVista search on April 12, 2000 using the keyword "acupuncture" brought up 162,615 web pages.

Much of what you find using a search engine like AltaVista will be marketing and media reports. You can scan these for references to research documentation. Some web pages will describe the treatment, what it involves, and where to learn more about it. You are more likely to find recent updates of information on the Internet than in distributed materials.

You will also find many examples of the "red flags" mentioned earlier. Anyone can put information on the Internet. Always look to see who is providing the information and why.

Databases

MEDLINE, the best-known online database of medical journal abstracts at *http://www.medlineplus.gov*, searches only a few select alternative therapy journals. A few other databases specialize in cataloguing complementary and alternative literature. These are available as subscription-based services or on CD-ROMs. Both are very expensive for the individual consumer. Some academic and medical libraries as well as professional researchers subscribe to them and offer to search them for a fee. Some examples of such databases are the Allied and Complementary Medicine database (AMED), the Centralised Information Service for Complementary Medicine (CISCOM), and Alt-Health Watch.

National Center for Complementary and Alternative Medicine (NCCAM)

Mandated by Congress in 1991 as part of the National Institutes of Health, NCCAM currently includes nine specialized centers, each focused on evaluating the most promising forms of alternative and complementary therapy and conducting research to qualify their effectiveness as treatment options. See Appendix B for a list of these centers.

Clinical trials

The budget for the National Center for Complementary and Alternative Medicine (formerly the Office of Alternative Medicine) at the National Institutes of Health (NIH) has grown from $2 million in 1992 to $20 million in 1998. The NIH is expanding the number of clinical trials on treatments currently seen as alternative or complementary. You can check directly with the NIH or look through current clinical trial listings. Also check with practitioners to find out if there are ongoing trials. Be sure to check the credentials of any organization sponsoring or conducting a clinical trial. (See Chapter 8.)

Magazine and newsletter subscriptions

For timely, fully sourced information, look into the following magazines and newsletters: *Complementary and Alternative Medicine at the NIH*, *The Review of Natural Products*, and *Alternative Therapies in Health and Medicine*. Annotations on contents, costs, and contact information are listed in Appendix B.

Books

Books will give you the most comprehensive overview of an alternative practice. Always note the date of publication and look for updates as the field is changing rapidly. You will find a list of recommended titles in Appendix B.

European and Asian studies

Germany, India, China, and Japan have medical traditions that include healing practices considered to be alternative or complementary in the United

States. More peer-reviewed research on those practices is available in those countries. Keep an eye open for information from studies and trials going on in those countries.

Associations and agencies

Associations of alternative care practitioners can help you find more information on their particular mode of treatment. Some have licensing programs and practitioner lists. Government and state agencies offer consumer information on regulatory policies and licensing.

CHAPTER 10

Support: Learning from Others

WHETHER YOU UNDERGO STANDARD TREATMENT, complementary or alternative treatment, or participate in a clinical trial, the experience of illness creates a need for new kinds of coping skills and support. Family and friends are essential, but additional social and emotional support can enhance healing and even longevity. There are many types of individual and group support for those facing difficult illnesses and for those who are caregivers.

Participating in support groups can give you the benefit of others' experiences when you're considering treatment options or coping with treatment. You might learn about new treatments, resources available to you, or how someone else made treatment decisions or coped with side effects. Considering the experiential side of the treatment decisions that you're making—whether you're asking questions in a support group or asking questions of yourself while working one-on-one with a therapist or counselor—can give you valuable information and help you feel more in control. The perspectives you gain can help you make better decisions.

In this chapter you find examples of many types of coping skills including how to find personal support, professional support, and support organizations. You also find questions you can ask to determine if a particular support group is for you. Finally, this chapter covers access to online support and the benefits of this new and powerful type of support.

Benefits of social networks

Humans are social beings. Throughout history societies have thrived when there are strong communities. Individuals live longer when they have support networks of family, friends, and even pets.

Several important studies have shown a connection between social networks and longer life:

- In one study of 7,000 people across the United States over ten years, epidemiologists Lisa Berkman and Leonard Syme found that individuals with poor social bonds had a 250 percent higher mortality rate than those with a good support system of friends and relatives. These findings held true even when they adjusted for poor health habits such as smoking, high alcohol use, and obesity.[1]

- Another study in Michigan found that in a nine- to twelve-year period, socially active men were two to three times less likely to die and socially active women were almost two times less likely to die than their more isolated peers.[2]

- Two studies involving pets also showed remarkable findings. In a 1980 study people discharged from a coronary care unit had a significantly higher survival rate if they had pets waiting for them at home. Another study in 1990 found that elderly people with pets had fewer doctor visits. Of course only those who loved their pets showed any benefit.

- One landmark study conducted by David Spiegel, MD at Stanford University found that women in an active support group for metastatic breast cancer lived 18 months longer than women with a similar diagnosis who did not participate in a group. Dr. Spiegel and his colleagues' primary focus was the emotional, not necessarily the physical, effects of support groups. In a follow-up study, they were amazed to find that the members of the support group had not only greater emotional stability but also improved health and longevity.[3]

Illness sets you apart from your friends and family. Feeling different from your social network carries a heavy psychological burden. Many individuals facing serious illness feel isolated and alone and even banished. Our mobile society challenges individuals to find and form new social groups as they move around the country and the world. This mobility can leave you without traditional social networks when you need help in coping with illness and need some type of support, whether it is physical, emotional, or both. Even when you have strong social ties, families and friends may be so worried about you that they find it difficult to listen when you need to talk openly about your own fears and hopes.

Often the best person to talk to is another person who has been there, someone who has faced the medical ordeal you are now facing and has come through it. Talking to others who have lived through a serious medical diagnosis similar to yours can help you feel more in control. Facing the illness with the support of others gives you strength.

A woman with colitis tells how information given by someone who had already gone through surgery helped her:

> For me, the most helpful thing was to be given information by other people who were actually going through it. Colitis is a terrible disease. It just devastates your life on a daily basis and it usually goes on for a long time.
>
> The best thing that was ever given to me was a diary by a patient who had the surgery I was going to have. He was a young policeman, 28 years old. It was so helpful to read this guy's story and realize he was healthy after…and to realize that he went through the same emotional stuff that I did, worrying that it was something I was doing, that caused my colitis. I worried that if I had just lived my life in a certain way, eaten certain foods, and had a certain lifestyle, that I wouldn't have this illness. Unfortunately, with colitis, it's just not true.

The human perspective

Acquiring medical information and research can be empowering. But medical facts deal primarily with physical aspects of disease: surgery, blood counts, antibiotics, etc. These facts alone are not enough for full decision-making. The missing piece is the human factor—the emotional and spiritual aspects of healing. How have others with your diagnosis made their decisions? Given various medical choices, what has their experience been? Would they do something differently, now that they have been down this path? What will it feel like for you, the patient? Where will you find support, and courage, and even peace? How will you live your life—the life you had before dealing with illness?

Your illness touches others as well. How will your friends and families cope with this illness that touches all of you? Will they need counseling and support in order to help you?

You can't try out medical procedures such as heart bypass or radiation therapy. But you can ask others how it feels, how they coped with side effects, how their lives have changed as a result.

Humans learn from each other. This concept applies to medical experiences as much as it does to housing, consumer choices, and other areas of life that we're accustomed to discussing openly. In the following sections, you'll find some of the ways you can stay connected to emotional and spiritual support and use these connections as part of your therapy.

What kind of support do you want?

Each individual has different needs and personality traits, although we all live healthier lives with good social connections. You may be a very private person and would benefit most from one-to-one interaction. You may thrive in a group. There are as many types of support and support groups as there are human needs. You know yourself best and you probably have a pretty good idea of the kind of help or support you would find useful.

You may choose one or several types of one-to-one support, group support, online support, peer support, and/or professional support including the following:

- Making personal contacts with individuals who have experienced the same illness and therapies

- Consulting counselors such as psychologists, psychiatrists, and social workers who are experienced in assisting people facing serious illnesses

- Accessing spiritual support and counselors such as ministers, priests, rabbis, and others who are experienced in helping people find spiritual support in facing a life crisis

- Joining formal or informal groups whose members lend support to each other and provide a forum for exploring options and voicing fears and hopes

- Learning to utilize yoga, meditation groups, and other supportive activities

- Joining an online support group

- Obtaining assistance for the activities of daily living such as child care, grocery shopping, house cleaning, transportation, friends to accompany you to medical appointments, etc.

- Asking friends to act as buffers or coordinators for well-wishers

Personal contacts

Ideally, you can locate people with similar medical experiences close to your home. The first place to start is right in your doctor's office and your hospital. Does your doctor know of any other patients who would be willing to talk with you? Can the nursing and social staff recommend other patients who have had similar treatments who are willing to share their experiences? Are social workers on staff aware of individuals and groups who share your experience?

A woman who was unsure of the impact that a surgery would have on her life recounts:

> The best thing is to talk with people who have had the illness. The therapists, whom I came to adore here at the hospital, would refer me to people who had just had the surgery or had it in the past. The people who had just had this surgery would answer questions. They are the ones living through it. Asking the doctors wasn't real helpful to me because they didn't know what it was like…what it's like to live with it every day.

Friends, coworkers, or family members may know of others who are willing to talk about their experiences. Because you're dealing with an unknown and fearful experience, it can be very grounding and reassuring to talk to others who have had the same experiences. You may be astonished at the outpouring of support from friends—especially those who you never imagined had faced serious illness themselves. One person expressed this feeling beautifully when she said, "I felt like my friends wrapped themselves around me like a warm blanket."

Friends may also be able to help in tangible ways such as donating blood or being tested for a tissue match. A woman talks about friends' response to a request for blood:

> A few days before my surgery, a nurse came in late at night and said, "I see on your chart that you're going to have blood with the surgery." I said, "Yeah."

We'd talked with the doctor. This was 1980s. We'd talked about the blood supply, the blood bank, AIDS, and everything. They'd assured us that there was no problem. This nurse said, "I could lose my job, but I hear doctors in the hall all the time saying they wouldn't give this blood to their own kids." My husband and I just looked at each other.

We called one of the parents at our children's preschool where there are 44 families. We asked them to donate because we know these families pretty well, and we're going to assume that if they think they're at risk, they won't donate. We figured we're just going to cut our chances as much as we could.

The next day it was overwhelming—they were turning people away. They had more blood than I could ever use.

Consulting counselors

Finding a psychologist, psychiatrist, or other counselor is a very personal choice. You can ask your doctor and other caregivers for the names of those experienced in helping people deal with illness. You can also ask your friends for recommendations. Another option is to call some of the local agencies such as the American Cancer Society or Hospice to see if they have names of therapists especially trained in helping people cope with serious illness. Your area may have an association of psychologists who can also make recommendations. You're looking for someone who has experience and a proven track record.

Usually the same few names will keep appearing and you can call one or two of them for an initial visit. It's a good idea to interview the therapist before you make a choice. Ask how they work, how long they think the therapy will take, and what fees they charge. Usually an introductory visit is offered at low cost or even free. Take some time in finding a therapist who you feel comfortable with and who really understands your needs. You want to have a sense of trust because you will be sharing some of your deepest feelings, hopes, and fears.

If you're not familiar with the therapist's background, you can check her credentials with the state licensing boards of your state. The contact numbers for these boards are in the "Government" sections of your telephone book or in the yellow pages. If your state does have a separate licensing board, you can contact the National Board for Certified Counselors at (336) 547-0607. The National Board for Certified Counselors also has an excellent web site at *http://www.nbcc.org*. This national board has information on individual state credential requirements as well as a section where you can request a list of certified counselors in your area. If the therapist you are considering is a psychiatrist, her credentials will be listed in the *American Board of Medical Specialists Directory.*

Some people avoid therapy because of the fear of the image of being crazy or the fear they'll have to face uncontrollable emotions. Remember that you're in control and you set the limits. Therapists are trained to create a safe environment for expressing emotions. Good therapists will be both compassionate and energizing and will help you sort through the myriad of feelings brought on by illness. Another fear might be that you'll be seen as weak if you can't solve your own problems. In reality, a good therapist helps you develop coping skills and acts as an advocate for you so that you become stronger.

Most health insurance plans cover at least some therapy. Some plans limit your choices to a certain "preferred" list of care providers. Friends or those in a support group may be able to help you narrow the list. One patient facing serious illness recounts how she found a therapist:

> *I was given the names of three "acceptable" therapists listed in my HMO when I told my primary care physician that I really needed help with the stress. I had no idea who any of these people were. So I called a friend who knows most of the psychologists in the area because she used to work for a social services agency.*
>
> *On the list, she pointed to one name that she said was one of the best in town. She didn't criticize the others, but she didn't recommend them either. So I made an appointment and did get some help from a therapist I felt I could trust.*

If your insurer does not cover therapy, or if the therapist you want to meet with is not on your insurer's list, you can ask if they have a sliding fee schedule. Many do. There also may be counseling through your work, usually called employee assistance programs. There may also be a foundation or agency that is available free of charge. Sometimes the therapists at these agencies are in an internship, gaining supervised experience for their licenses. You may want to speak with those in charge to make sure anyone you see does indeed have experience in dealing with clients with serious illness. Another possibility is to talk to those who lead support groups to see if they can spend some individual time with you.

Accessing spiritual counselors

Ministers, priests, rabbis, and other spiritual leaders are also experienced counselors. You may feel more comfortable working with a leader of your church. If you have a religious or spiritual tradition, prayer and religious ritual can give you much comfort and assistance. There have been several studies linking prayer and meditation with healing. One recent study has shown that those attending church regularly had fewer hospital admissions.[4] Another randomized, double-blind study of patients with advanced AIDS found that "distant healing" including prayer and psychic healing had a profound effect on the AIDS patients. While the AIDS viral load counts of the two groups remained the same, the subjects receiving distant healing had fewer hospitalizations, fewer doctor visits, and significantly fewer AIDS related illness.[5]

Regardless of your religious affiliation, spiritual support can add to your quality of life. You will likely see more formal studies on the spiritual aspects of healing as consumers push medical caregivers to include consideration of a patient's spirit along with treatment of the body.

As one woman undergoing cancer treatment relates:

> I think that addressing the spiritual side is what ultimately helps you to combat fear because once you really address that, what is there to fear?

> To me, facing the spiritual side includes asking the big questions such as, What is the meaning of life? What might the end of life mean? What is the value of what I am doing? But the spiritual side also goes into the power of who you are. You are not just your physical appearance or your name, but an energy, a force—a spirit.

> I don't know if this is something that was delivered to me because of my spiritual searching or it was already in my nature and facing cancer brought out this inner strength. I genuinely feel that I managed to conquer the fear and was totally sure that I was going to be fine. I just knew that I was going to be okay.

Support groups

There are support groups for virtually every condition or illness. Formal support groups are led by trained professionals such as psychologists and social workers to help people deal with similar concerns. Informal support groups are organized and led by the actual members of the group. Informal support groups are often called "self-help" groups.

Both types of groups benefit you primarily by helping you to overcome feelings of isolation and by helping you face issues that would be more difficult to cope with if you were alone. Usually a group will be made up of individuals facing a shared concern such as prostate cancer, leukemia, Alzheimer's, etc., and the members of the group already share many common experiences.

Besides the shared bond of a particular experience, there are many ways that you can benefit from support groups:

- Exchange information about new treatments and about ways others have found to cope with problems similar to yours.

- Find a safe place to share fears knowing others face those same concerns.

- Help and support each other, regaining a sense of purpose, usefulness and value as one who is helping others.

- Share the combined strength of all of the members of the group and this support helps you to establish control over your life.

Your doctors, nurses, or friends can often recommend support groups. Public libraries and information agencies in communities can also make recommendations. National organizations such as the American Heart Association or the American Cancer Society will often have a local chapter that sponsors support groups. There are also organizations that maintain directories of support groups locally and throughout the country. Two of the national support organizations are:

- The National Self-Help Clearinghouse, (212) 354-8525 or *http://www. selfhelpweb.org*, shares information about self-help and support groups and helps individuals find groups that share similar concerns.

- The American Self-Help Clearinghouse, (201) 625-7107, provides information on existing groups and offers training and assistance to existing and new self-help groups. They also publish the *Self-Help Sourcebook* and provide information on many groups including both health-related groups and social support groups such as Violence Anonymous.

Types of support groups

There are several types of support groups, and you may want to consider which format would be best for you. The basic types are listed below, but there are many variations in actual format:

- Time-limited, formal groups have set length of sessions such as eight weeks and a limited number of participants. A trained psychologist, social worker, or other professional usually leads these groups and the members of the group are screened for compatibility.

- Drop-in groups are also led by trained professionals and are ongoing. Participants may join or drop out at any time. Many return for a tune-up from time to time.

- Members of the group, usually on a rotating basis, lead self-help groups. These are often informal groups and may have grown out of a formal group that has disbanded or through the energies of several individuals who share a common concern.

Evaluating support groups

When you are choosing a support group, you are still vulnerable and you want to be sure that the group actually does support you and helps you deal with each day and each challenge. In evaluating a support group, consider the following questions:

- Does the group focus on the needs of the members of the group or does the leader of the group act as a teacher or recommend a specific therapy?

- Is there a companion group for caregivers and family members?

- Do the people in the group have some agenda that may not reflect your own feelings? For example, are they all rejecting mainstream treatments in favor of alternative medicine, or are they all expressing anger or critical of each other?

- Is this a place where you feel safe to express your fears, share your triumphs, cry, and learn to face what is ahead of you?

Support groups are not for everyone. You might not find a group for your particular concern or you may be a very private person who copes more effectively using different types of assistance. It is always your choice to select the type of support that meets your particular needs.

Other healing group activities

Often a yoga or meditation group will become an informal support group when one of its members is facing a serious illness. Sometimes, however, a yoga or meditation group will be created specifically for the purposes of healing. You may be able to find a yoga group specifically for people facing cancer or arthritis or some other condition. Yoga and meditation can help you stay in touch with your body. Many of the breathing exercises of both yoga and meditation are extremely beneficial and have a calming effect.

As one woman who found such a yoga group describes:

> I was very fortunate. My surgeon's nurse told me about a yoga group specifically for women with mastectomies. The stretches were gentle, the classes were relaxing, the teacher was knowledgeable, and the fees were low. It was a wonderful, safe place to start feeling at home in my body again.
>
> When the yoga class ended, several of us started an informal support group, and we're still going strong more than four years later. Although we now have a broader range of topics than cancer, it's a place we can always bring research findings, fears of relapse, and other health concerns.

In selecting a yoga or meditation group, you can use the same strategies as you would when you select a counselor. Ask others whom they would recommend. You can contact the teacher of any group you might join and ask how much experience he has with people facing serious illness. Ask if there are any groups specifically dedicated to the healing process. If you can't find a group, you may find a good teacher and create your own group. You can also benefit from some excellent audiotapes and videotapes that can provide yoga or meditation instruction. Local video and New Age stores often rent these, or you may buy them from a catalog.

Often a social group such as a book group or bridge club will take on the characteristics of a support group if one of their members is going through difficult times:

> Our book group meets once a month to discuss a particular book we have chosen. I've been surprised to see that it functions informally as a support group too. We have come to know each other over the years and keep up with what is happening in each member's life. We have shared support for those caring for elderly parents and have been there for those who have had to face the death of a loved one. We've also helped each other when dealing with illnesses and accidents and have cheered on those who need encouragement coping with the decision to quit smoking or losing ten pounds or changing employment or returning to graduate school.
>
> Although we're just a book group, we care about each other and support each other when one of us has an immediate need.

Online support groups

Online support groups, often called discussion groups, offer possibilities for sharing and types of support available nowhere else. Online support groups have made an impact on medicine and healing that many see as the greatest change in medicine in recent years. Tom Ferguson, MD, author of *Health Online: How to Find Health Information, Support Groups and Self-Help Communities in Cyberspace* uses the word "magic" to describe the innovations possible for those reaching out for help and reaching out to help others in an Internet based community.[6]

Online support groups have several unique advantages: When you're in an online community, you can reach people at any time of the day or night, an important concept for anyone facing illness. You never know when you'll wake up in the middle of the night and want to talk to someone, or times when you want to share some new treatment that has improved your health.

Online support groups are international and this adds strength to all in the group. Individuals from Japan or Europe may have information about therapies and drugs not yet used in the United States or Canada, and vice versa. Patients all over the world are sharing information about clinical trials, medical centers, research findings, and general supportive information such as diet, exercise, ways to locate clinical trials, quality of life advice, and much,

much more. Since choices in care differ in regions of the country and the world, it is the patients who have become an informal forum on the success and failure of certain treatments.

Online groups are a safe place to share thoughts, fears, joys, and those little steps back to wellness. Since members of an online support group are not your immediate family or neighbors, you don't need to worry about their reactions to the things you say and you can be very open in your communications. Members of online support groups often become so close that they make an effort to meet each other face to face.

One woman whose participation in an online group impacted her treatment decisions recounts:

> Initially, when I was first diagnosed in 1994 with LCIS (lobular carcinoma in situ), I had to make a decision about what I want to do in terms of treatment. This could have been do nothing, at one extreme, or undergo bilateral mastectomies at the other.
>
> On the Internet I found the National Institute of Health and the National Cancer Institute sites and got some information from them. But these organizations didn't really answer my questions which were more personal. I wanted to know what treatments mean to an individual. What is a mastectomy like, and what do you look like afterwards? How do you find clothes? I had read about discussion groups or mail lists.
>
> Just after I had the mastectomy I wrote a message to the Breast Cancer List and told what had happened to me. Then I asked my basic question, "What about reconstruction?" I also asked about buying prosthetics. I wasn't convinced that if I bought them I'd wear them—they're quite expensive.
>
> What I got back was incredibly valuable—personal feelings from women about why they were glad they were wearing prosthetics as well as personal communications from women who chose not to wear prosthetics, even one-breasted women.
>
> That was encouraging to me that both options were livable. I also got very practical advice saying "Don't buy the cheap ones (prosthetics), buy the expensive ones"—and they were right. The expensive ones feel natural and act as a protective shield. No one at the store shared any information like that. Another women wrote and said that the prosthetics kept her

warm. I did decide to get prosthetics. That was my initial experience with the list. I stayed on it for two years, interacting daily.

This same woman grew to feel very close to others in the online group in which she was participating, and got long-term support:

> *I felt really close to people on the list. You tend to share incidents that you don't share with your closest friends. There's a safe distancing when you don't see the other person's reactions.*

> *There was one woman who talked about having had a mastectomy and how it had changed her sex life. She then said, "I can't believe I'm talking about this with 900 people and I haven't even shared it with my closest friends." Many people wrote to support her and told her they had many of the same experiences, including being surprised how open they were on the list. There's that sense of distancing and safety that allows you to talk about things you wouldn't discuss with people you see every day. I don't know if you would share those kinds of things in a support group with people you might see at the grocery store, but you do share them online.*

> *One friend I had made on the list came to visit because she was going to give a workshop in a nearby town. We met at the airport and were surprised that we didn't look like the mental picture we each had of each other. One evening we were sitting talking about extremely personal things and then we both started laughing because while we hadn't known what each other looked like, we knew each other's personal lives and thoughts intimately.*

To access online support groups, you need only a computer with a modem and access to the Internet through an Internet service provider. Often online discussion groups are called listservs because that is the name of one of the most popular software programs used as a platform for discussion groups.

Some online support groups are moderated (i.e., edited) and some are open. Most discussion lists have basic guidelines for the members on the list. Guidelines usually include restrictions against commercial advertising, no posting of messages like "ditto" or "me too" that will clutter up the list without adding any real content. All lists exclude "flaming" such as the use of profanity or personal criticism of one of the members of the list.

Finding and joining a discussion list is quite easy:

- Medical organizations can often refer you to online discussion groups.

- There is also a web site that specializes in locating mailing lists and discussion groups. The URL for the web site that helps you locate a discussion list is *http://www.liszt.com*. This web site lists over 300 medical and health lists, as well as thousands that are not medical. You simply connect to their home page and either type in the subject of a list you are seeking, or click on the health category and look for a group that is discussing your concerns.

- Another web site that can be useful is the archives of cancer lists. It is sponsored by the Association of Cancer Online Resources, Inc. and includes discussions by date from nearly 70 cancer related discussion lists. By reading the archives you can evaluate the kinds of information people are sharing and determine if the list would be useful for you. The URL for the Association of Cancer Online Resources is *http://www.acor.org*.

Once you have found a discussion list that looks like it deals with your own concerns, you can subscribe to it and then just read the comments and get a sense of the group. There is no requirement that you participate by sending a message. Most new members "lurk" in the background at the beginning. Those who read comments of members of the list but never send messages are indeed called "lurkers" in the jargon of online discussion groups.

Some cautions about participating in an online support and discussion group include confidentiality and loss of your time, i.e., using hours each day to sort through the messages from a large group. You might also start feeling like a victim if the more outspoken contributors to a list have a strong point of view that differs from your own.

Confidentiality is an issue since many lists save archives; your communications and feelings at a moment in time may be saved for years. You might, for example, share that today you hate your children for being selfish or that you no longer enjoy sex. Those feelings pass, but may be saved for posterity. Anyone joining the list will have access to the messages you have shared in the past. Often online chats and discussions are archived as transcripts and searchable under your name. Also, you should be cautious about web "bulletin boards" where your message is posted on a web-based discussion site. Search engines simply are looking for matching terms and someone may inadvertently stumble across a message you sent long ago since it's on the Web. For many, confidentiality is essential. Those who have AIDS or cancer may face discrimination from employers or insurance companies if their condition were known.

There is a web site that specializes in assisting people who want to share openly, but worry about the social and financial consequences of sharing on the Internet. People who feel that they need to know that their messages are private can use a service called a "remailer." The URL for a web site keeping track of those who provide remailer services is the Anonymous Remailer FAQ, at *http://www.andrebacard.com/remail.html*. The Anonymous Remailer FAQ web site contains frequently asked questions about remailers and keeps track of web sites that offer this service. They do state they will not protect anyone who is involved in illegal acts such as terrorism, embezzlement, or organized crime.

Friends for support

Friends help each other and help support the families of people going through treatment for a serious condition. The types of support people extend to each other when they are in need is testimony to the kindness and creativity of man.

As a friend of a woman undergoing treatment for cancer recalls:

When my friend was going through chemotherapy, she needed a lot of rest and she needed her husband to be free from the constant ringing of the telephone. We organized a telephone tree and assigned one friend to be the coordinator.

Her husband made one phone call each time there was any change in her condition and that friend got the information to others who cared for her. Her husband also set up a notebook when she was in the hospital, so that those dropping by could leave her a message if she was asleep when they came to visit.

We knew she really needed and wanted all of the support and love that her friends could provide and that she also needed to be quiet and to reserve her energy for healing.

One doctor recommends letting friends become advocates and logistics coordinators:

> People need to make lists not only of questions for their doctors, but also they need to make lists of things they need from friends. They can give this list to a friend who volunteers to become their coordinator. Spouses don't often do this well, but close friends are remarkable. This friend can sit with them and make a list of all of the logistical things they need such as rides, errands, food, etc. That friend can call other people and say "Mary needs this, can you help her with that?" I've seen support like this lighten people's lives so they can concentrate on healing.

Obtaining and giving assistance

Sometimes you just need help such as picking up dry cleaning or going to the bank. Often friends are more than willing to help you out if you only make it known that you could use help in a certain area. When friends ask you what they can do for you, it can be helpful if you have an actual specific list of activities that would assist you and help you cope with your illness, job, or family concerns.

A woman recuperating with a full-leg cast learned to be specific in her requests:

> I've learned a lot about asking for help in the past two months. When you're asking for help, you have to be really clear about what help you need. At first it's hard to be "bossy," because you're so happy to see your friends and you want them to come back again. But you have to learn to tell them, "No, that's not helping, please do it this way."
>
> At first I wouldn't do that. My friends would leave and I would be in this bind of having something out of reach. So I started getting clearer and saying a lot more, "Do this, do that, don't do that."
>
> If you haven't tried to get in bed with a long leg cast, you don't know that it's almost impossible to pull the covers back. You can't slide under the covers if you can't bend anything. I had several friends willing to come and change my bed and it took some learning to get real specific and ask my wonderful friends to "fanfold" the covers so I could just pull them up easily. It made such a difference!

Once I learned how to ask for specific help I would call friends and ask for one thing like "Please bring sushi" or "Could you find a back-scratcher when you're out shopping?" It was great. They knew they were helping and I got exactly what I needed!

Think of the special skills of some of your friends. Some may have financial or legal expertise; others may know every take-out food menu in your area. Others may be great with children.

If you are a friend interested in assisting, you can offer specific rather than general help. Suggestions of what to ask from groups of friends include the following:

- Call to say you'll be in the neighborhood and you'd like to bring over a dinner. Ask if there is any particular food that sounds good.

- Tell your friend you need to show off your new vacuum cleaner and ask if you could use it at her house.

- Announce that you're taking your children to the park or the beach or the zoo and ask if you can take her children as well. Also ask if she wants to come along.

Sometimes the support you need is not easy to find or readily available. More likely, you need many different types of support. One woman created her own personal "army" to help her face a family crisis:

I don't exactly know where the ideas came from or where I found the energy to set up my "army of support." I reached deep into myself and somehow figured out what I needed to keep me going. I appointed myself General, because I knew I needed to be "in charge." I then appointed two lieutenants, one was to watch my emotional health and the other lieutenant was to assist me with my education. (I was finishing college and planning to attend graduate school and I didn't want to lose sight of that goal.)

Among my friends I found one who was expert at finance and one who was appointed legal advisor. Others in my army included walking companions, including my loyal dog, and eating companions to be sure I was eating properly. Through a coworker I found someone to make sure my house was in repair, etc.

I asked for extra time in my meditation group every now and then if I had had a setback or needed to cope with some overpowering emotional

challenge. I had a group of women friends who had been together forever,
since our now-grown children were babies. They were assigned to keep me
laughing and take me shopping. When I was finally through the crisis I
had a big party for my "army." Many of them didn't even know each
other but became instant friends.

One woman shared an especially wonderful type of support that her husband's friends created when they heard he had to drive a long distance each day for radiation treatments:

> *He had to go every day for five weeks for radiation treatments…*
> *every day to UCLA. That's a 100-mile drive each way. I thought, "Oh my*
> *gosh, this is going to be awful." Well, one of our friends talked to us about*
> *it. He had gotten a calendar and had called all my husband's friends.*
> *Each of those guys had taken days off that whole month to take him to*
> *UCLA. It was wonderful. I had them drive my car because it was more*
> *comfortable. He had his appointment at two o'clock every day, so they*
> *would just pick him up. Every day was a new guy, a new visit. He was so*
> *up because of those guys. If I had taken him each time, he would have*
> *gotten into this mode of "This is so tiring," which we all do. But because*
> *he was with a new guy each time, and they could swap stories each time,*
> *it was wonderful. He's such a private person. He experienced so much*
> *love from those guys. He hadn't ever known that could happen with*
> *guys—it was just wonderful.*

Why find support?

Although instinctively people know that participating in support groups helped them emotionally and spiritually, recent findings show that support groups help you physically as well. Science is learning more and more about how the mind affects the body, including the immune system. Human support and interaction are being found to uplift our spirits and ease some of the fears, loneliness, and difficulties in dealing with serious illness. It's exciting now to learn that support can actually help in healing, including strengthening the ability to fight disease.

CHAPTER 11

Evaluating and Using Statistics

IN THE COURSE OF MAKING TREATMENT DECISIONS, you may encounter statistics in a variety of ways:

- You might be considering preventive treatment measures based on your estimated risk for a particular disease.

- You might have already been diagnosed with a disease and need to decide whether to have treatment now or watch and wait.

- You might be trying to decide between two or more proposed treatments.

In these situations, your initial gut instinct about what's right for you might be very wrong. Perhaps your perception of the risk you are trying to prevent is overblown, or the degree to which you think the treatment will help is mistaken. Your perception of the risk of mortality if you do not act and the risk of side effects if you do, may be skewed. The overall statistics may not provide an accurate picture of your individual situation. Digging a little deeper into the studies—to look at sample size and characteristics of patients studied—could uncover information that is not reflected by the simple numbers themselves.

You don't need to be a mathematician to learn how to evaluate the numbers. This chapter addresses why you should be familiar with statistics; how misperceptions of risk can cloud your judgement; what you should know about medical tests, disease rates, and risk; how to use statistics to help evaluate your treatment options; how to read a medical research paper; and what statistics can and cannot tell you.

Why you should be familiar with statistics

There is no escaping the onslaught of statistics that comes with the diagnosis of a disease. One woman explains the statistics she was given just after her initial biopsy proved cancerous, but before any staging of the cancer was done:

> I was hit with statistics from the very beginning, from the moment I talked to the surgeon. We weren't even sure if my cancer was invasive or noninvasive and he was throwing statistics at me.

> He told me that I had a 90 percent chance with chemotherapy if the lymph nodes were negative and a 70 percent chance if the lymph nodes were positive. Immediately, there's 20 percent gone, depending on the results of a test.

> You are given statistics very quickly up front. That seems to be what's directing your decisions—the recurrence rates and this percentage or that percentage for treatment response rates.

Most people assume that medical statistics are carefully compiled and rigorously tested. This is not always true. Many medical statistics are preliminary or are initially explained by theories that do not hold up after further testing.

You may be surprised to learn that the use of medical statistics is a relatively new practice. It was not until the latter part of the twentieth century that widespread use of computers gave statisticians the means to gather and manipulate huge amounts of study data. The application of statistics to medical treatment decisions is a new field for everyone. You are not alone if you are feeling inexperienced and confused. Researchers, doctors, and patients are all learning how to evaluate and use statistics appropriately.

Medical statistics provide useful tools for overall disease prevention planning, diagnosis, and disease management. But they are also sometimes used to promote a product or support a theory. It's important to look at the source of the statistic to separate those that should be looked at skeptically from those that deserve more attention. After years of researching his condition, one man describes his approach to the statistics he finds in studies:

> I think it is just a matter of saying, "Based on everything else I have read, this procedure is nonsense. Or based on everything I have read, this one has possibilities." You develop some level of internal wisdom.

Medical statistics are calculated for a variety of purposes:

- Medical researchers analyze statistics to calculate the risk of disease within a population, verify and compare the benefits and risks of a proposed treatment, and make inferences about potential causes of disease.

- Government and public health officials use statistics to track outbreaks of disease and develop public health policies to reduce the incidence of disease.

- News writers use statistics to alert the public to life-threatening dangers and to support announcements of new discoveries or advances in medical treatment.

- Product manufacturers use statistics to promote the benefits of their products.

- Doctors use statistics to evaluate the extent of an individual's disease, to estimate the likelihood of recurrence, and to compare the potential risks and benefits of specific treatment options.

Medical statistics are sometimes presented as more certain than they actually are. A research scientist explains why he feels it is important to look beyond the simple numbers to see how and why the results were calculated:

> Scientists can't be objective. They have to make hyperbolic claims to get their research funded. Even in a purely academic career, you're not going to get tenure very fast unless you can make a case that you are doing cutting-edge breakthrough research.
>
> If you look through the research, you can see the researchers are shading certain things in their favor, like using extremes instead of the averages, or maybe there's something a little funny about the population. Once you've read through a few research reports, you accumulate a catalog of things that raise flags. The ultimate antidote is education and critical thinking.

Medical statistics are subject to the same flaws, uncertainties, and misinterpretations as any other type of statistical measurement or prediction. As one patient notes about his experience:

> We like to have clear-cut answers. But if things go wrong with the outcome of a treatment, you can't blame yourself, because it does happen.

> *It's very important to know something about the odds and uncertainties before you make your decisions. Then if something does go wrong, you won't feel betrayed, because you were aware of the risks when you made your decision.*

Approach a medical statistic the way you approach tomorrow's weather prediction. You may take your umbrella, but you won't be surprised if it doesn't rain.

Misperceptions of risk

Misperceptions of risk can cloud your judgement. You use statistics every day to guide your actions. You probably can't quote the exact risk statistics for being in a plane crash, having a bicycle accident, or being hit by a meteor, but you make decisions based on the likelihood that any of those events could occur. You look both ways before you cross the street to reduce the risk of being hit by a car.

Risks in daily life

One of the difficulties in understanding medical statistics is that they are seldom put into the context of the risks we address in our daily lives. What is the likelihood of dying of heart disease versus dying in a plane crash or auto accident? Table 11-1 provides some baseline levels of risk to give you an idea of how some disease risks compare to risks you consider on a more frequent basis.

Table 11-1. Deaths in 1994 According to the National Center for Health Statistics [1]

1994 US Deaths from the Following Causes	Deaths (pop. 260,372,000)	Proportion of 1994 Deaths
Heart disease	732,409	1 in 3
Cancer	534,310	1 in 4
Pneumonia and influenza	81,473	1 in 28
Diabetes mellitus	56,692	1 in 40
HIV	42,114	1 in 54
Motor vehicle accidents	42,524	1 in 54
Assault by firearms	17,527	1 in 130
Fall	13,450	1 in 169
Air and space transport	1,075	1 in 2,120
Drowning in bathtub	301	1 in 7,571
Lightning	84	1 in 27,131
Snakes, lizards, spiders	6	1 in 379,832

Risk distribution

Risk distribution figures are appropriate to use when you are looking at prevention options for the whole population, but the probabilities change substantially when you take individual profiles into account. For example, the probability of dying in an auto accident is far greater for someone who spends a major part of the day on the road than for someone who sits at a desk in an office all day.

Lightning causes about 90 deaths per year in the US. A person hiking in the mountains of southern California during an electrical storm is at the about same risk of being struck by lightning as a person hiking in North Carolina during a storm. However, the average person living in North Carolina, where lightning storms are frequent, will be more at risk for death from lightning than the average person in southern California, where such storms are rare.

Factors that affect your sense of risk

Your intuitive sense of risk can be skewed in the following ways:

- Familiar risks are less threatening. People often feel more at risk flying on a plane than doing more familiar things like riding a bike or driving a car. The risk of being killed in a plane crash, however, is much lower than the risk of being killed in a car or bicycle accident.

- Drama and imagery increase our sense of danger. Newspaper journalists and marketing experts know that drama and imagery have a major effect on public perception of risk. The likelihood of a plane landing on the freeway is very small, but when TV viewers see it happen right before their eyes, they will be less likely to dismiss the possibility in the future. Similarly, after a major earthquake in California, drivers avoided stopping under the freeway overpasses. Vivid imagery of twisted concrete overpasses increases the sense of risk associated with time spent under an overpass.

- Risks you can control are less frightening even when the risk is greater. Cold weather is usually predictable, so we have time to find shelter and warmth. Earthquakes happen without warning. Even though the toll is greater from cold weather, earthquakes are more feared.

The added impact of medical statistics

Medical statistics can feel very personal. You may begin to feel your strength and well-being are dependent on statistical risk predictions and the results of ongoing medical tests. One patient tells about the difficulty of absorbing statistics as they applied to her:

> I knew that my doctor was a good "numbers" guy. I had checked out his qualifications. I knew he had done research at NCI and I had asked an expert doctor about him.
>
> I didn't think I wanted chemotherapy. However, he told me I had a 60 percent chance of dying within five years if I didn't have it, and 40 percent chance of dying in the same time period, if I did. I made him repeat it: did I have a 40 percent chance of dying with no further treatment or a 40 percent of living? I couldn't take it in. I've always been a pretty lucky person. I couldn't believe how bad my numbers were.

Your doctor gives you an incidence or survival figure and tells you that your choices can increase or decrease that figure. Remember that the statistics define the overall probability of an event; they do not define your personal future.

Treat medical statistics like you treat normal daily choices, such as driving a car or taking a plane flight. Evaluate the statistics and prioritize your willingness to take specific risks. Some risks you can or must live with, some you choose to take, and some you will choose to minimize in whatever way possible.

Question medical statistics in the same ways you question any nonmedical statistic. Ask for information that tells you how and why it was calculated, look for other possible interpretations, and identify the characteristics of the individual who is most likely to fall into the population described. Medical statistics are guidelines, not guarantees. As a pathologist explains about trying to predict cancer response:

> There are so many possibilities. Everyone is different and everyone's immune system is different, everyone's genetics are a little different. If every human being when they are normal is genetically different, then why shouldn't every tumor be potentially different?

Medical tests

Medical tests are used to screen for inapparent disease, rule out disease, classify and measure disease, and monitor the course of illness or treatment. A test should only be done when the results will affect your healthcare program, namely the diagnosis, prognosis, or therapy or well-being.

In *Working with Your Doctor* (O'Reilly & Associates, Inc.), Nancy Keene describes reasons why you might want to refuse a test if its potential value is negligible:

> Many tests, once given routinely, have been shown to be unnecessary or even harmful. One recent study found that $30 billion is spent on preoperative tests in the US each year, 60 percent of which are unnecessary. In addition, injury can result from the further evaluation and treatment of false-positive results.[2]

One patient recalls finding an alternative to the diagnostic test first recommended, after expressing her concerns about the safety of the test:

> When I had an ultrasound to look for gallstones, the radiologist saw several tiny cysts on my pancreas. My doctor ordered a pancreatic CT scan, which showed more cysts. She sent me to a specialist who wanted me to have a pancreatic endoscopy to rule out pancreatic cancer. He told me that the procedure had risks so I should go to a regional center where it is performed more often.
>
> The more I read about the procedure, the more concerned I became about the likelihood of the procedure causing pancreatitis, an extremely painful, sometimes long-lasting condition. The cysts, themselves, were not painful. I asked for a consultation with the regional expert before I agreed to have the procedure.
>
> The expert told me that the risk of pancreatitis was higher for people with my profile and that the purpose of the test would be only to rule out pancreatic cancer, not to treat the cysts. He agreed that the endoscopy was premature in this situation and told me about a MRI procedure that he felt was better for identifying cancer and had no risk of causing pancreatitis. I chose the MRI.

For more information on evaluating the need for a test, see Chapter 2, *Knowing Your Rights*.

Accuracy of tests

An effective medical test is one that yields a positive result when it should be positive (true positive) and a negative result when it should be negative (true negative). Despite the fact that tests and test technology are always evolving, no test is perfectly accurate. The result could conceivably be a false positive—you might be told you have x, when in fact you don't. The result might also be a false negative—you might be told you don't have y when in fact you do. Tests are rated for their ability to detect disease (sensitivity) with true positives and their ability to rule out disease (specificity) with true negatives.

The rarer a condition or disease, the higher the proportion of false positive test readings when the test is used for screening the general population. For example, a 99 percent accurate test for pheochromocytoma (a rare adrenal gland tumor) when used to screen 1000 people in the general population, would yield approximately 1 true positive (.99), and almost 10 false positives (9.99). There would be 989 true negatives and 0.01 false negatives (1 out of 100,000). Table 11-2 illustrates these results.

This test would be very good for assuring you that you do not have this rare disease (true negatives), but about 10 out of 1000 people could be diagnosed with a disease they don't have (false positives). For this reason, tests for such rare conditions should not be used for screening the general population. Even a very accurate test for a rare disease should be reserved for cases where there is already reason to suspect that the patient has the disease.

Table 11-2. Accuracy of a Test for a Rare Condition (1 case per 1,000)

	Disease	No Disease	Total
Positive Test	0.99 (true positives)	9.99 (false positives)	10.98
Negative Test	0.01 (false negatives)	989 (true negatives)	989.02
Actual Incidence	1	999	1,000

The importance of the level of accuracy depends on the situation. As Victor Cohn notes in his book on statistics in reporting, *News and Numbers*:

> How well should a test do in avoiding false negatives and false positives? That may depend on its goal. If the main aim is not to miss some serious condition, it may shoot for high sensitivity to pick up every

possible case. If the main concern is to avoid false positives in a disease doctors can't do much about anyway, one may opt for more specificity.[3]

Some tests with rather poor accuracy may replace more accurate tests because of factors of convenience, cost, invasiveness, or risk. For example, a test that has high accuracy but that requires a painful, expensive, dangerous, or time-consuming procedure such as a stomach biopsy to diagnose celiac disease, may be foregone in favor of a simple blood screening test that is not as accurate. The less expensive or less accurate test might be the most appropriate for screening and the more accurate test used later for verification if the screening shows a positive result.

A patient talks about learning to put her test results in perspective:

> *I was treated for cancer and was in remission. Every six months, I would have blood tests before visiting my doctor for a checkup. I was always in a sweat about those tests and any slight variation in the counts.*
>
> *One checkup, I asked my doctor how accurate the tests were. He said that tumor marker counts would predict a recurrence about one third of the time; they would miss a recurrence about one third of the time; and one third of the time an elevation of counts would be a false positive. I asked why he even used the tests at all? He replied that a pattern of elevated counts would indicate that he should use other physical screening tests to see if cancer had returned.*
>
> *From that description, I decided I could relax a little about the test results. They weren't going to prove anything, once and for all, in a single office visit.*

An evaluation of a test result most properly rests within the entire context of a patient's health, most commonly in conjunction with the history (interview), physical examination, and assessment of risk for a variety of other possible illnesses. If a test result does not seem compatible with a patient's other findings, it should be questioned and repeated. A doctor gives an example where his clinical observations would outweigh the accuracy of a test:

> *If a previously healthy 15-year-old boy comes into my office with complaint of a two-day sore throat, I do a clinical exam. If he has no fever or significantly enlarged lymph nodes in his neck, but he has a*

mildly red throat and profuse clear nasal discharge, he is most likely to have a viral cold. No further evaluation at that time is necessary.

On the other hand, if he had a fever of 102 degrees, prominent lymph nodes, and a white coating on his throat, my presumptive diagnosis would be a strep infection. Antibiotic treatment would be indicated. In this case, the likelihood of a strep infection exceeds the sensitivity of the throat culture for detecting strep. If the boy's symptoms were less clinically well defined, the test would be more useful in discriminating.

When you are basing an important decision on the results of a test, you might want to verify the accuracy of the test. Ask a technologist at the lab where the test was done about the percentage of true positives (sensitivity) or the percentage of true negatives (specificity) for that particular test.

Normal results

Normal ranges usually represent the distribution of results in 95 to 97 percent of a total patient population. Abnormalities (the 3 to 5 percent outside the normal range) may represent clerical error such as mislabeling or machine or human error. Abnormal results can also be caused by non-disease factors (pregnancy alters a number of laboratory values), normal variation, interaction with medications (prescribed, alternative or self-prescribed, or illicit), or true disease. Sometimes the results can vary from laboratory to laboratory as this woman explains:

One of my enzyme tests kept coming back slightly elevated. My doctor mentioned that the lab I was going to uses a different test than the other labs in town. The next time I went to a lab that uses the more familiar test and my results came back in the normal range. He suggested that the difference might be in the calibration of the test, not a change in my enzyme level.

The normal range for a test may even vary from lab to lab using the same test. A lab technologist explains:

When we start using a new test, use new equipment, or change a reagent, we draw blood from a group of healthy people to establish our normal range for that test. We draw blood from each other and use samples from people coming in for annual checkups. Usually it comes out to be the same as the range in the published insert, but sometimes our *population is just a little bit different. We establish the normal range every time we make a change.*

If you have a series of positive tests or show a greater magnitude of variance from normal, that is more likely to reflect true disease.

Radiologists refer to a patient's previous x-ray as the "world's greatest consultant." The previous x-ray may be scrutinized for any change or stability of findings when compared with a current film. A patient describes how an x-ray taken a year before saved him from a possible biopsy:

> *While I was in the hospital for rectal bleeding they did a CT scan. The radiologist came in afterwards and said, "We found a nodule on your lung that we'd like to explore. We've set you up for a follow-up CT scan of the lungs."*

> *When I went down to the CT scan, I pulled the technician aside and said, "I want you to be aware, that four years ago I had a severe case of pneumonia and I have also been exposed to Valley Fever. What you're seeing was seen on a previous x-ray by my physician."*

> *The radiologist got the previous x-ray and saw the same thing in the x-ray that he saw in the CT scan. He came back and said, "We're not concerned. We might do another x-ray or CT scan in four or five months to make sure there is no activity, but we're confident that it has been there and, as you say, it's probably just a granuloma due to the pneumonia or cocci from Valley Fever."*

Panels of tests

A doctor may order a panel of tests, each of which has some predictive value. The results from that group of tests give more useful information than a single test could.

According to an article in the *American Journal of Medicine*:

> *The probability of any given test being abnormal is about 2 to 5 percent, and the probability of disease if a screening test is abnormal is generally low (0 to 15 percent). The frequency of abnormal single tests is 1.5 percent (albumin) to 5.9 percent (glucose) and up to 16.6 percent (sodium). Based on statistical expectations, when a panel of 8 tests is performed in a multiphasic health program, 25 percent of the patients have*

one or more abnormal results, and when the panel includes 20 tests, 55
percent have one or more test abnormalities.[4]

Panel testing usually includes groups of lab tests, whose elements are most often determined by Health Care Financing Administration (HCFA). (The US HCFA has defined which panels will be reimbursed by Medicare and private and public providers have followed suit.) The strict groups of tests determined by HCFA are purportedly designed to most economically detect and follow disease and treatment. Standard panels include a comprehensive metabolic panel, basic metabolic panel, complete blood count, lipid panel, urinalysis, etc.

How disease rates are measured

Disease statistics were first gathered in an effort to understand, manage, and prevent outbreaks of disease at the community level. Official registration of deaths in both the US and the United Kingdom began in some urban communities in the mid-1800s. Full national death registration began in the US in 1933. Today we look at disease and death rates in the general population to measure progress in prevention or treatment of disease, identify areas of increase, and as the basis for predicting risk in the general population.

Incidence, prevalence, and death rates

In the course of researching your disease, you will see incidence, prevalence, and mortality rates mentioned. These rates describe large groups of people. The variation among individuals within a large group is averaged into a group rate. Using a single number gives the impression that the group is homogenous. It is not. The rate of a disease or event describes a group, not an individual. Rates include:

- **Incidence.** Incidence is the number of new cases of a disease in a population during a specified time period, usually one year. The *incidence rate* is the proportion of new cases in the total population. There is no formalized process of registration for all diseases. Incidence rates are compiled from many sources, such as emergency room records or disease tracking agencies such as cancer registries or the Centers for Disease Control and Prevention (CDC). They can also be compiled from insurance or disability claims or from health surveys.

- **Prevalence.** Prevalence is sometimes confused with incidence, but it is different in two ways. Prevalence includes all cases, not just newly diagnosed cases of a disease. Prevalence is measured at a particular point in time, not over a period of time.

- **Mortality.** Mortality refers to the number of deaths during a specified time period, usually a year. The *mortality rate* is the proportion of deaths out of the total population during that period.

Adjusting the rates

Incidence, prevalence, and death rates are usually given per 100,000 people to provide a common denominator for comparisons of different sized populations. Statistics used in comparisons often need mathematical adjustments to correct for other variables that can affect the rates.

For example, census information may be age-adjusted to equalize the distribution of age groups in two census years. Many of the life-threatening diseases occur more often in older age groups. An age-adjusted comparison reduces the effect of an aging population to see what other factors might be affecting the disease rate. While carefully adjusted statistics are useful for comparison, it is important to remember that mathematical adjustments introduce more potential for error and distortion, particularly when comparing very dissimilar groups.

Separating out subgroups

Incidence and mortality rates are usually broken into subgroups by disease category or type, such as all cancers or a cancer type such as prostate cancer. Mortality and incidence tables are used to show distribution of disease by age, gender, ethnic group, and combinations of these, such as black men aged 35 years to 40 years.

These rates and groupings help to identify differences between groups and to measure national progress in the prevention and treatment of specific diseases. These numbers help to set goals for healthcare policy within a community and for the country.

Timeliness

Gathering and compiling huge amounts of data into meaningful reports is time consuming. In 1999 most of the latest disease rate reports available from government agencies and national organizations were based on 1996 figures.

Survival rates

Survival rates are most frequently given in one-year, five-year, and ten-year increments. The populations used for these rates are groups of people diagnosed with a particular disease.

The accuracy of survival rates depends on careful follow-up. Some members of the study population will be lost to follow-up, often because they move away from the area where they were treated. A general rule of thumb is that less than a 20 percent loss to follow-up is desirable. The impact of loss to follow-up will also be affected by the size of the group being studied. A 20 percent loss in a group of 10 would have more affect on the reliability of the survival data than a 20 percent follow-up loss in a group of 10,000.

National incidence and survival rates are extrapolated from sample populations. Survival rates are estimated from sample groups. No national agency currently follows all people diagnosed with a disease to record the final date and cause of each one's death. Even the National Cancer Institute's Surveillance Epidemiology and End Results (SEER) cancer data is compiled from cancer registries which cover only about 14 percent of the US population.[5]

For prognostic purposes, you might be quoted either a *mean* or a *median* survival rate. The *mean survival rate* is the average number of years a sample population has survived after initial diagnosis (the total years divided by the number of people in the sample). The *median survival rate* indicates that half the people in the group survived longer and half survived less than the given median number of years.

The *absolute survival rate* measures the proportion of people followed who are alive a specified number of years from diagnosis. In her book *Non-Hodgkin's Lymphomas*, Lorraine Johnston describes some of the limitations of survival statistics:

> *Survival statistics are developed using groups of people, many of whom are not very much like you, even if they appear to have the same disease, categorized using the same system or by a single research center. Your chances may be considerably better, for example, than those of someone who has several chronic illnesses such as heart disease or lupus along with NHL [non-Hodgkin's lymphoma]. In addition, many of those whose cases find their way into medical journals, and who become the basis for statistics regarding the success of one technique versus another, are those*

who have had many different treatments and who may have one or more organ systems compromised owing to repeated toxic treatments.[6]

Statistics can also be misleading if you are a younger person looking at long-term survival rates of diseases that occur more often in older people. More than 80 percent of men diagnosed with prostate cancer are at least 65 years old. A 75-year-old man is more likely to die in the ten years after treatment than a 40-year-old man who undergoes the same treatment, but the older man may die from something other than prostate cancer. The *relative survival rate* is adjusted to exclude people who died from other causes.

Never hesitate to ask how the data was obtained and calculated when you are given a survival rate. It is also meaningful to know size and the characteristics of the population studied. What was the age distribution or the severity of disease at diagnosis? What is the proportion of people whose disease recurred after initial diagnosis?

Risk calculation

Prediction of disease incidence, recurrence, and mortality are based on the historic rates of disease and mortality for a population. Those *rates* are used to calculate *risk.* Prediction requires guesswork to account for unknowns, assumes similarities between a study population and the general population, and assumes the future will mimic the patterns observed in the past. (Risk predictions would be much more accurate if nothing ever changed.)

In *Working with Your Doctor*, Nancy Keene writes:

> *If you choose to learn about the probabilities associated with your medical treatment, make sure that the numbers cited are current for your age, disease, amount of disease at diagnosis, condition, and proposed treatment. (If you are going to participate in an experimental treatment, there may be no statistics on success rates.) Also, consider the qualifications of the person providing the numbers.*[7]

Recent and future changes in treatments will affect disease rates and need to be considered when looking at risks based on historic rates.

Understanding probability

Probability is the basis of risk prediction. Probability ranges from 0 (certainty that the event will not occur) to 1.0 (certainty that the event will occur). Everything in between represents some level of uncertainty. A probability of 0.5 means an event has as much chance of occurring as not.

To express a probability as a percentage, multiply the probability by 100. For example, a probability of 0.5 is 50 percent. Expressed as a fraction, 0.5 is 5/10 or 1/2. This proportion can also be represented as 1 out of 2. More examples are shown in Table 11-3.

Table 11-3. Equivalent Ways to Express Probability

Probability	Percentage	Fraction	Risk
0.0	0%		None
.01	1%	1/100	1 in 100
0.1	10%	1/10	1 in 10
0.5	50%	1/2	1 in 2
.75	75%	3/4	3 in 4
1.0	100%		All

Remember that even though risk is often presented as a single number, like 60 percent, it is always a proportion.

The *law of large numbers* says that the larger the sample, the more probable the accuracy of the result. The probability of a coin landing heads up is one chance out of two, but you will probably toss a lot of coins before you begin to see a clear 50 percent distribution between heads and tails. Two people out of ten or 2000 people out of 10,000 can both be expressed as 20 percent, but the second proportion is much less prone to error. The sample size used to calculate the probability is critical to your evaluation of the reliability of the result.

Accumulating lifetime risk

One of the most controversial predictive risk measures is cumulative lifetime risk, not because it is inaccurate, but because it is misleading. This risk measure lumps together all age groups and views risk from an end-of-life perspective.

Most women hearing they have a 1 in 8 lifetime risk of developing breast cancer, assume that means that is their risk at any point in time. But the 1-in-8 figure only applies to a woman who has lived to be 95 to 110 years old. It means that she had a 12.5 percent probability of developing breast cancer at some time during her life. A woman who lives to 75 would have had a 1 in 11 probability of developing breast cancer. Table 11-4 shows a woman's cumulative risk of developing breast cancer by a specific age.

Table 11-4. Cumulative Lifetime Risk of Breast Cancer According to the NCI Surveillance Program[8]

Age	Cumulative Risk
25	1 in 19,608
35	1 in 622
45	1 in 93
55	1 in 33
65	1 in 17
75	1 in 11
85	1 in 9
Ever	1 in 8

Eight girl babies in a newborn nursery have no accumulated lifetime risk of breast cancer. If all eight lived past 95, probability predicts that one of them would have developed breast cancer at some point during her life. The law of large numbers tells us that it would take many groups of eight babies for the frequency to settle around 1 in 8. We are also assuming that the incidence of the disease will remain stable throughout the 95 years.

Risk divided into shorter time periods is more meaningful. According to the American Cancer Society's *Breast Cancer Facts and Figures 1999-2000*, if you were age 20 in 1999 and breast cancer free, your risk of developing breast cancer by the age of 30 would be only 0.05 percent. If, however, you were 50 and breast cancer free, your risk of developing breast cancer by the time you were age 60 would be 2.67 percent. The risk levels from the previous periods do not carry over to the next period. Even though your cumulative lifetime risk (1 in 8) is 12.5 percent, your risk from age 70 to 80 is only the 4.01 percent risk during that ten-year period.[9]

Lifetime risks can be used to compare the risk of one disease to another such as breast cancer incidence to heart disease incidence, but always make sure you are comparing statistics based on the same assumed life span (i.e., by age 75, 95, or whatever maximum lifetime is chosen).

Estimating life expectancy

A child born in 1995 had an estimated life expectancy of 75.8 years. That child will probably live longer, given the future medical advances not factored into this estimate. The average life span when you were born was lower than the average life expectancy if you are living today.

Using life expectancy as a base for historic comparison can be misleading. If you were born in 1900, your estimated life expectancy was 47.3 years. The number of childhood deaths in the previous century brought the average life expectancy to a low that does not reflect the fact that a person who survived into adulthood could expect to live to what even today is considered old age. If you were age 65 in 1900, your projected life span was 76.9 years. If you were 65 in 1995, your projected life span would be 82.4 years.[10]

Life expectancy is the baseline figure used for calculating the number of years lost to disease or gained by treatment. Being an average, this number does not reflect specific variables such as the effect of age at diagnosis. And since most statistics are taken from data three or more years old, they won't reflect recent changes in treatment.

Calculating annual risk

Annual risks of incidence and mortality are used primarily to raise awareness about the toll that a particular disease is taking in the population and to encourage people to take preventive action. The American Cancer Society predicted 175,000 new cases of breast cancer for the year 1999 and 43,700 deaths.[11] These numbers were estimated from previous years' rates and the current rate of yearly increase or decrease.

Since the population of the United States was approximately 272,300,000 in 1999, the risk of death from breast cancer during 1999 would be 43,700 out of 272,300,000, or about .016 percent.

This number is not terribly useful to an individual since it assumes that all members of the population are at equal risk. In fact, most of those deaths will be women's. Far more deaths will occur in women over the age of 50 years than under age 50. The likelihood of death from breast cancer from birth to 25 years is comparatively small. Tables of risk by age and gender are more informative, but are still far too general for individual risk assessment.

Predicting mortality by the minute

The 2000 Heart and Stroke Statistical Update from the American Heart Association states that more than 2,600 Americans die each day from cardiovascular diseases.[12] If you divide that by 24 hours, that's about three deaths a minute or 1 every 33 seconds. This type of measure is commonly used in advertising and for awareness-raising talks and literature. It is used to illustrate incidence as well as mortality levels.

Note that the size of the population affects this measure dramatically since the denominator will always be 365 days. The larger the population, the more urgent the message. Worldwide estimates are even more frightening. But if the incidence in your community is five deaths per day, that would be about one every three hours. The community statistic is somewhat more meaningful to you, but the national or worldwide statistics are far more impressive and more likely to be used.

Using statistics to evaluate treatment options

Some people feel statistics are of little value in decision-making. A patient describes why she decided not to give statistics too much sway in her decision making:

> I really did not put too much weight on the statistics. The statistics I saw were based on studies of very small groups of people who were studied for a very short period of time. But mainly, I really didn't think about statistics because it is too much like politics, I don't believe the polls either. It's like smoke and mirrors or political spin—you can switch them around until you find a statistic to fit whatever you want to say.

When used carefully and thoughtfully, however, statistics can help you quantify and prioritize your options and evaluate the likelihood that a treatment might be of benefit to you. One woman explains that she picks and chooses among the statistical input:

> I have certain things that I look at. The rest I ignore. With all the statistics you receive, you get to be like a pilot on an airplane that gets instrument fatigue. Airline manufacturers have so many things that a pilot can look at, but they've determined that pilots can't fly and look at all those things at the same time. So they have to decide which things to put in the cockpit because pilots get information fatigue.

Some statistical measures are better than others for evaluating treatment options.

Absolute and relative risk

Absolute risk compares the percentage of new cases that occurred in each group in the study. If 5 cases of heart disease developed in a treatment group of 100 participants, the absolute risk for that group is 5 percent (5/100). If the control group developed 10 cases out of 100, the absolute risk for that group is 10 percent (10/100). The absolute risk reduction (ARR) is 5 percent (10 percent minus 5 percent).

The relative risk (or risk ratio) is a much more dramatic way to compare the differences between the two groups. Like absolute risk, *relative risk* compares the percentage of new cases in each group. But rather than reporting the *mathematical difference* in incidence rates between the two groups (subtraction), the relative risk gives you the *proportional relationship* (division). In the previous example, the 5 percent incidence in the treatment group would be divided by 10 percent incidence in the control group, so while the absolute risk reduction would be 5 percent, the relative risk would show a 50 percent reduction.

In case-control studies (where the incidence of disease in one group is 100 percent and zero percent in the other) and sometimes in studies where the incidence of a disease is rare, the odds ratio is used in the place of the relative risk. There is a slight difference in the way they are calculated, but they are both used to show proportional differences between groups.

A relative risk or odds ratio of 1.0 means that the intervention or risk factor being studied has no measurable effect on the study group. A ratio greater than 1.0 indicates a positive effect, and less than 1.0 indicates a negative effect. A 2.0 ratio means the study group showed a two-fold, or 200 percent, increase. A ratio of 0.5 indicates a 50 percent decrease.

Beware of relative risk. The increase or decrease in the relative risk ratio may not give you a clear picture of the actual number of cases affected. A decrease of the incidence in a group of 100 people from 2 percent to 1 percent can be referred to as a 50 percent relative risk reduction, but the absolute risk has only been reduced by 1 percent. Table 11-5 illustrates how important it is to look at the actual numbers when relative risk is used to describe treatment benefits.

Table 11-5. Relative Risk in Perspective

Incidence Rate in Placebo Group	Incidence Rate in Treatment Group	Relative Risk Reduction	Absolute Risk Reduction
2 in 10,000 (.0002)	1 in 10,000 (.0001)	50%	.01%
2 in 100 (.02)	1 in 100 (.01)	50%	1%
2 in 10 (.2)	1 in 10 (.1)	50%	10%
2 in 2 (1.0)	1 in 2 (0.5)	50%	50%

In *PDQ Evidence-Based Medicine Principles and Practice*, Ann McKibbon says:

> *Relative differences are always bigger than absolute differences, and often tend to inflate perceptions of what the results of the study truly are. Some clinicians admit using relative numbers (the larger numbers) when they want the patient to choose the treatment, and using absolute numbers (the smaller numbers) when they would like them not to.*[13]

Relative risk and odds ratios are best used for showing the strength of particular risk factors. Absolute risk is more useful for making clinical treatment decisions because it is more reflective of the number of cases and the actual impact of a proposed treatment.

Number needed to treat (NNT)

The number needed to treat (NNT) is another way to measure the effectiveness of a particular treatment. The NNT tells you the number of people who would need to be treated for one additional person to be helped by the treatment. The smaller the NNT, the more effective the treatment is for the population.

The NNT is the inverse of the absolute risk reduction (1/ARR). It is often given in published studies that evaluate the effectiveness of a treatment. If not, you can calculate it based on the absolute risk reduction between the two groups.

If the absolute risk reduction provided by a treatment were 2 percent over 5 years, then the number needed to treat (1/.02) would be 50. That means that the clinician would need to treat 50 people for 5 years to achieve one additional positive outcome. Be sure to look at the length of time the treatment was studied, the profile of the participants, and size of the study.

Cost versus benefit

Cost of treatment is an economic variation of the number needed to treat. In this case, you look at the dosage used in the study. Multiply the daily dosage by the number of years of treatment. So if a 2 percent reduction required three pills a day for five years, that would be 1,095 pills per person (3 × 365) per year. Over a period of five years, that would come to 5,475 (5 × 1,095) pills per person. Fifty people would purchase 275,750 pills (50 × 5,475) with the hope that they would be the one to see a favorable outcome. If each pill cost $.50, the total cost for one positive outcome would be $137,875. One lucky individual will benefit from a $2,757.50 investment over five years. The rest will lose their money to the house. You may or may not be that individual.

While these calculations may make the cost-to-benefit ratio of many treatments look bleak, there are some important questions to ask yourself when you consider the value of a treatment. Does the treatment reduce incidence or does it reduce mortality? Are there factors that make you more or less likely to respond to the treatment? Is the disease you are hoping to prevent especially aggressive? Is the mortality rate high? How long should you take the medication? Does it continue working or is there a threshold on its effectiveness? A woman considering chemotherapy to prevent recurrence of her cancer explains why she would consider the optional chemotherapy:

> My oncologist lamented the tragedy that 100 patients have to be treated to save five. But I'd have to go into it assuming that I was going to be one of those five, because the risk of it coming back is just too high.

Risk factors

All of the statistics we have mentioned so far are population averages. Population averages do not define your personal risk. There are really only two groups: those who get a disease or respond to a treatment (100 percent occurrence) and those who don't (0 percent occurrence). The risk statistic just tells you how the population is split between those two groups. As one man explains:

> As far as I'm concerned, I'm n=1. There is nobody else involved. So I don't really care what the percentages are. I'm a new study and we're flipping the coin again. I have a 50/50 chance of it either being good or bad.

What you want to know is whether you will be in that subset of people likely to get the disease or for whom the treatment is beneficial? Do the benefits outweigh risks for you as an individual? Are there any other treatments or lifestyle changes that might reduce your risk with fewer potential adverse effects?

A woman describes her concern about the possible long-term effects of a treatment tested primarily on high-risk women:

> It's the long-term effects that really worry me because I am a low-risk patient. An older person or a person with advanced disease isn't as worried about that. But I'm 46, so what will happen 30 years down the line is a big issue for me.

Population averages will not tell you how a treatment will affect you as an individual. You want to know what factors characterize the people in each of the two groups. Comparing the characteristics of the people in each group can help you to infer which group you might fit into.

Stephen Jay Gould describes this process in his essay "The Median Isn't the Message," which can be found on Steve Dunn's CancerGuide web site at *http://www.cancerguide.org/median_not_msg.html*. When Mr. Gould was diagnosed with incurable mesothelioma, he was told that the median mortality was eight months. He knew that median meant that half of those diagnosed live less than eight months and half live longer. He says:

> When I learned about the eight-month median, my first intellectual reaction was: fine, half the people will live longer; now what are my chances of being in that half. I read for a furious and nervous hour and concluded, with relief: damned good. I possessed every one of the characteristics conferring a probability of longer life: I was young; my disease had been recognized in a relatively early stage; I would receive the nation's best medical treatment; I had the world to live for; I knew how to read the data properly and did not despair.[14]

Identifying risk factors

Observational studies compare populations to identify groups that show excess risk for particular diseases. For example, when a disease rate is higher in one country, researchers look at factors such as food, environment, genetics, and behavior to try to find a pattern that differs from countries where the rate is lower. Follow-up studies are done to identify factors that might make the individuals in one group more or less susceptible to the disease than those in another group. When you look at risk factor data, ask about the type and level of treatment or exposure as well as the length of time the groups were followed.

Adding up your risk factors

Avoid the urge to add up the percentages or probabilities associated with your risk factors. By the same token, factors that are said to provide protection (protective factors) cannot simply be subtracted. For example, if one factor increases risk by 50 percent and another reduces risk by 80 percent, you are not at a −30 percent risk of developing the disease if you have both factors. The percentage described as the level of risk is usually a relative risk. That means that the people in the group that had a particular exposure or behavior were 50 percent more likely to get the disease, not that a person with that risk factor is at a 50 percent risk.

Probabilities can be confusing too. For example, an independent event, one that is not altered by previous events, has the same level of risk at each possible occurrence. As this woman explains about genetic risks for inheriting a condition:

> My husband and I are both carriers of a rare genetic disorder. Our chance of having a child with this disorder is 1 in 4. I participate in an Internet discussion group where people often write, "How could this happen? I have four children and three of them have this disorder. The risk is only 1 in 4." They don't understand that each time they have a child, the risk is 1 in 4 that that child will have the disorder.

In this example, the likelihood of a second child being affected by the disorder is not related to whether or not the first child was affected. Each birth is an independent event.

One risk factor might make you more susceptible to the effects of another risk factor. For example, a person with the ataxia-telangiectasia genetic disorder may be more vulnerable to cell damage from x-ray exposure. Or a group of risk factors might be listed as separate factors, which are actually all different ways of measuring one underlying risk factor. For example, beginning menstrual cycles at an early age and experiencing menopause at a late age are both given as risk factors for breast cancer. Each of these criteria helps to identify a woman's lifetime exposure to estrogen. The underlying risk factor is her total estrogen exposure, but we list the measurement criteria as separate factors.

Look at risk factors as an attempt to help you identify whether or not you fit into the group of higher risk individuals who might be more likely to benefit from further treatment. But do not feel condemned to some inevitable outcome. Many people in a high-risk group will never get the associated disease. That's the nature of statistics. No one knows all of the risk factors or protective factors for any one disease. It's educated guesswork, but it's still guesswork.

A man talks about risk factors for his pancreatitis:

> There were a few things my doctors said I had to stop, like I can't drink alcohol. They didn't seem as emphatic about fats, they just said to watch it—not to eat any greasy burgers. They felt my prognosis was good. Alcohol seems to have a high correlation, although pancreatitis is idiopathic in about 10 to 20 percent of the cases. Even with alcoholic pancreatitis, they don't know why alcohol causes it or what the mechanism is. They may have found out more in the last eight or ten years, but my feeling is that it's sufficiently complicated.

Strength of association

New associations, or *correlations*, are announced daily between behavior, exposure, or genetic mutations and development of specific diseases. A link by association does not mean that a behavior, exposure, or condition causes that disease. One woman expresses frustration with the never-ending list of risks announced by the media:

> My mother tries very hard to do what's healthy. The problem is she believes what she reads in the news. Foods are, by turn, good and bad for the various body systems or preventing disease. She interprets those risks as absolute pronouncements. I felt sorry for her when a study showed produce with the highest pesticide residue included some of her favorite fruits.

Medical researchers look for the root causes and development path of a disease. The identification and study of environmental, behavioral, and genetic factors associated with the disease helps researchers characterize higher risk groups. An associated risk factor is a stepping stone to identifying causal relationships. Scientists hope that by studying high-risk individuals, they will be able to identify the mechanisms of disease development. The ultimate goal is to find ways to counteract or correct the steps that lead to disease development.

Preliminary associations make exciting headlines, but many of these associations will be discarded as further research disproves them. Read the text beneath the headline carefully for the details that can help you evaluate the strength of an association. Sometimes the search for correlations is referred to as data mining—the search for something publishable in a study. Watch for qualifying phrases like, "appears to be associated with," "has been linked to," or "up to."

It took years of study before tobacco was actually shown to be a leading cause of lung cancer. Once an association has been refined and observed in multiple studies, it is subjected to further study to try to determine if the strength of the association points toward a causal relationship with the disease. In the case of tobacco and lung disease, the US Surgeon General assigned a committee to review the evidence of the causal link between smoking and lung cancer. The following are some of the questions they included in their inquiry and are good questions to ask about any new association:[15]

- Does the exposure always precede the disease?

- How strong is the association (e.g., a 50 percent increase in risk or a 3 percent increase)?

- How much exposure is required?

- How many other studies have shown the similar results?

- What other variables might explain this association? For example, it has been observed that pet owners are more likely to develop multiple sclerosis (MS) than those who do not own pets. Researchers could look further to see if there is a connection between exposure to fleas and MS or to the pesticide used in flea collars. They could also take a closer look at the characteristics of people who own pets. Are they in a particular age range; are they more or less likely to have children?

- Is there a biological explanation for the increase in risk?

- If the exposure is withdrawn or eliminated, does the disease diminish or disappear?

Reading a medical research paper

Treatment statistics and risk factors are identified in medical research papers and usually published in medical journals. Even a medical research paper must be read with care. In her book, *Advanced Breast Cancer*, Musa Mayer points out some caveats about researching a life-threatening condition:

> *Reading the medical literature published for physicians means you will run across tables of mortality statistics as they apply to differing treatments and the various stages of the disease. Since the temptation will be to apply the statistics you find to your own situation, you must look carefully to see that the treatments are not outdated (with poorer results) and that you've interpreted the prognostic factors accurately.*[16]

Medical research papers have a standard format regardless of the journal publishing them. Familiarity with the function of each section and with statistics cited in a paper will help you read them more effectively.

Abstract

The first thing you usually see when you look at a clinical trial or other research in a published medical journal is the abstract. An abstract is a *summary* of the article. The abstract will tell you a great deal about the reliability of the study and its usefulness to you personally.

Nearly 75 percent of the medical studies indexed in MEDLINE since 1985 have abstracts. MEDLINE can be freely accessed through Internet in several formats. MEDLINE abstracts allow you to get a sense of the soundness of a study even if you don't have access to the full text of the given study.

The large number of medical research studies published each year has led to an effort to standardize the format of an abstract to make it more informative. Abstracts of medical studies usually contain short explanations of each of the following elements of study or clinical trial:

- Objective/background/purpose
- Methods (including design of the study, the setting, participants, and interventions)
- Results/measurements
- Conclusion(s)/implications

Be aware that in a recent study of six major medical journals, the study authors found many cases where the data in the abstract was different from the data in the paper or that sometimes data appeared in the abstract that was not found in the actual paper. The percentages of abstracts found "deficient" in one or both categories varied from 18 percent in one journal to a high of 68 percent in another.[17]

In spite of these alarming findings, abstracts provide a valuable first step, an overview of the study. As always, you must look at all information critically. This is especially true if you are making medical choices based on the information you find. One humorist remarked that researchers sometimes put information in the abstracts of their articles that they think they put in the actual study.

Even with these caveats, understanding each segment of an abstract can give you enough of an overview to decide whether or not the full study might help you understand a topic more completely and/or help you make decisions. Most abstracts are divided into sections that correspond with sections in the paper.

Objective section

The objective (background or purpose) defines the reasons for the study and explains the importance of the investigation. Often the objective or background will present a new study or the study of the outcomes of some older therapy. It may also present the necessity of further investigation into the beneficial and/or adverse effects of some new drug or surgical or medical intervention. Simply put, the researchers will tell you why they felt compelled to undertake this particular medical research.

Methods

The methods section of an abstract is the most important section for determining its value to you as a medical consumer. This section sets out the design of the study, defines the group of patients studied, and the time periods of the study. The methods section of the abstract also provides important clues as to the strength of the study.

In the methods section, the investigators will define who was eligible to participate in the study. Selection of subjects, by age, sex, and other characteristics such as ethnic background are defined. The authors will also explain whether or not there was a control group (a group of patients similar to those in the study but not receiving treatment or receiving a placebo).

The methods section identifies the methods used to collect data, such as by evaluating medical records, conducting patient interviews, or recording measurable physical responses to specific interventions.

In her book *Non-Hodgkin's Lymphomas* (O'Reilly), Lorraine Johnston describes the importance of looking at the statistical model:

> *Those of you who studied statistics in school are aware that many different statistical methods exist to manipulate data, any two of which may in some cases give differing results. Statistical analysis is really just a method for making sense of large amounts of otherwise incomprehensible data. Consequently, sometimes the statistical model chosen represents science's closest guess regarding how to analyze the outcome of treatment. Some statistical models chosen may not be a good fit for some collections of data. In spite of the best faith on the part of researchers and statisticians, these inconsistencies may creep into research papers.*[18]

The methods section also helps you determine the type of study being reported. Is it a clinical trial that studies an actual treatment or intervention, or is it simply an observational study?

In an *interventional study*, a treatment is given or performed on patients and their response to this treatment is followed closely. The strongest type of interventional study, the "gold standard" for medical research, is the prospective randomized double-blind controlled clinical trial.

An *observational study* follows groups of patients, but does not intervene or treat them. One of the best known of these studies is the Framingham Heart Study that began in the 1940s in Framingham, Massachusetts. This study followed 5,209 adults between the ages of 18 and 62. Participants had medical examinations every two years to determine and study risk factors for heart disease. Another example of a large observational study is the Nurses' Health Study that included 121,700 women. This study identified an increased risk of breast cancer in women taking estrogen and progesterone.

In an observational study such as the two mentioned, researchers conduct large-scale surveys and/or examinations and evaluate the information found as it is generated. This is a *prospective* study. In a *retrospective* study, researchers gather facts from medical records, looking backward in time to determine similarities among patients who undergo certain treatments, etc.

The strength of observational studies is that it is easier to involve large groups of people. One weakness of an observational study is that survey participants may interpret questions quite differently or the medical records may be dissimilar enough that the researcher may not be able to find clear comparison groups.

There are many subsets of these study types, and the methods section of the abstract should clearly define what type of study is being utilized. You should also find clear descriptions of the interventions used, if any, and the setting or location for the study.

Results

The results section of the abstract gives you additional insight into the strength of the study. This is the statistics section of the abstract. Here, you will usually find the numbers of subjects who participated in as well as the number who actually completed the study. You also find the numbers of subjects who dropped out of the study before it was concluded and how long the follow-up period lasted.

The results section will refer to a statistical term called the *p-value* (the probability value). The p-value is used to quantify the probability that the same results could be obtained randomly or with no intervention. Traditionally, the p-value should be less than .05 for the results to be considered statistically significant. If a p-value is expressed as p<.05, it means that there are 5 or fewer chances in 100 that the same results could be obtained by chance. A low p-value like p<.001 means that there is an even smaller chance that the results could have been obtained by chance (i.e., less than one in 1,000).

Another statistic used to measure the reliability of the results is the *confidence interval* or *CI*. The size of the group studied and the frequency of the disease affect the confidence interval. The confidence interval uses the margin of error to compute a range within which the true results might fall if multiple studies of the same size were performed.

The standard confidence interval is based on 95 percent confidence that the true result falls within the given range. The confidence interval is usually shown in parentheses. For example, an estimate of mortality after coronary artery bypass surgery or (CABG) can be expressed as (95 percent CI=1.26–4). This would mean that the researcher is 95 percent confident that mortality in the 36 months following CABG will fall into the 1.26 percent to 4 percent range.

Another way to express this is if the study were repeated 100 times, the result can be expected to fall between 1.26 percent and 4 percent in 95 of the studies. In the other five studies, it might fall outside that range.

The rule of thumb for looking at the range in a confidence interval is "wider is weaker." The tighter the range, the less variation can be expected from study to study.

Most confidence intervals show the 95 percent confidence range for relative risk results. The confidence interval range for a relative risk should not include 1.0. A range that crosses 1.0 indicates that subsequent studies could show positive effects, negative effects, or no change. The confidence interval should fall either completely above 1.0 or completely below 1.0.

The results section of the abstract will also contain any statistically significant subgroups discovered in the study. This includes any findings that differed widely for some definable group such as a group of low-income participants or a group of participants from a specific ethnic group.

Conclusion

In the conclusion section, the authors present their interpretation of the meaning and/or implications of the results obtained in their research. A conclusion might be that smokers have a greater chance of dying of lung cancer than nonsmokers, or that men taking one aspirin per day have less heart disease. Sometimes researchers indicate that the conclusions are tentative and that a broader study or a follow-up study is needed to verify the results.

One woman explains how she depends on the conclusion section to decipher a medical article:

> *You don't have to understand every single word in an article to read it. You can certainly understand enough to make sense of it. You don't need to know all of the chemistry details and formulas. You see what the conclusions were and how they arrived at them.*

The body of a paper

The body of the paper explains more fully how the study was conducted and how the researchers arrived at their conclusions. In the body of the paper you'll usually find useful tables, graphs, and diagrams that help explain more completely the range of the study and its conclusions. Each of the sections of the abstract is presented, but with much more detail.

In the body of the paper, look for clear descriptions of the study participants, including a full disclosure of the numbers of participants who may have dropped out of a study and the reasons for these dropouts.

Techniques for critical review of a study

All studies are not created the same. Researchers usually begin a study to test a hypothesis or expectation. That's why clinical trial designers use randomization and blinding to minimize the possibility that their expectations will bias the results. Be on the lookout for potential bias.

Interpretation bias

Determine for yourself whether or not the conclusions reached by the author actually make sense. Could other conclusions be drawn from the same numbers? Could some other factor besides those mentioned be responsible for the findings?

Note that statistical significance does not always mean that a conclusion has real practical medical significance. A reduction in symptoms from 2 to 1 in 100,000 persons taking a prescribed drug could be described as a 50 percent increase in cure rate, but only 1 person out of 100,000 would actually be helped!

The last issue of the *British Medical Journal* (BMJ) each year contains many humorous articles that have been written scientifically but have often arrived at absurd or irrelevant conclusions.

Selection bias

Selection bias occurs when the researchers select certain people over others without acknowledging that fact. For example, if all of the participants in a given study were from the same rural area of the country, there could be genetic and environmental factors that would influence any medical conclusions. Selection bias may exist if a given group has some common traits which are not taken into account before the study.

A woman describes how she later realized she had been part of a study that showed selection bias.

> *I joined an osteoporosis study through my aerobics class. Our health-conscious teacher arranged reduced cost for bone-density screenings for all of her students over 40.*

The physician who administered the bone density evaluations was astounded at the results. He said that the bone densities of ALL of the 75 women in the study were "over the top." Every one of our bone densities were higher than the norms for our age groups.

The physician then observed that most of the other women he had tested had been referred to him because they were at high risk for osteoporosis. He realized that the data he was used to seeing was for women who were selected for him because they probably had low bone density.

He had never seen this many women at one time who all had such strong bones. We were proud of ourselves and vowed to keep attending our aerobics classes. Our teacher walked around with an "I told you so" smile for weeks.

Both the exercising group and the high-risk group could be looked at as examples of selection bias. Neither group represented a true cross section of the population.

Recall bias

In a retrospective study, the researcher may have to depend on the subjects' recall of prior exposure or previous behavior. Sometimes the risk factor being studied had not been identified at the time the subject was treated so the answer is not in the subject's medical records. A subject's memory of what happened prior to his illness may be influenced by the length of time since the experience as well as what he personally thinks might have caused his illness.

Hearsay bias

In a study based on surveys or interviews, the researchers may interview relatives if the patient is deceased. Relatives sometimes remember things that might not quite be true, such as "Joe loved to eat my pies," or "Virginia never touched a drop of liquor." These statements may not be factual and the researcher should acknowledge this possibility if the studies include interviews of those other than the patient. Studies like this take place when the patients suffering from a given condition become too sick or die too quickly to be interviewed themselves, or they may be the only way to follow up a retrospective study based on old medical records.

Reporting bias

Studies with positive results tend to be reported and published more than those whose hypotheses weren't proven. For some reason—probably because we all want to hear good news—articles are selected by the editors of journals more often if they show the drug or treatment made a positive difference. We often never know what treatments have been found to fail or were discontinued because of serious side effects.[19]

Look at who participated in the study

Note the number of withdrawals or dropouts from the study. Were there more than 10 percent in a study that lasted less than three months, or less than 20 percent in a long-term study? A large number of dropouts weakens the strength of the study and may alter the findings. If a large number of study participants dropped out, that could point to adverse drug reactions, poor follow-up by the researchers, or many other causes such as a group of subjects who would be difficult to follow in any case, such as homeless individuals. A large number of dropouts should be a warning sign that something in the study needs further checking. The rule-of-thumb for an acceptable drop-out rate is about 20 to 30 percent.

Study evaluation checklist

When you are considering treatment options based in part on the results of a study, ask the following questions about the study:

- Is the data in the abstract different from the data in the body of the paper?
- Is the data in the abstract explained in the paper itself?
- Is the study observational, i.e., is it a study of information collected through medical records, interviews, or surveying other studies? If yes:
  - Is it a case record of a specific patient?
  - Is it a consolidation of many studies (i.e., a meta-analysis) and are those studies similar enough to be combined?
  - Is the study anecdotal or based on opinion (e.g., "I remember many patients who reacted positively to…")?

- Is the study a treatment study? If "yes" answer the following questions:

  - Did the researchers clearly define the population being studied?

  - Is the size of the group being studied large enough to draw a conclusion? (Any study with less than 100 participants should be questioned and confirmed by later studies. Groups larger than 1,000 are considered reliable enough to be statistically significant if they are randomly selected.)

  - Is the control group well matched to the treatment group or is there a statistical adjustment?

  - Is the group representative of the general population—or were they selected for certain characteristics (e.g., previous stroke victims, diabetics, etc.)?

  - Were there many dropouts from the study and are specific numbers given?

  - Do the conclusions seem logical based on the results, or could they be attributed to other factors?

- Is there bias in the selection of the study population?

- Is there a recent and comprehensive bibliography supporting the findings?

- Were any researchers able to duplicate the results in subsequent studies?

- Is the study funded by a commercial organization such as a drug company or manufacturer or by an independent organization such as the National Institutes of Health or the National Cancer Institute?

- Does the funding source stand to profit from the results of the study? (Usually these are drug studies or studies discussing new high-tech equipment.)

- Is the author an authority in the area covered by the study?

- Are the results clear and understandable—can you determine how the researchers came to their conclusions?

- Are all of the measurements objective? Subjective measures (i.e., the "participant seemed depressed" or "acted fatigued") are unreliable.

- Were any important findings overlooked or unexplained (i.e., several of the participants developed a slight cough, but this was not pertinent to the study...)?

- Even if the results are "statistically significant," are they actually relevant or useful in making treatment decisions (e.g., 30 percent reduction in mortality only actually saved 1 life in 5,000)?
- Is the confidence interval (CI) narrow or wide? (A wide CI indicates a wider variation in response or a small sample size.)
- Was the study published in a peer-reviewed journal?

What statistics can and cannot tell you

Statistics can't predict what will happen to you but they can give you a sense of perspective. A woman whose son was diagnosed with diabetes recalls the reassurance that statistics gave her:

> One thing I found out right away was that because of the development of the electronic blood monitor, my son's life span was probably going to be within the normal range. I was very relieved to learn that.

A cancer patient tells about making the decision to go ahead with chemotherapy treatment after surgery:

> I assigned a value to my treatments based on the 20 percent risk reduction they represented. Intellectually, I know you either have a recurrence or you don't (100 percent or 0 percent), but it helped me cope with the chemotherapy to tell myself that each treatment increased my expected life span.
>
> I didn't dig for more precise statistics. I just wanted some reassurance.

Remember that even when statistics are used to promote a sense of certainty (or inevitability), they also are a measure of the level of uncertainty. It's important to remember to look at risk statistics from both directions. If you are at 60 percent risk of a particular outcome, there is still a 40 percent chance that it won't happen to you.

When you were diagnosed, somehow you made it into the smaller percentage of people diagnosed with a particular chronic or life-threatening disease. But now you are told your decisions will affect the progression or regression of your disease and you are offered statistics that assume you will fall into the larger percentage of people treated. You may or may not.

In his book *Confronting the Big C*, Henry Weaver says this about basing his life on statistics after being diagnosed with a secondary cancer in his spine:

> The neurologist who examined me early in the illness indicated that there was a 1 percent chance that my problem could be caused by cancer. That is a chance of 1 in 100, but it was true in my case. Any individual case may fall within the upper and lower limits of a statistical range. If they told me that my life expectancy was six months or two years or five years, I would be tempted to plan and expect accordingly. I felt it was better to know that some cases are essentially cured and I would work on the hope and expectation that in my case this would be true.[20]

It's up to you to sort through the assumptions these risk statistics are based on, look for risk factors that make you more or less likely to be in a higher risk category, and weigh the risk, benefits, and costs of the treatment.

Use statistics as guides, but also acknowledge your own sense of urgency or comfort with the options available to you. Statistics are just one part of the decision-making picture.

CHAPTER 12

Reviewing Information with Your Doctor

IN CHAPTER 1, *PREPARING FOR RESEARCH*, we talked about gathering enough information from your doctor to begin your research. In this chapter, we discuss coming back to your doctor with the information you have found and integrating the information into the treatment plan discussion.

We describe the elements of a mutually beneficial doctor-patient relationship as well as some of the time and communication barriers that affect doctor-patient dialogue. We address how to use a research-enhanced understanding of your condition and treatment choices to fine-tune your questions, strengthen your role in the doctor-patient dialogue, make the time you spend with your doctor more efficient, and focus on choosing the most appropriate diagnostics and treatments for your situation. We end the chapter with a discussion of ways to handle insurance reimbursement restrictions on doctor-patient conference time.

Elements of a working relationship

A good working relationship with your primary care doctor and/or treating specialist is important if you plan to be an active participant in the decision-making process. With today's medical structure, however, you are not always given as much control over your choice of physicians or as much time with your physician as you might like.

You may not find a perfect fit with a doctor. But you can look for the best fit if you keep in mind the elements of a good relationship between patient and doctor: mutual respect, shared responsibility, trust, honesty, consideration of emotional and physical well-being, and availability.

Mutual respect

Mutual respect means that you respect each other's intelligence and have confidence you are both working to find the best possible solution to the problem at hand. This does not mean that you always agree, but that you are comfortable sometimes agreeing to disagree and can find ways to move forward from that position. A doctor describes his response when a patient wanted to try a treatment he doubted would work:

> I saw a patient recently who is very intelligent. I explained why I didn't think the approach he wanted to try would work, but I knew he was going to try it anyway. I said, "If you understand all these things and that's still what you want to do, then I'll figure out how to monitor your response to see if it is working or not." He agreed.

Shared responsibility

If both parties agree to share in the decision-making, negative outcomes will not result in blame or a sense of betrayal. A woman who chose to try an herbal approach to treatment describes how her doctor supported her:

> My doctor was wonderful because he respected my wishes as a human being. He knew I'd had this condition for a long time and I'd been on all the standard drugs before. He respected my desire to try something else. It meant a lot to me and made it easier for me to accept when it came time for me to go back on the drugs and then eventually have a risky surgery. I considered surgery to be my last resort. When it came time to have the surgery, I knew I'd tried everything else. I was ready and I was ready to deal with whatever happened afterwards.

Another woman describes her willingness to accept the consequences of an informed decision she made with her doctor's guidance:

> When I was diagnosed with breast cancer, people started second-guessing what might have contributed to my getting it. Friends have said to me, "Oh you've been taking hormone replacement therapy for ten years, that may be what caused your cancer."
>
> Even my primary care doctor asked me how I felt about the decision to go on hormone replacement therapy, looking back on it.

I told him that I feel fine about it. He and I had discussed the decision ad infinitum, weighing benefits and risk according to the information we had at the time. A definite link between that therapy and breast cancer is still not clear and I feel totally okay with that decision.

Trust

Since you cannot possibly learn all there is to know about your condition, you need to feel confident in your physician's level of knowledge and skill. Here's how one woman addresses this:

Even with a background in science, I realize I can't learn everything I need to know. So I do enough research to be able to recognize my doctor's level of knowledge and skill, then I choose a doctor I trust and don't worry as much about checking everything out.

Likewise, your doctor needs to be able to trust that you will do your part in any agreed upon course of action. That includes letting him know if you note unexpected changes or if you change your mind.

Honesty

You need to feel comfortable expressing your preferences, concerns, and expectations with your doctor. You and your doctor don't need to share the same point of view, but you should feel confident that your evaluation of what is important or not important to you will be acknowledged, not judged. By the same token, when you ask for your doctor's opinion, you can expect it to reflect her view on things such as quality of life.

If both patient and doctor feel comfortable expressing themselves and are aware that no single point of view is more right than another, there will be less conflict over unspoken assumptions. A woman describes one of her questions in looking for an internist:

My husband and I are in our sixties. We expect that whomever we choose as an internist will stay with us for a long time. One of the things we wanted to know, in interviewing doctors, was how they felt about euthanasia, because that could be a critical issue and we wanted our feelings about it to be understood.

Your doctor should also feel comfortable saying "I don't know," if she doesn't have an immediate answer to your questions or "We don't know," if there is uncertainty within the medical community. One patient explains that he is comfortable with that kind of honesty:

> Given the state of information we have now, I'm happy if my doctor says, "Here is what we know, and here is what we can infer. And next week it may all change." I understand that. However, I get the feeling that some doctors are hesitant to say they don't know or are noncommittal because they are afraid you will call them on it later.

Attention to emotional and physical well-being

You need to feel listened to and acknowledged when you express your concerns and fears, not placated or dismissed. Emotions are an important part of well-being and should be explored, not ignored. Emotions can mask what actually could be a physical response. A doctor describes how a symptom of a suspected emotional issue could actually be a physical warning sign:

> An elderly man who has recently lost his spouse of many years comes to my office and I note a fifteen-pound weight loss. He may be suffering from grief and depression alone or there might be another more life-threatening cause. I could delay investigating this symptom until a more ominous symptom such as bone pain, a blood clot, or a severe weakness occurs. Or I might do further tests to see if something else could be causing the weight loss, such as a metastatic colon cancer. The patient's survival time might not actually be significantly different, but ignoring the complaint would be considered neglectful.

A woman who has had some difficult-to-diagnose problems describes what she expects in a doctor's approach:

> I've been to doctors who were perfectly nice people or highly respected in certain areas, but who simply didn't clue into what was going on with me, no matter how much information I gave them. Why should I waste my money with someone who's so glued to a textbook they ignore the individual patient?

Availability

Your doctor needs to be reasonably accessible. You need to feel assured that in an emergency situation, your doctor or an equally competent colleague will be available to help you.

It's also important to be respectful of your physician's personal privacy. Determine up front when and how it is best to contact her to discuss concerns or ask questions. One woman trying to get answers about her mother's condition talks about placing calls to the doctors:

> I called both my mom's doctors in the morning and again in the afternoon. I waited all day for them to call me back. Her primary care doctor called me back in the evening, which I realized afterwards was actually a better time for discussion because she wasn't running between appointments.

Another woman emphasizes the element of accessibility:

> My husband and I have come to the conclusion that you can research, ask questions, and be assertive, but a lot depends on the personalities of the doctors, how much they are willing to cooperate with you, how busy they are, and whether they listen to you. I hate to say that so much responsibility is theirs, but it is. They control the time and the place.

The doctor's role and contribution

Your doctor can be your most valuable resource. Not everything you need to know is written on paper. In addition to having a background in the study of medicine, your doctor can offer you insight, perspective, and the intuition that comes from experience.

Training and experience

Training and experience are, of course, fundamental to what your physician brings to the table. Your physician is trained to serve your vital medical interests, which include prolonging life, relieving symptoms, and restoring function. As a medical student he survived a number of intellectual challenges with a heavy emphasis on rote learning and memorization, moving from intensive classroom training into intensive clinical training.

Established physicians rely first on past experience, and next on teaching or advice of colleagues, the medical literature, and other areas of continuing education. While an older physician might not have the highly detailed information base of a more recently trained physician, his clinical acumen from years of experience may be so well tuned that he can sense when a patient looks ill or when a clinical pattern does not fit.

A specialist completes the standard three to five year medical, surgical or other residency program and then may train a further one to three years in a fellowship to complete subspecialty training. Upon completion of the residency or fellowship, he is eligible to take a board certification examination in that specialty (after a residency), or in that subspecialty (after a fellowship). About 55 to 60 percent of applicants pass the board certification examination to become board certified or a "diplomate" of that specialty. A primary care physician can have specially focused training in primary care, but not have formal recognition by the board of medical specialties. A physician does not actually need to be board certified to claim a specialty or be a specialist.

Overview of body systems

Even if you have done a lot of focused research into your particular condition, your doctor will have a broader sense of how one body system relates to another. As you look at risks and benefits, you will be looking at how a treatment for one thing might affect the balance in another part of the body. For example, an article on hormone replacement therapy might stress the benefits to your heart without mentioning that it might increase your risk of breast cancer. Your doctor can look at the overall picture of your family history and your personal risk factors for breast cancer and heart disease and help you identify your personal risks and possible benefits, should you choose to take or not take hormone supplements.

History and controversy

Your doctor can offer historical perspective on treatments that have changed or been replaced by newer more effective treatments. A doctor explains how things have changed during his career:

> *Many disease such as hypertension, diabetes, and AIDS, which had lethal prognoses are now becoming controllable long-term. Age-associated*

conditions such as Alzheimer's, cataracts, and osteoarthritis are now considered distinct diseases, which are considered manageable, rather than an inevitable part of the aging process.

As we learn more about diseases, differences in degrees often become differences in kind. Or a given disease may have subtypes that are eventually determined to actually be discrete diseases.

An oncologist describes trying to help his clients put information offered to them by well-meaning friends into perspective:

Chemotherapy has a well-deserved reputation as a harsh treatment. Patients come in apprehensive about advice given to them by a neighbor whose mother was treated twenty years ago. I need to explain what has changed in the past twenty years.

In addition, your doctor can identify areas of controversy and uncertainty currently under debate within the medical community that may affect the information you are reading. He may be able to point out subtleties in the literature that might not be obvious to a less experienced reader. A doctor speaks about this from personal experience:

All careful observers of medical literature have witnessed sudden reversals in which a once wildly popular therapy is discredited. One of the strengths of medical literature is that it is vigorously debated.

Another doctor recommends:

With all these recent "medical breakthroughs," I recommend cautious optimism.

Referral

Your doctor can also direct you to a subspecialist with more expertise than he might have in a particular area or he can contact the specialist himself to augment or update the information you have. A doctor explains why this is so important:

The best system allows physicians to maintain good communications with each other. A specialist arguably manages problems such as congestive heart failure, psoriasis, or rheumatoid arthritis more successfully and cost-effectively for the patient. A primary care doctor manages the more

common conditions and refers the patient to the appropriate specialist for
more complex conditions. The days of the super-doctor are gone. A physi-
cian who claims to be a specialist in everything is delusional.

If you request it, he can also introduce you to other patients who have made the decisions that you are considering. Former patients are often willing to share their thoughts and answer questions about their experience after making a particularly difficult choice.

Coordinator and advocate

As your treatment coordinator, your doctor also acts as your advocate, ordering tests, making changes in the treatment plan as needed. He will facilitate and monitor the connections between members of your medical team—technicians, radiologists, pathologists and other specialists. He will also define the structure of your treatment plan and identify appropriate progress markers and re-evaluation points. He knows what to look for and the questions to ask when evaluating the progress of a treatment. In this example, a doctor describes the things he considers when he recommends a treatment:

> *When you are thinking about doing a treatment or not doing a treat-*
> *ment, especially if it is very iffy and there's a high toxicity or limited bene-*
> *fit, the importance of establishing baselines and criteria for measurement*
> *are really important. You especially try to find quantitative things to mea-*
> *sure. Sometimes, at the very least, that's just talking to the patient and*
> *trying to see what the patient thinks is going on, how he or she feels, and*
> *how you see the patient doing. Once you can establish those indicators,*
> *you can both monitor the therapy to decide if it is helping or not.*

Not all of your doctors will play the same role. You will usually have one primary doctor or specialist with whom you spend your decision-making time. One woman describes a conversation with her surgeon about his role in her treatment:

> *I said to him, "You know, I don't want to feel like a piece of meat on a*
> *conveyor belt." I just didn't want to feel like another faceless body under*
> *the knife.*
>
> *His response was amazing. He said, "People never think of it being*
> *the reverse. I'm like a top car mechanic. Wealthy men bring me their*

Mercedes—their wives, and say they need service. Then I fix them and they take them away and that's the end of it."

I thought about it. Of course, if he does a good job, he never gets to see the person again. What is the point of there being any personal connection? You meet, he agrees to do the surgery, you agree to undergo it, and that is the end. There is no need for an ongoing relationship.

Your role and contribution

Your physician is a guide and facilitator, but you are the ultimate decision-maker. This represents a shift in the traditional patient role, as one woman explains:

Our generation is taking more responsibility for these decisions. I think it has to do with the fact that women are working now. They are supporting their families, and they don't feel comfortable letting other people make these kinds of choices for them anymore.

A man involved in his own decision-making points out that we can't do it alone:

I want to be involved in the decision-making. On the other hand, I don't want my doctor to say, "Well you decide," when I haven't gotten full information.

Another woman offers her perspective:

I can see how people would be scared of the whole medical system. This is not part of our background, but things are changing. You do have to partner with the medical people. You have to, because it's your body.

Quality decision-making requires a partnership. Everything your doctor needs to know about you and your condition is not written on paper in the form of lab results or research studies. You are unique and your physical response to treatment will be unique.

Your input, feedback, understanding of your medical situation and your help as an information gatherer all contribute to your doctor's success in treating your condition.

Symptoms

Keep your doctor updated on your symptoms—a sudden increase or decrease in old symptoms, or any new symptoms. It's sometimes difficult to identify which changes might be important, especially if they are transitory. It's helpful to keep a journal during both the diagnostic and treatment phases, to remind you of things you should mention and also for recognizing trends or patterns in response.

In her book, *Working with Your Doctor* (O'Reilly), Nancy Keene emphasizes the importance of your side of the dialogue:

> *What you tell your doctor is the foundation on which diagnosis and treatment rest. Clear explanation of symptoms, combined with relevant context from your personal life, allow the doctor to begin his examination armed with all pertinent data. You are the expert on your symptoms, feelings, and medical history. Without this vital information, the doctor, despite the availability of a high-tech arsenal, cannot give you the best possible care.[1]*

Concerns and values

Legitimate fears and concerns are triggered when your health and future are in question. It's important to express these feelings. Otherwise, they may make you appear resistant in ways that are difficult for your doctor to understand. One woman explains why she was resistant to the suggestion of chemotherapy:

> *With chemo, it was really the fertility issue—that I could become sterile. I didn't care if I was going to lose my hair or any of the other things. Those were just unpleasant side effects. But I wanted to have kids, so that issue that made it really hard for me to decide.*

A woman talks about her resistance to taking medication during a period of severe depression:

> *I had mixed feelings about drugs. I'm one of those children of the sixties. The one thing I knew about myself was that I'd been drugging myself daily with the one legal drug that gives momentary cessation of pain: alcohol. So why would another drug be better? Couldn't I just stiff upper lip it out of this pain, with therapy and truth?*

I'd made so many jokes about Prozac in my life that taking it seems to be not only capitulation, but selling out. Selling out—the worst phrase that could be assigned to a child of the sixties.

My psychiatrist understood my fears, but she told me about how antidepressants work. She even drew pictures for me. After taking it for about six weeks, I remember the change I felt so vividly. Everything had been gray, colorless, as if I was staring into a pit of mud. One day on a walk, I realized I was seeing colors, really seeing them for the first time in two years.

I'm not wedded to taking any drug forever, but after working with my doctor, I realized that right now, for where I am at this time in my life and work, this medication helps me.

Family and finances

Your family responsibilities and your financial situation will also affect your decision-making. Don't be shy about discussing these conditions with your doctor. They affect both your ability and your willingness to make certain decisions. The mother of a 6-year-old girl talks about her decision to reschedule the start of her chemotherapy:

I was scheduled to begin my chemotherapy right before my daughter's seventh birthday. We had been planning the birthday party and my daughter was very excited. I was concerned about how I was going to be feeling just a few days after my first chemotherapy. I decided to discuss this with my doctor to find out if the delay of a week would make a significant difference in my treatment. He felt it would be fine, so I started therapy a week after the party.

A woman who has grown children explains how her family situation affects her evaluation of treatment choices:

I think if I were under 50, I would make different decisions and the difference would have been because I would have younger children and more responsibilities.

Financial discussions are sometimes uncomfortable in a medical setting, but if you are responsible for paying the bill, you need to know ahead whether or not you can afford the option being recommended. A man describes his concern about the cost of an upcoming series of radiation treatments:

> I asked the doctor how much the radiation treatment was going to cost. He's a very dedicated doctor. He said, "I don't deal with the billing part, I want to provide the best treatment." I explained that we needed to know because we have a very large deductible and we needed to figure this out. I don't think that the financial part of the treatment should be so concealed.

If you find that personal or financial responsibilities are affecting your decision, they should be discussed. The possibility of an alternate solution might not be addressed if the problem is not presented.

Research

In the role of information gatherer, you have the opportunity to focus in on specific areas of disease that your physician might not have the time to address without your help. In a typical day, the amount of time your primary care doctor or specialist has to look at any particular case in depth and ferret out new research is minimal. As one patient notes about her surgeon's case load:

> While I was waiting in the examining room, I heard my surgeon moving from room to room, from personal crisis to personal crisis. Mine was only one of many different types of surgery that he does in a single week. I realized how quickly he has to change gears to give my condition his attention. When it was my turn, he spent time explaining his basic concerns with me and then he told me where to go to find more information.

Dr. Susan Love, a noted breast cancer surgeon, says the following about the patient's contribution to information gathering and how it aids the decision-making process:

> I've learned from years of working with breast cancer advocates that no one is more motivated to become an expert on one disease than the person who has it. Doctors can use this to their advantage. The doctor's job is not to know everything, but to come up with the treatment that is most appropriate for each patient. Through research, the patients gain a much better understanding of their options and more realistic

*expectations for therapy. Together, doctor and patient can share both deci-
sion-making and responsibility.*[2]

Treatment feedback

It is your job as the patient to understand what needs to be communicated
and to make sure it gets communicated. For example, if you are a diabetic
who takes insulin, you will be the one who monitors your blood sugar and
reports significant changes.

Over time you develop an intuitive or experience-based awareness of when
your body is or isn't functioning properly. Trust this and share it with your
doctor. After a few days in the hospital with intestinal bleeding, this man
recognized a change that hadn't yet shown up in his lab reports:

> *I felt the bleeding had stopped, but there was no way to tell. It was
> just intuition. I was still passing blood, but it could have been from previ-
> ous bleeding. One of the diagnostic tests we were considering would only
> be useful if I was still bleeding. We decided to wait.*
>
> *You develop an awareness. During the bleeding, I experienced a taste
> and aroma that was so strong and pungent. I talked to my doctor about it.
> He said, "Oh yes, that's something I always look for." He said that he, too,
> can recognize the smell of internal bleeding.*

Preparing for your appointment

Unfortunately, doctors no longer have time to make house calls. In the clinical setting, they don't have time to get to know their patients on a more personal level. You and your doctor have a lot to accomplish during your six to
fifteen minute office visit. The better prepared you both are, the more satisfying the exchange will be. You can deepen the level of communication by
thinking through and outlining what needs to be accomplished during your
visit.

First of all, find out how long your appointment is scheduled to last. This
will help you organize your time better. You might want to inquire if you
should send your questions or pertinent information ahead of time rather
than try to present it all during your appointment. If the time allotted seems
inadequate, consider scheduling another appointment a few days later to
discuss the rest of your questions, if possible.

Make a list

It's helpful to keep a list of things to discuss at your next appointment. A list serves two purposes—it helps you prioritize and remember the things you want to discuss and it gives your doctor an idea of what you hope to cover during the visit. One patient explains her approach:

> I go in with my questions written and I give the doctor a copy. I realize it takes time to hear what patients are saying and give them information, but a doctor can say, "I don't have this information right now, can I send it or email it to you?"

A doctor explains how a written list helps him allocate his time during the appointment:

> If my patients have a number of questions and concerns, I like them to bring me a list so I can give appropriate attention to each item. If a patient expresses the most important concern at the last moment, as I am moving toward the door, it will not get the attention it deserves.

Include symptoms, medications, concerns, and questions in your list.

Bring medications

If you are taking more than one medication and have concerns about side effects or interactions, bring the medications to your visit. A primary care doctor explains why he prefers seeing the actual medications:

> Frequently people are not able to name all their medicines and dosages. Often I don't know all the things that my patients are taking if they are seeing other doctors. And sometimes the pharmacist changes the medications to whatever is covered by the patient's insurance plan formulary. The insurer recommended medication might be similar, but not identical. I can also look for possible interactions, confirm that the correct medications were dispensed at the pharmacy, and verify the dosages.

A woman helping her mother through an illness gives an example of how two medications given by different doctors were interacting and causing problems:

> My mother had been put on a diuretic when she was having heart problems. Another doctor put her on prednisone for an inflammation in her lungs. Apparently both medications make you eliminate water. Mom

was constantly having to use the bathroom and she had no energy. After I explained the symptoms and told the primary care doctor what my mom was taking, she adjusted the medications.

The bag of medications you bring in should also include vitamins, over-the-counter medications, and supplements that you take on a regular basis.

Take a friend and a tape recorder

In addition to taking your list of discussion items and your medications, consider taking a friend and/or a tape recorder. Some doctors are not as comfortable talking with a tape recorder, but most will agree if you explain the purpose. One doctor explains his feelings:

A tape recorder is a good idea. The only thing about tape recorders is that I feel like I have to speak with really good diction because whatever I say is going to get played back.

There are several good reasons to use a tape recorder:

- It frees you to participate in the conversation rather than having to take notes.

- Listening to a tape later often corrects misunderstandings. What you expected to hear is sometimes what you thought you heard rather than what was actually said.

- A tape is a much more accurate way to share information with other family members who are helping out but might not have been able to go to the appointment with you. You can also use it to clear up disagreements between family members or friends who did go to the same appointment and understood things differently.

Taking a friend or family member with you to an appointment can be especially helpful if that person agrees to act as a note taker and extra listener. Again, that frees you to participate more fully in the discussion.

Exchanging information with your doctor

Patient use of the Internet to find medical information has increased patient understanding and involvement in treatment planning. Doctors, however, are overwhelmed by patients who come into their offices with 200 pages of information that they have downloaded from the Internet for the doctor to read.

Doctors struggle to stay up-to-date on conventional literature in their own specific fields of practice. A large pile of papers from an unknown variety of sources is not likely to be welcomed. However, an informed patient who can ask thoughtful questions and provide appropriate input is a blessing to a busy doctor.

Take your doctor a summary of the information you have reviewed, with references to supporting information. Bring documentation, not advertising. Do the legwork. Find the supporting articles, the original articles, not someone else's interpretation of them or the abstracts.

Risks and benefits

Ask your physician for the full range of standard treatment options. Make sure risks and expected outcomes are clearly identified and explained. A man explains what he would like to hear from his doctor:

> I can summarize what I would have liked. I'd like the doctor to say, "This is what I know about your disease status. This is what I think can possibly happen, these are the percentages for what I can do and how much it will help you, and this is how I will let you know how you are doing."

One of the most confusing and frustrating parts of decision-making for patients is conflicting opinions from their doctors about which treatment choice is recommended. One woman describes her experience:

> My gynecologist said tamoxifen can cause endometrial cancer. He said he wanted to do an endometrial biopsy as a baseline test so if there were any changes, we could reconsider my continued use of the tamoxifen. When I told my oncologist, he said, "Oh, he's not up-to-date."

Don't be afraid to point out such conflicts and ask for a more specific explanation. Sometimes the conflict stems from a specialist's familiarity with a particular treatment modality, and sometimes it's a personal preference.

In the previous case, the oncologist probably meant that he didn't think a biopsy would be necessary because there are less invasive ways to monitor the uterine lining. But his comment could easily be interpreted that he thinks that endometrial cancer is no longer a concern.

It's reasonable to ask a doctor, "What would you prefer if you or your spouse were the patient?" But be sure to ask the doctor to explain why. The explanation will help you to understand the values that prompt the recommendation.

Asking comprehensive questions

Try to identify the critical factors that will affect your decisions before you go to your visit. If you are seeing a specialist, identify the area of your treatment in which the doctor is most likely to have experience and expertise. A woman describes how she was able to make maximum use of a fifteen-minute visit with a specialist:

> I went to see a gastroenterologist whom my doctor had recommended to perform a test my doctor thought necessary. I had scheduled time for consultation only, since the test was risky. I first needed to decide if I would do the test.
>
> I drove two hours to get to the specialist's office. Mine was the first appointment after lunch. He was late and his waiting room was full when I got called in.
>
> I sat in the examining room wondering how I was possibly going to get enough information to make the decision about whether or not to have the test scheduled for the next day. As it got later and later, I realized that he was going to be under pressure to rush through my appointment to get to the next patient.
>
> But my prior research paid off. When he came in, he did not need to explain the procedure to me. I knew my concerns. I told him I had come to him for his experience. I wanted to know the purpose of the test in my case, the frequency and severity of adverse effects he observed in his practice, and if he had an intuitive sense of the patient profile he found most likely to experience them.
>
> Based on those criteria, we were able to make the decision well within the fifteen minutes and even do a physical exam.

Providing additional relevant information

In addition to reviewing your list of questions, concerns, and symptoms, the office visit is the time to provide family history and previous medical history. This is also the time to talk about your personal attitudes toward quality of life, including physical and emotional comfort. All of these factors affect your treatment decisions.

One woman gets a quick idea of where she needs to fill in gaps by asking the doctor, "What do you know about me?" She explains:

> They tell me what they know about my medical situation, but they don't
> often ask me questions that would establish who I am as a person. What
> they see is a plump 60-year-old woman—they have no idea about me.

Creating a plan of action

The ultimate goal of informed decision making is to agree on a treatment plan. The objective of a single office visit is often only to identify the next steps toward that goal.

Remember that even when you do make a treatment choice, it is not set in stone. Most often the choice will rest on variables identified as you work with your doctor. The optimum treatment varies according to the situation. A doctor gives an example:

> If a person develops appendicitis, the safest course of action would be
> to go directly to the hospital to have his appendix removed. If, however, he
> were in an undeveloped country with poor medical facilities at the time,
> the safest course of action might be to go directly to the airport to catch a
> flight home.

About making a complicated treatment decision, a woman noted:

> I learned that what we think we know changes with every passing
> conversation, whether it's with our doctors, our therapists, or our
> children.

Many cases do not offer a clear best choice. In cases of diagnostic uncertainty, you may be choosing: 1) watchful waiting, 2) further testing, or 3) treatment to see if a response occurs. Sometimes you will combine two or all three of these approaches.

It is critical to build re-evaluation points into your treatment plan. To do this, you will need to address the following:

- Realistic expectations for your treatment options
- The criteria you will use to evaluate your response to the chosen treatment
- What feedback you can provide to monitor treatment progress
- Keeping careful records of all of your therapies, symptoms, and signs of improvement while you are in active treatment

If you and your doctor are both clear about the steps, the re-evaluation points, and how to communicate if a problem arises, you have both done your jobs well. A woman offers a realistic perspective on her expectations and relationship with her doctor:

> I had to be kind to myself going through all of this testing, diagnosis, and treatments. There was so much confusion. I sometimes felt overpowered by doctors who seemed to know everything and then disappointed that they didn't know enough. But I could never resent my doctor because he had so much compassion. I knew this man was on my side.

Handling potential problems

While informed consent requires that your doctor inform you of risks, benefits, and alternatives to a recommended treatment, informed decision making includes you as an active participant in the information gathering, processing, and decision making. Informed decision making takes more time for both doctor and patient.

In today's medical setting, appointment time and sometimes access to a doctor is limited. Both patient and doctor are caught in this dilemma. This section discusses the problems that can occur and suggests ways to handle them.

Insurance restriction

In the latter part of the twentieth century, healthcare costs skyrocketed. Patients have come to depend on health insurance to bridge the gap between the costs and what they can afford. Doctors also depend on insurance to protect them from malpractice suits. As a result, insurance companies exercise a lot of influence over the current practice of medicine. A primary care doctor talks about how this has changed the doctor-patient relationship:

> *The worst of managed care is overly restricted care, when zealous providers or cost conscious insurers, motivated by cost containment, limit care. In the past, the doctor was the primary patient advocate, unrestricted in ability to test or treat. In the early age of managed care, physicians were placed in the role of limiting care. When physicians are expected to limit care solely to save money, a wedge is driven between doctor and patient.*

Physician referral and treatment restrictions

Some insurance plans have a limited pool of contracted doctors. If you go to a doctor outside the plan you pay more, sometimes a lot more. A doctor who is a contracted provider for that plan may risk losing her contract if she refers you to a specialist outside the plan.

If your doctor feels that you will be best served by seeing a specialist outside the plan and you agree, there are a couple of approaches you can try. You can talk with the specialist about the problem and pay out of pocket, or you can make a request to your insurance company, explaining why that particular specialist is important to your care. If you can justify the need, the denial may be overridden.

Do not hesitate to ask when a treatment is recommended if it is the best treatment for your condition or if it is the best treatment available under your insurance plan. You can also make an appeal to the insurance company to pay for treatments that are not covered. It may take some research on your part and support from your doctor to show that this treatment is a reasonable request.

In the case of prescription drugs, sometimes your insurance company will recommend a lower cost substitute for a drug your doctor has prescribed. In some cases, that drug might not be as effective as the prescribed drug. If the pharmacist suggests a substitution, ask if the prescribed drug is covered by your insurance. Sometimes the substitution is only a recommendation. If your insurance does not cover the prescribed medication and your doctor feels that medication is significantly better, you can consider paying for it out of pocket and re-evaluate whether or not your current insurance plan is meeting your needs.

Restrictions on billable time

The time your doctor dedicates to working with you and researching your case outside of your office visit is rarely, if ever, covered by an insurance company. Face-to-face time is billable, but restricted. If your doctor spends two hours with you, chances are that only an hour at most will be paid for by insurance. Phone calls are usually not billable. The time spent reading through articles about your condition or treatment options is not billable. Many doctors will do research anyhow because they take their responsibility for your well-being seriously. But they are doing it on their own time.

A primary care doctor explains her dilemma:

> People are used to paying other professionals for services as they are needed, but not physicians. They'll pay an attorney or a car mechanic or a complementary therapist for each extra service, but they see healthcare as a right.
>
> It's nice if a patient says, "I'm willing to pay for the extra time I need," but if I am contracted with their company, I may not be able to accept it.
>
> The insurance companies I contract with have codes for patient consultation. You have to look up the code to see the fee that your contract allows you to bill. Some insurers have a code number for patient conferences, but don't pay for that service. If a patient with that insurance pays me out of pocket for a conference visit, I'm at risk of losing my contract if I accept the money.
>
> I often spend lots of extra time with a patient in crisis or one who has an immediate decision to make. I want to support them. Physicians want to provide enough information to help make choices, but it takes time. I spend evenings researching options for my patients. Right now I have a couple of manila envelopes full of information from two patients. I keep the envelopes in the car so that I can try to read the information during my children's piano lessons or dental appointments.

Another doctor talks about how administrative requirements can impact his available time:

> The level of complexity for a busy practitioner may approach that of an air traffic controller as he juggles patients in the office and hospital,

phone calls from patients, lab and x-ray reports, and the administrative burdens imposed by insurers and hospitals.

Doctors are plagued with endless submissions of copies of patient notes, justifications for treatment, and treatment denials.

Understanding the time problem helps. When possible, you can offer to reimburse your doctor for extra time spent. You can also plan to break your visits up into several appointments. And most important, come to your appointments prepared with a sense of what you can realistically expect to cover in the allotted time.

Who is my doctor?

When multiple doctors are working on a case, particularly in a hospital setting, it can become confusing. Sometimes it is not clear who is in charge of what or if everyone is talking with each other. One woman describes her concern that no one seemed to be monitoring her mother's condition:

My sister called to tell me Mom was not doing well. When I got there what I saw was Mom on full-time oxygen in her home, too weak to get herself out of bed or to the bathroom, too weak to transition from the wheelchair without my help. She was eating nothing except a few sips of chocolate shake.

I was thinking the primary care physician was monitoring all this. I think that's true but she had sent Mom to a pulmonary specialist and probably figured she would take care of whatever needed to be done.

But looking at the situation, I realized that no one was looking at the whole picture.

It's important to be clear about who is in charge of what. If you have come into the hospital as an emergency and your primary care doctor is not there, talk with the nurses to find out who is in charge of your care. A man hospitalized describes a well-coordinated situation:

I was impressed that all three of the specialists seemed to be working together as a team. I hadn't seen a situation like that before where you have an expert in each one of the areas trying to cover it from all corners. I think my primary care doctor arranged it that way.

Being labeled non-compliant

Many patients worry that if they disagree with their doctor's recommendation, they will be labeled as non-compliant. If you have developed a good working relationship with your doctor, that should not be a problem, but in some cases you must be assertive even when the doctor is resistant. A woman describes her surgeon's reaction to her request for a second opinion on a pathology report:

> I asked for a second opinion on my pathology report because the first was unclear. It hinted at in situ cancer but didn't confirm it. I could tell the surgeon saw me as something of a pest.
>
> He sent me a copy of his letter to the pathologist requesting that the samples be sent elsewhere. He had obviously added a comments slip to the original letter. He had dug in so deeply with his pen that I could read the imprint on the copy he sent me. It said, "Apologies for this, but patient is very (underlined three times) persistent." Like only "very persistent" patients have the gall to ask for a second opinion.

Eventually, this patient turned out to have invasive cancer, so her persistence paid off. It's better to be persistent when it could be a matter of life or death.

A woman describes her approach to getting the help she needed:

> I think that a lot of working your way through the system has to do with confidence. There's a nasty way to go about it, and you'll get attention, but I never was nasty...just dogged.
>
> I enlisted the nurses' involvement, was friendly with them, and clear about what I needed. I used words like "I am very concerned." If I had said, "I'm under stress," I would have gotten a different kind of attention. I could feel the word "concern" work when I was using it.

Another woman talks about how she let her doctors know what she had decided:

> I told my primary care doctor that I'd decided to have the surgery because it seemed clear to me that it needed to be done, but I didn't want to decide about the radiation and chemotherapy immediately. I was going to go hike.

I wrote to all the doctors concerned and said, "I appreciate your good intentions, but this is what I'm going to do." My doctors were very supportive. They said there was no immediate hurry. So I took three weeks and hiked. I was able to think and make decisions in a much more sensible frame of mind when I came back.

While an assertive patient may be higher maintenance than a passive one, most doctors appreciate a patient who is understanding and shares the decision-making responsibility.

CHAPTER 13

Making Your Decision

IF YOU WANT TO MAINTAIN CONTROL over the direction of your healthcare, you will have to make some decisions, or they may be made for you. In this chapter you'll find summaries of many of the concepts from earlier chapters on patients' rights, the power of information, and the fact that all decisions regarding your healthcare are yours to make. You can find information on your illness, learn from your physician(s) what the prognosis may be, and what you may experience with each type of treatment. When you integrate these facts with your own feelings and choices, you can make the decisions most appropriate to you, since the choices are ultimately yours. Included will be some questions to ask and some guidelines for making sure your wishes are followed if you are incapacitated in any way.

Difficulties of medical decisions

Learning to make daily decisions is a part of the life process. You make decisions such as what school to attend, what career to follow, where to live, which car to buy, which entrée to order at your favorite restaurant or what to wear to work. You're also experienced at making simple medical decisions such as when to go to the doctor or dentist for routine examinations and what kind of insurance to carry. When coping with a serious illness, the medical decisions feel different and they are much more difficult than the decisions and choices you make almost instinctively day-to-day. The uniqueness, and indeed seriousness, of medical decisions can be defined by five "I's": Irreversibility, Immediacy, Incomplete Information, Insurability, and Instinct.

- Irreversibility. Many medical decisions are irreversible. Each surgery or drug regimen may have a permanent or very long-term effect on your life and physical and mental well-being. Also, each step in treatment may eliminate options for further treatment of that condition or cause other symptoms to arise from a given course of therapy.

- **Immediacy.** The consequences of delaying a medical decision can be fatal or cause some deterioration in your condition that limits your options. The pressure to make a choice quickly adds to your stress at a time when you're just coping with a frightening diagnosis and not feeling you're strong enough to make difficult decisions. You may also be taking medications that complicate clear decision-making.

- **Incomplete information (or, information overload).** You may find in your experience and research that physicians interpret information differently, or that there are no clear-cut answers or studies covering long term prognosis for some of the medical or alternative therapies you are considering. There is a great deal of uncertainty in many of the new therapies and new drug treatments, yet these are the ones that carry the most hope. With the newest drugs, however, long-term adverse effects are not known.

- **Insurability and/or cost considerations.** You may have determined that a certain therapy or certain specialist is the optimum choice for your illness, but your insurance won't cover this therapy or specialist. Additionally, you may find that the most effective therapies are taking place across the country or outside the country, at some clinic you could not afford, or even spend the time to visit. Another very real "insurability" fear is that your insurance may be canceled due to some findings of an experimental diagnostic test or treatment. Actual cost versus cost of treatment is another important consideration. Insurance does not pay for everything. Even when a generous policy may pay for treatment at a distant medical center, it would not pay for your housing or the costs of childcare and house sitters, etc. As one patient who checked herself out of an observation stay at a hospital against her doctor's wishes put it, "Who is going to feed my children and cats and water my houseplants while you observe me?"

- **Instinct and intuition.** After hearing your physician(s) recommend one therapy over another, you may feel that you only want part of that therapy or that you specifically want to follow an entirely different course of treatment. You may have a strong feeling or intuition that one therapy is right for you. There may be quality of life considerations or a strong desire to be treated near your home and support network. Additionally, you may have found that a great deal of the research supports a different treatment path.

Components of a medical decision

To arrive at a medical decision, you would consider each fact, assumption, recommendation, and personal preference for your own treatment plan.

One woman dealing with decisions about her cancer therapy emphasizes the importance of taking some time to make these decisions:

> I think the decision-making is crucial. People think about getting medical leave for treatment, but I think you need it from the moment you know you have cancer. You need time to analyze your situation. If it's at all possible, you need to take time right away so you can evaluate things.

Basic elements to be factored into your medical decision include consideration of the following components:

- **The diagnosis.** What is the diagnosis and has it been confirmed?

- **Treatment recommendations from physicians.** What treatments are recommended and is there a second opinion favoring one course of treatment over another? Are there conflicting recommendations?

- **Preferences.** What are your preferences for recommended treatments based on the possible outcomes. How do you feel about the range of outcomes? How can you assure that your preferences will be followed?

- **Complementary/alternative treatments.** Are there alternative and/or complementary treatments that may be viable but have not been recommended?

- **Trade-offs and results.** What do you give up in selecting one option over another? Do the results of one treatment preclude following with another?

- **Risk and uncertainty.** What are the risks associated with each treatment and what are the uncertainties? Are you comfortable with risk-taking and uncertainty? You may be a risk taker or you may not. If none of the standard therapies appear to be effective in your situation, you may be willing to try riskier or unproved therapies.

- **Cooperation.** Will your physician and healthcare providers honor your decisions and work with you even if they don't fully agree with your choices?

Let's look at each of these components of a medical decision or choice and see how these can be implemented into your own decision-making process.

The diagnosis

If the diagnosis is serious, such as determination that a condition such as diabetes is nonreversible, or that a tumor is malignant, or your condition necessitates surgery, you would want to get a second opinion or verification of the diagnosis. In fact, some insurers and HMOs require a second opinion for any costly or long-term treatments. You may want a specialist to confirm the diagnosis, especially if a specialist did not make the initial diagnosis. You want to know exactly what you are facing.

A breast cancer patient found several opinions before making her own decisions:

> I think you need to feel that you've made an informed decision. I think it's absolutely crucial, given the state of breast cancer therapy today, and that means seeing more than one doctor. If I'd gone with the opinion of my surgeon, the first oncologist, and the first radiation therapist, I would have done a lumpectomy and radiation therapy and that would have been the wrong decision. I ended up seeing nine different doctors. I may not have needed nine, but the thing is when you see only one doctor, you don't see the confusion in the field. If you talk to more than one, you find out the going opinion will vary.

Treatment recommendations

If several treatment options are discussed, which are you most comfortable with? You can draw up a list of pros and cons for different treatments. You might also make a list which puts each suggestion in a hierarchy from the least invasive (do nothing) to most invasive (surgery with adjunctive therapies) and list the positive aspects and drawbacks of each. For every therapy there is usually a hierarchy of treatment protocols. These increase in complexity and possible complications as the treatment gets more aggressive. Think of the treatment choices and how you feel about each one.

Sometimes the most invasive approach will give you more peace of mind, knowing that you have taken the most complete approach. Sometimes selecting the path of doing nothing will seem appropriate—especially if none of the treatments have a good prognosis or if your diagnosis is uncertain.

Some therapies bring on such drastic side effects that they may be worse than the disease you are trying to defeat.

A woman with MS tried the new drug Betaseron but finally abandoned that treatment:

> I took Betaseron for seven months. It involves giving yourself an injection every other day, and so I was sick every other day. I was home and could do nothing. I would just lie around, watch the OJ trial, and wish I wasn't sick. I discontinued it after seven months because the side effects were so significant. Luckily, I was on a medical leave because I could never have worked while I took that drug and I've never been sorry I stopped.

While the physician, often a specialist, will treat the specific disease, she may not consider your full medical history. The physician may not know, for example, that your father suffered from a rare blood disease when she recommends Coumadin, which might bring on the disease for you. Most of the drug references have lists of contra-indications which spell out the conditions and parallel drug therapies that would cause problems and drug interactions with a given medication.

One cancer survivor tells about her experience terminating one drug therapy because it caused another serious medical problem:

> There were important considerations that affected my decisions since I have a co-existing autoimmune disease about which only I have full perspective. It is an inherited problem—my mother died of lupus at 50 and I have similar autoimmune mechanisms. Instead of lupus, I have autoimmune problems with my liver. They manifest as chronic active hepatitis, for which I have spent many days being hospitalized. My oncologist was hesitant about my rejecting an additional 4 cycles of Taxol when I found a large number of articles on the adverse effects of Taxol in relation to liver disease. I was very fearful that my cancer would be dealt with, but I would be left with irreversible liver disease. I have changed oncologists and now have a much more receptive one.

Occasionally, the physician, often a general practitioner provided by your HMO, will not have enough experience to make fully informed decisions. David Eddy, in his book *Clinical Decision Making*, makes some excellent points. He notes that physicians must make decisions about very complex problems and that they need more solid information about the consequences of clinical choices. Outside sources such as insurance companies cannot effectively make medical decisions, since they look primarily at the bottom line. He advocates that "we must build processes that support, not dictate, decisions."[12-1]

Preferences

Once you know your diagnosis, treatment recommendations, and you have an expectation of given outcomes, you can stop for a moment and look at your personal preferences. What do you know about each type of treatment and its impact? What is the most desirable outcome you can expect? Would you avoid surgery, even if the nonsurgical options usually result in poor outcomes? Are there less invasive types of surgery such as laparoscopic or endoscopic surgery that have similar outcomes to traditional surgery? Even if you have always thought you would never spend a day in a hospital, does this diagnosis change your mind? Do you have religious or spiritual values that impact medical preferences? Is your family or circle of friends urging you to undergo treatments that go against your wishes? Often family and friends urge you to choose one option over another out of their fears and concerns for you or even for themselves. They don't want to lose you and may urge you to try absolutely every therapy there is. You are the one who knows the chances of success of each option and it is you who will live with the side effects.

One woman gives her reasons for choosing a difficult therapy:

> *The decision was hard because treatment options are such a gray area but I would have done whatever it took at that point. I also felt that I was likely to feel pretty unwell for quite some time whichever treatment I was on. Actually, I imagined chemo as far worse than it really was. I decided as long as I was going to feel ill, I might as well be getting something that might work. Quality of life was something I could put on hold for awhile. In a way I thought of the approaching six months of treatment as hibernation.*

You are the one person who must personally live with the consequences of any treatment. You have many considerations besides the actual treatment of a specific disease to contend with.

One man shares his experience of having many friends advise him to take many different paths to treatment:

> I have a good friend who gave me a bunch of books on cancer and its healing which helped my decision process. As I began to make my decisions, some friends really wanted me to have surgery, some wanted me to have radiation, some wanted me to have both. It seemed that whatever I did, I would disappoint somebody. Then this good friend who had given me the books came through with a wonderful gift of wisdom. She said "Well, when they have their cancer, they can decide what to do for themselves. This is yours and you get to choose."

While many treatments may be proposed, each will impact your quality of life. Will you be incapacitated for a long time or in pain long after the treatments have ended if you choose a certain course of treatment? Is that acceptable to you? Will you be able to participate in life with your family, or be able to work, or even be conscious enough to enjoy music and interactions with friends and family?

Complexity/disruption of life

Hand in hand with quality of life are the considerations surrounding the complexity of treatment choices and the disruptions they may require. For example, you may have to drive 100 miles one way to participate in a clinical trial at a university. Or you may have to actually move to a distant locale such as the Mayo Clinic in Rochester, Minnesota, or Memorial Sloan-Kettering in New York, if you want a particular therapy available only at one of these centers. Who will handle your obligations at home if you make one of these choices? If your family cannot come with you, can you face treatment without their support?

Complementary/alternative treatments

Have any complementary and/or alternative treatments been recommended or have some been overlooked? Have you found that an alternative therapy is being used successfully as the primary treatment for a given condition or is it being used as a complementary therapy to augment and support traditional treatment? Alternative and complementary therapies include acupuncture, massage, diet therapy, yoga, and stress reduction techniques and a host of other therapies. These are seldom recommended as the only treatment, but they can make traditional therapies more effective and certainly more tolerable. You can choose to include them in your own treatment plan even if your physician has not recommended them. It is always important to tell your physician about any complementary therapy to be sure that the treatments are supportive of each other and not conflicting. There is much more on this in Chapter 9, *Complementary and Alternative Therapies*.

One woman who was dealing with intractable pain tells about her experience trying hypnosis:

> I was so excited when I heard about this psychologist who has excellent results using hypnosis to deal with pain. I remember going back to my doctor and telling him I wouldn't need to keep taking the numerous pain medications we were trying. He's usually so positive, but instead of saying "Stop everything," he said "This is wonderful. Let's cut back a little and wait and see." That was lucky for me because even though I learned to hypnotize myself, I was not able to make a difference with this kind of pain.

Trade-offs and results

What are the trade-offs or results of each treatment being proposed? If you were told you should have a hysterectomy, your ability to bear children would be ended. You would also enter what is known as "surgical menopause" and may have to deal with hormone imbalance immediately, instead of gradually at a later date. If you have heart bypass surgery, will your physical activities be limited or will they be enhanced? Each treatment will have some impact and force some changes in your life. You want to be clear about the results of each type of treatment including the complementary and alternative treatments. Trade-offs and results often limit future medical options. If you have chemotherapy, you may not be able to enter a clinical trial at a later date. If you have your spleen removed, you won't be able to take certain medications that may become important to you. If you are taking Coumadin or other blood thinner to prevent blood clots, you would be at high risk for emergency surgery.

Ask your physician and other caregivers about these results and trade-offs. You don't want to blindly follow some treatment path only to find out at a later date that one treatment precludes another effective therapy. You can also consult many of the medical texts and databases mentioned in earlier chapters to search for prognosis, adverse effects, complications, and long-term success of a given treatment.

Risks and uncertainty

All choices, even for the most proven therapies, have unknowns and associated uncertainties. Your own inherited physical makeup and your medical history will impact your therapy. You may have a strong family history of heart disease, so you would be very careful about trying some therapy that is known to exacerbate heart conditions. You may have undergone some drug therapy or developed an unknown concurrent disease that could cause serious complications in a normally routine therapy at a later date. Other co-existing conditions will alter your prognosis. For example, if you are diabetic, you may be more prone to postoperative infections than someone who does not have diabetes. Patients with very low or very high blood pressure are considered to be more of a risk in surgery.

If exact outcomes could be determined, medical decisions would be easy for you, as well as for your caregivers. The more experimental a treatment is, the more uncertain the outcome. Each person is unique and few experience the same exact outcomes for a given treatment. Psychologically, you may be able to handle uncertainty and risk more easily than another patient. You may be the "Evil Knievel" of medicine—ready and willing to try anything, with no risk too frightening. If traditional therapies become ineffective, you might be willing to try riskier or less proven therapies. Both you and your physician can look at as many of the outcomes as possible to determine the most acceptable course of treatment.

A woman describes how she weighed the risks and benefits of keeping her ovaries before her hysterectomy:

> I did not want to make a drastic change to my system, unless there had been enough research done to state statistically if you have a non-cancerous fibroid or ovarian cyst, you are at higher risk for ovarian cancer. I was perfectly happy in giving up my period, but the ovaries were another story as they regulate the hormones and I really wanted to go through a natural, normal menopause. So I called my doctor and asked

her two questions. The first was: "Is there any evidence in the research to show that a person with my condition is at higher risk for ovarian cancer than a person who does not have this condition?" She said there was no evidence to suggest that. The second question was, "If you were me, would you want to give up your ovaries?" She said, "I am not sure."

You are probably already familiar with basic decision making tools such as the simple two-column list of pros and cons or assigning a numerical score to each option in selecting the best option for you. Medical decision-making can be more complex because there are many individuals involved in the decisions and also because the consequences of each decision are more permanent. Another tool is called a "decision tree", which is simply a way to visualize a medical decision and look at the process (see Figure 13-1). A good explanation of decision trees and clinical decision making is in the JAMA "Users Guide to the Medical Literature" series.[12-2] A decision tree is actually a flow chart showing your medical options and indicating where each may lead.

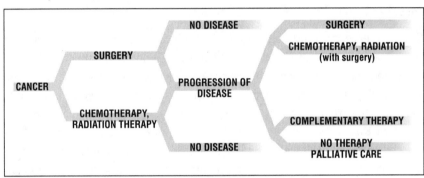

Figure 13-1. Sample decision tree for cancer treatment

In drawing a decision tree, you want to know if all of the realistic clinical strategies were compared, and if all of the clinically relevant outcomes were considered. The visual mapping out each of the options can help you see each choice and where it may lead.

Cooperation

You will want and need the cooperation of your physician and caregivers to implement your choices. Many people interview physicians to be sure they have the same values that you do regarding treatment. Most doctors are willing to work with patients and encourage and support them when they add complementary therapies such as meditation and/or acupuncture into their treatment plans. Other physicians may not support such choices. It's important to feel that you can work with your doctor and that you understand each other. You might create a list of a few questions to help you determine your potential doctor's philosophy of practice. Some sample questions are:

- How long does an average patient visit last?
- Do you work with patients over the telephone?
- Who covers your practice when you're away?
- Are you comfortable with patients who want to act as healthcare partners, or do you feel more paternalistic towards patients?
- Are you willing to spend some time answering questions?
- How do you feel about complementary and alternative medicine? Could you discuss these types of therapies comfortably?

In the event of more serious illness, Dr. George Burnell, in his book *Final Choices*,[12-3] lists some questions you can ask your physician. It's always a good idea to ask questions about end of life issues while you are still healthy.

Questions about treatment of pain, life support equipment, and hospice care can help you determine if you and your doctor share the same philosophy. If you sense condescension or your doctor laughs at your questions, you can feel warned that you may not get the cooperation you need if you are truly facing serious illness. The most effective doctor-patient relationship is one based on trust and respect.

Decision, choice, and responsibility

You may be overwhelmed by information and conflicting findings and decide to let your medical team make decisions for you. If these are people you have come to trust, this may be the best situation for you. In another situation, you may want to control each choice. You may want to choose an alternative therapy or choose to abandon one course of therapy once it has begun. All of these options are yours to take.

Do you have to make decisions?

Actually, you don't have to make your own decisions. You may be more comfortable allowing the doctors and medical personal to make recommendations and treatment choices. You can find lots of people ready and willing to decide for you, from physicians and hospital personnel to family and friends. However, if you want your wishes followed, you'll probably have to be alert and make your own decisions.

You can appoint someone familiar with your wishes to decide for you if you are incapacitated. In the sixteenth Century, Alexander Pope wrote in his *Moral Essays III*, "Who shall decide when the doctors disagree?" Today there are many more opinions than those of doctors. With the advent of managed care, insurers may insist on the least-costly options, while your physician and the research may show that the more complicated and costly therapies have fewer side effects and greater long term benefit. Hospitals often have their own restrictions regarding which therapies they are prepared to support, and indeed, which therapies they must administer despite your wishes. These agencies and individuals may conflict with your own preferences.

The final decision is still always yours. If you do not take charge, the person or corporation making medical decisions for you may make your interests and preferences a secondary concern.

Deciding *not* to have treatment

You may not want anyone to choose for you, but decide NOT to take any action. By deciding not to undergo treatment, your medical condition may become more severe and your options will be much more limited if you finally do decide on a treatment course. Deciding not to have treatment is your right, but you will have to be very clear about this.

Physicians, nurses, and hospitals have a commitment to saving lives and our current healthcare system is dedicated to keeping people alive even if it results in a poor quality of life. In fact, physicians and hospitals are under pressure from the fear of malpractice lawsuits to show they have done everything possible to save each patient. Hospitals will usually have release forms you can sign. Your physician may understand your wishes and want to cooperate with you, but still worry about a malpractice lawsuit at a later date if you change your mind or if your relatives feel your physician withheld treatment. You can write a simple letter to your physician absolving him of responsibility for your decision and yet encouraging him to remain as your advisor. Following is an example of such a letter.

Sample letter:

> *Dear Dr. Jones,*
>
> *After reviewing the long-term effects of the radiation treatment you have recommended, I have decided to refuse this treatment. I understand that you have given me the advantage of your best medical insights and that I have weighed and considered each recommendation.*
>
> *I hold you and your clinic harmless for any consequences of my decision to refuse treatment, including my premature death if it should come to that. I have also instructed my family to hold you and your clinic harmless for a decision that is mine alone.*
>
> *I'm having this letter witnessed and notarized so that it will protect you legally from any consequence of my actions. I have valued your caring concern and advice during each step of my treatment, and I sincerely hope that you will continue to be my medical advisor, since we have many medical decisions yet to make. Thank you and your staff for your very kind and patient care. It means a great deal to me.*
>
> *Sincerely,*
>
> *Jane Doe*
>
> *Date:_____ Witnesses:_____*
>
> *Date:_____ Notary:_____*

Deciding to stop treatment once it has started

Along with choosing not to have a certain treatment, it is your right to stop a treatment after it has started. Some therapies may have such debilitating side effects, that it is just not worth having the treatment. Your quality of life may have become worse than certain death and you do have the right to abandon a certain therapy. You should make a decision like this in consultation with your physician in case there might be some problems of withdrawal from a certain medication or if you needed some other drug to help you cope with the side effects. You could modify the sample letter in the previous section, if your physician doesn't fully agree with your decision.

One woman talks about listening to her intuition when she just knew it was time to stop chemotherapy:

> On the fifth month of chemo, I went to have my blood work done and my white cells were way below 1,000. I went to the grocery store, and at the grocery store, I suddenly, it was like I was paralyzed, I could not move. We called my husband and he picked me up and we called the doctor's office. The doctor's office thought it might be flu, and prescribed antibiotics.
>
> I said to my husband "You know, it is not the flu." My intuition and that spiritual energy that helps me to make decisions felt really strong all of a sudden and I said, "You know what, I have a feeling my body is telling me it has had enough." I mean, they say "Six months of chemo." Why? It is just a totally arbitrary number.
>
> Anyway, I decided that I would not do any more chemo. I just knew it was time to stop. So the next day I called the oncologist's office and said that I wanted to speak with the doctor. His nurse said he was busy but that she could relay a message. I told them my body had gone into a crisis and I decided I would not do any more chemotherapy. I told them I felt that it was probably my body's way of telling me that it was enough. The doctor relayed the message back that it was fine to stop the chemo. I was annoyed that he didn't talk to me personally, though.

Arranging for others to carry out your decisions

You never know when you might need to make a medical decision. It's a good idea to make your feelings and preferences for care known to your family and friends as well as your doctor, in case you are involved in an accident or experience some acute or life-threatening situation. Of course, it's always wise to think of these things when you are physically and mentally in good health. It's not easy to think of yourself in a helpless situation where you couldn't communicate your wishes, but that is a possibility.

What happens when you can't make a decision?

In medicine there are acute or immediate emergencies, and there are chronic conditions or long-term care decisions. When the condition is acute, there is often no time for decision. If you are delivered comatose to the hospital emergency room in an ambulance, the emergency physicians will probably be making your medical care decisions. Types of acute situations are a heart attack, burst appendix, a stroke, an automobile accident involving traumatic injuries, or even a fall from a swing set. Often emergency service workers help you or your family select the facility best equipped to deal with your emergency.

One way you can become involved in even emergency medical decisions is to have Advance Directives, including a "medical durable power of attorney" and a "living will." The medical durable power of attorney authorizes an individual to make decisions for you if you are incapacitated. The living will spells out your own preferences for resuscitation, interventions, and other important guidelines such as blood transfusion. Since 1991 federal law has required that all healthcare institutions and agencies provide you with information about Advance Directives.

You don't need a lawyer to make out a living will, but it must be signed by you in front of two witnesses who are eighteen years of age or older and who are not related to you or employees of any facility where you are a patient. Of course, the witnesses must also sign and date the living will. If you include directions regarding the specific types of treatments you wish to include or restrict, you will make the living will more useful. Such treatment that may concern you can include tube feeding, CPR or cardiac resuscitation, antibiotics, dialysis, blood transfusions, and any other medical intervention about which you feel strongly.

The medical durable power of attorney document actually authorizes someone to act as your agent or attorney-in-fact to communicate your wishes in the event that you are hospitalized due to a temporary or permanent illness or injury. The medical durable power of attorney helps you retain some control over medical decisions so that caregivers and family members do not have to guess about your wishes. This document, like the living will, can include specific instructions on specific treatments such as CPR. One nurse, who had seen many patients resuscitated when it was their wish to refuse this treatment, jokingly remarked that she was going to have DNR or "Do Not Resuscitate" tattooed on her chest, so that the caregivers would have a clear direction. She had taken care of so many people who could not communicate their wishes, she wanted to be absolutely clear about her own.

It's important to make your living will and medical durable power of attorney documents readily available in the event they are needed. One way to make them available is to make several copies and leave them with your family, your doctor, your attorney, and even your local hospital if they are prepared to keep such documents well in advance of an admission. The original copy should be filed with other important papers.

If the person you would select to act in your behalf is not a direct relative, it is even more important that you have a legal medical durable power of attorney. You may choose a close friend because they know your wishes, or you may choose someone living near you if all of your relatives live a great distance away. If there is no formal legal connection, your close friend or partner may not be able to voice your wishes over those of distant blood relatives or even over those of hospital administrators.

One woman tells of her "just in time" decision to sign advance directives and durable powers of attorney:

> My partner and I went to an attorney and had living wills and durable powers of attorney forms made up. We had been together a long time and were somewhat estranged from our respective families. I wanted someone I could trust, someone who knew my wishes, to be my spokesman if I ever had a medical emergency—not some relative I hadn't spoken to in years. I was always glad we had decided to sign those documents. It was hard at the time—facing the fact that you might be so sick you couldn't make your wishes known.
>
> But what happened, was two months after we had gotten those documents, my partner got seriously ill and had to go to the emergency room and then was in Intensive Care for three days. I was so relieved to know I could be sure that his preferences were honored, even when he was too sick to talk. I think everyone should have those advance directives, even if they are pretty young. None of us will live forever.

Currently each state has different laws regarding living wills and medical durable powers of attorney. An excellent organization that keeps track of the current legislation and even can provide documents that meet the advance directive requirements for different states is Choice in Dying. Their web site is *http://www.choices.org*, and their telephone number is (800) 989-WILL or (800) 989-9455.

After you've done everything you can to communicate your decisions about medical care, you can trust you've done all you can for the moment. Even seemingly acute situations may allow some time for decision-making. A diagnosis like a malignant tumor, a gall bladder attack, or cataracts will necessitate treatment, but not usually in the emergency room. With these types of problems, there is some time to gather information and make treatment choices. For example, after the emergency room treatment of a heart attack, there may be recommendations for open-heart surgery or balloon angioplasty or even a heart transplant. Each of these options can be considered and decided upon. Later there will certainly be some recommendations for lifestyle changes involving diet, exercise, and stress reduction. When dealing with medical conditions and treatment, there are always decisions to make.

Always your choice

It is important for you to remember that most choices will always be yours to make. Your right to make medical choices pertaining to your own body is supported by law and by your own force of will. Choices, which are always yours, include the following:

- You control your own diet and exercise unless you are being fed intravenously.

- You can control your own attitude towards dealing with an illness or condition. You can take a proactive and positive point of view and make decisions for your care that encompass hope. This can often be difficult and you can ask for help in keeping your attitude positive.

- You can choose to be a part of each decision in your treatment plan.

- You can choose to include supportive therapies such as massage, meditation, and counseling to help you cope with your illness.

- You can choose to forego some or all of a therapeutic process. For example, you might accept radiation but not chemotherapy, or you might work with a physical therapist to alleviate some type of joint pain, but refuse surgery when it is recommended for the same condition. You might also at some point refuse all treatment if the treatments are ineffective or the adverse effects are intolerable, or just because you feel that your quality of life is so diminished that it is better to allow nature to take over.

- You can choose to change doctors or clinics. These are not realistic options for all patients, but many individuals change doctors right in the middle of therapy. They find that they have better rapport with one doctor over another or that one clinic or hospital will support complementary and alternative therapies that they wish to follow. It's your body.

- You can choose to ask for assistance from friends and family. While you may be too weak to do many of these things for yourself, your loved ones will appreciate your direction in allowing them to help you focus on your healing.

- Finally, you can choose to learn all you can about your condition so that you will make decisions on your care based on facts rather than fears and misconceptions. Your knowledge will give you strength in deciding the course of your treatment and give you a voice in your own care.

One individual emphasized how individual and personal medical decisions are:

> When you make a decision you are prepared to live with it or die with it. I say to people, "There is nothing you can say until it happens to you." You cannot say, "I would have done this, or I would not do that, if I had it." There is no way to know, for all your bravery, and belief system and whatever, until it happens to you. Then you make your decision. You can't know what you will finally do, when you are making choices that may mean life or death.

A woman tells about knowing when it was time to stop looking for newer and better therapies and to just be. She compares her choices to poker:

> One of the things I'm finding is you have to know when to hold. In other words, don't bet higher. There's a temptation to get the most aggressive care to take care of the cancer. When I considered joining the study group, I finally had to say, "hold."

> Two of the three doctors I talked to said the drug combination would probably be better in terms of its effectiveness. But in my case, the chances of metastasis are small, so the absolute advantage might be only 1 to 2 percent benefit. Although if the cancer comes back, I'm sure I'll wonder whether I should have decided to "hold."

The frustrating reality is, of course, that you can only decide with the facts available at the moment. Medical history encompasses a series of breakthroughs that have permanently altered the current course of therapy. What if there had been penicillin in the First World War? What if the smallpox vaccine had been discovered in Roman times, and what if bacterial infection and disinfecting practices had been widely known during the plagues of the Middle Ages? One sad fact of medical decision-making is that you usually cannot wait for the breakthrough treatment to be discovered. Most often, you need to take action quickly or your condition may deteriorate and even become untreatable.

So you make your decisions with the best information you can get from all of the sources you can find and just accept the fact that you've done what you can do. Then it's time to let go and focus on your healing.

One woman eloquently describes the point when she was ready to make decisions:

> There was a point where you have read so much, and talked to so many people. You do become familiar with it, you become knowledgeable and informed. There is definitely a saturation point, where you just don't want to read one more book or article about it. It's like you simply come to understand that "I know what I need to know to make my choice."

Patient Questionnaire

THE FOLLOWING QUESTIONNAIRE will help both the patient and the friend or family member offering research assistance to identify research goals and guidelines.

Have the person for whom you are researching answer these questions about what's most important for him at this time. Needs and interests do change, sometimes rapidly. We suggest you copy this blank form and reuse it as needed. (As mentioned in Chapter 2, if you're researching treatments, you'll need the exact description of the condition—from a doctor, pathology report, etc.—and an exact description of recommended treatment or options.) Be sure to discuss any questions or answers you do not understand clearly.

The kind of information I'm interested in

- Contact names _____.
- A comprehensive list of information you find, so I can point out what I'm interested in.
- A recommendation (e.g., for what treatment or other topic) along with brief reasons why and who/what you consulted in forming this opinion.
- I need this information by (if there's a date) _____.

The level of information I would like to read

- Full text of what you find (books, journal articles, clinical trial listings).
- A summary only of what you find.
- Source materials aimed at physicians, including statistics.
- Digests of technical information, e.g., review articles or in-depth patient information.
- Graphic descriptions of treatments or possible outcomes.
- Only information that can give me hope and comfort. Spare me statistics of how well an "average" patient might do.
- No technical terms; material written for lay people, but in detail.
- Material written for lay people, in very abbreviated form.
- Specific answers to specific questions, only.

Standard medical care

- What is the standard accepted level of care?
- What are the current treatment controversies?
- Are there other medical treatments in use by some doctors or at some facilities with advantages of higher cure rates or fewer side effects?
- Are there any clinical trials for my disease? What are they testing?
- Other issues? (These might include knowing what insurance will cover; how to request a second opinion; how to obtain medical records; how to fill out an advance directive or medical power of attorney and what it means; and what it means to and how to refuse certain treatments.) _____

Doctors and treatment centers

- Who are the recognized experts on disease/procedure?
- Who are regarded as experts in this general area, i.e., whom could I see for a second opinion?
- Who are recognized as good, competent, local doctors?
- Which of the following doctors are highly regarded? What specialties, board certifications, and training do they have? Are there lawsuits pending or has disciplinary action been taken against them? _____

- Are there reasons I might want to consider going to a specialist or super-specialist for treatment?
- Which facilities are best suited for my treatment if travel is no object?
- Which of the following facilities would be best suited to my treatment needs? What is each of their expertise and reputation? _____

- Are there reasons why I might want to consider going to a particular type of facility for treatment?

Physical coping with condition or side effects

- What are possible side effects from the treatments that have been recommended to me or that you have researched?
- What methods of coping do doctors, nurses, and other healthcare providers suggest? Are there benefits for me having physical therapy, occupational therapy, or other follow-up care?

Complementary and alternative therapies

- Are there any complementary therapies that could help me cope with a condition or course of treatment? (Nutrition, vitamin supplements, stress reduction, acupuncture, massage, yoga, psychologic pain relief, therapeutic touch, visualization, biofeedback, chiropractic, herbal medicine, etc.). I'm particularly interested in: _____

- Therapies I don't want to consider:_____

_____

- Recommendations for complementary therapy practitioners.

Organizations, support groups, patients to talk to

- What national organizations provide information and support for patients in my situation? What services do they offer?
- What local or regional organizations offer information and support?
- What support group meetings are nearby? Who are they for? When/where do they meet? Who leads them?
- Are there other patients who've been through what I'm experiencing who are willing to talk to me? Characteristics I'd like that patient to have (e.g., close in diagnosis/treatment, same sex, close in age, someone with a positive experience, etc.): _____

_____

- Who are the contacts for support groups in my area?
- What books/articles deal with being a patient with this condition/treatment? Particulars to avoid/look for are: _____

_____

(For example, I don't want to read about anyone with my condition who dies; I don't want to read a particular religious interpretation; I don't want to be told that I caused my disease or can think it away; etc.)

Other factors important at this time

(Can rank as 1, 2, 3..., with 1 being most important.)

- Having someone listen to me and be with me.
- Receiving the most aggressive treatments to maximize chance of survival.
- Making sure I get a good standard of care.
- Understanding my options.
- Receiving standard medical treatments, proven by years of data for large groups of patients.
- Receiving emerging medical therapies with the best chance for success.
- Using complementary therapies that will not conflict with Western techniques.
- Making sure that my doctor is well-trained and experienced.
- Following what my doctor tells me, unless there's some compelling reason to make another decision.
- Experiencing humane, compassionate care from my medical care providers.
- Being treated close to home.
- Going to a local doctor.
- Going to a local hospital/treatment center.
- Conserving my energy.

- Keeping costs down.
- Making sure my insurance plan covers treatment.
- Getting physical support to deal with the condition/treatment.
- Minimizing the symptom/side effect: _____
- Retaining qualities of life I especially value (in my daily environment and activities):_____
- Receiving emotional support. I expect to get this support from my (doctor, nurses, friends, family, church, community, support group, therapist, etc.):____ _____
- Receiving spiritual support of the kind: _____
- Getting practical help at home (for example, getting meals on the table, laundry, taking care of children, taking care of pets, cleaning, yardwork, shopping, etc.):_____
- Receiving help getting to medical appointments.

  Getting help with finances (for example, figuring out insurance, filling out forms and calling about claims, battling for coverage, seeing if any group can help me pay for expenses, etc.): _____

Resources

THE LIST THAT FOLLOWS reiterates some of the groups, publications, services, and web tools discussed throughout this book, and includes additional resources that also may serve your needs. All entries in each category are listed in alphabetic order, not by importance. See the "Notes" section for more resources.

Knowing your rights

One of the first steps in making a medical decision is knowing that you are entitled to privacy, consent to all procedures, and to have copies of your medical records and tests. You also want to be certain that recommended physicians and caregivers are currently licensed and certified. The web sites, organizations, books and articles listed below can help you obtain the information you need in protecting your rights.

Organizations and web sites

Association for Responsible Medicine
http://www.a-r-m.org

The online medical malpractice magazine stating "if you must go into the hospital, go ARMed with the facts."

The American Board of Medical Specialists (ABMS)
47 Perimeter Center East, Suite 500
Atlanta, GA 30346
(800) 733-2267
http://www.certifieddoctor.com/verify.html

Publishers of *The Official ABMS Directory of Board Certified Medical Specialists,* a directory of board certified physicians who have chosen to specialize in a particular area of medicine. Use The ABMS to check specialists' credentials.

The American College of Surgeons (ACS)
633 North Saint Clair Street
Chicago, IL 60611
(312) 202-5000
http://www.facs.org

The American College of Surgeons can verify whether your surgeon is board certified in a surgical specialty. It also maintains a web site that lists other valuable information such as the ACS list of accredited cancer treatment centers.

MIB, Inc. (MIB)
Medical Insurance Board
P.O. Box 105
Essex Station
Boston, MA 02112
Phone: (617) 426-3660
FAX (781) 461-2453
http://www.mib.com

MIB is a voluntary membership association of life insurance companies in the US and Canada, with about 600 members. MIB maintains coded records that include resumes of medical conditions, tests, etc., on many individuals. You can request your own record to find out what is on file about you. The small fee for this and an application is on the MIB web site.

Books and articles

Alpers, A. "Respect for Patients Should Dominate Health Care Decisions." *Western Journal of Medicine* 170, no.5 (May 1999): 291–2.

Annas, G. J. "Informed Consent, Cancer, and Truth in Prognosis." *New England Journal of Medicine* 330 (1994): 223–5.

Beck, C. S. "The Needs of the Patient Come First." *Mayo Clinic Proceedings* 75, no.3 (March 2000): 224.

"Big Browser is Watching you!: Privacy Special Report, Part One," *Consumer Reports,* May 2000, 43–50.

Blau, Sheldon P., and Elaine F. Shimberg. *How to Get Out of the Hospital Alive: A Guide to Patient Power.* New York: Macmillan, 1997.

Dickey, N. W., and P. McMenamin. "Putting Power Into Patient Choice." *New England Journal of Medicine* 341, no.17 (21 October 1999): 1305–7.

Dickman, R. L. "Bending the Rules to Get a Medication." *American Family Physician* 61, no.5 (March 2000): 1563–4.

Ellig, David H. *A Patient's Survival Guide, Or, Never Get Naked On Your First Visit.* Mesa, AZ: Med. Ed. Inc., 1992.

Freeman, V. G., and others. "Lying For Patients: Physician Deception of Third Party Payers." *Archives of Internal Medicine.* 159, no.19 (25 October 1999): 2263–70.

Johnson, Diann, and Sidney M. Wolfe, MD. *Medical Records: Getting Yours A Consumer's Guide to Obtaining and Understanding Medical Records.* Washington, DC: Public Citizen's Health Research Group, 1995.

Keene, Nancy. *Working with Your Doctor: Getting the Healthcare You Deserve.* Sebastopol, CA: O'Reilly & Associates, Inc. 1997.

Napoli, Maryann, "A Second Opinion: How to Get One and Why You Should," *HealthFacts,* January 1999, 1–6.

Robson, R. "Debating the Patient's 'Right to Know.'" *Canadian Medical Association Journal* 160, no.9 (4 May 1999): 1321–4.

Medical tests

It is important to know what your medical tests reveal and how to interpret the results of those tests. You are, of course, entitled to copies of each test and it is a good idea to keep those copies with your medical records. You can use the organizations, web sites, books and articles below to assist you in deciphering test results as well as in determining that you are getting the appropriate test(s) for your situation.

Organizations and web sites

The Biology Project. University of Arizona: *http://www.biology.arizona.edu.*

Department of Pathology, University of Washington, Seattle: *http://www.pathology.washington.edu.*

The University of Michigan Pathology Laboratories Handbook. Enter the test name and click "search": *http://po.path.med.umich.edu/handbook.*

The University of Pennsylvania Cancer Center. Enter the test name and click "search": *http://www.oncolink.upenn.edu.*

Books and articles

Andrews, Maraca, and Michael Shaw. *Everything You Need to Know About Medical Tests.* Springhouse, PA: Springhouse Corp., 1996. An excellent comprehensive reference written for the patient in a readable and respectful style.

Brodin, Michael B. *The Encyclopedia of Medical Tests.* New York: Pocket Books, 1997.

Fischbach, Frances. *A Manual of Laboratory and Diagnostic Tests,* 6th ed. Philadelphia: Lippincott, Williams & Wilkins, 1999.

Griffith, H. Winter. *Women's Health: A Guide to Symptoms, Illness, Surgery, Medical Tests and Procedures.* New York: Perigree Books, 1999.

Stauffer, Joseph, and Joseph C. Segen. *The Patient's Guide to Medical Tests: Everything You Need to Know About the Tests Your Doctor Prescribes,* 4th ed. New York: Facts on File, 1998.

Zaret, Barry, L., MD, ed. *The Patient's Guide to Medical Tests.* Boston: Houghton Mifflin Co., 1997.

Information resources

The organizations, web sites, books and articles listed below include some of the most useful general medical resources. The information from these resources provides a good "first step" in finding information to support your medical decision making.

Organizations and web sites

General

Centers for Disease Control and Prevention (CDC)
1600 Clifton Road
Atlanta, GA 30333
(404) 639-3311
http://www.cdc.gov

EurekAlert
http://www.eurekalert.org
A clearinghouse of scientific, medical, and technological press releases.

US Food and Drug Administration (FDA)
http://www.fda.org

Internet Health Sites
http://www.silcom.com/~noster/wcindex.html
This is the list compiled and updated by Nancy Oster, with the help of Lucy Thomas and Darol Joseff, MD, from sites used to teach the Internet Health class mentioned in the Preface of this book. This web site is updated frequently and contains over 100 evaluated health links.

National Cancer Institute (NCI) Public Inquiries Office
Building 31, Room 10A03
31 Center Drive, MSC 2580
Bethesda, MD 20892
(800) 4-CANCER
http://www.nci.nih.gov

National Institutes of Health
Bethesda, Maryland 28092
http://www.nih.gov

National Library of Medicine (NLM)
US National Library of Medicine
8600 Rockville Pike
Bethesda, MD 20894
(800) 338-7657
http://www.nlm.nih.gov

The main NLM web site includes links to the MEDLINE database PubMed; MEDLINEplus, for consumer health; the "clinicaltrials.gov" database; and other valuable medical information. NLM is the world's largest medical library.

National Women's Health Information Center (NWHIC)
(800) 994-WOMAN
http://www.4women.gov

The National Women's Health Information Center is a free, one-stop gateway for women seeking health information. It is designed for consumers, researchers, health professionals, and educators. It includes health news, legislation, information in Spanish, a search engine, dictionaries, and much more.

US Patent Office Databases
http://www.uspto.gov/patft
Search for a chemical name or patent number. Entries include references submitted with the patent applications.

Doctors' web sites

There are many physician-sponsored web sites with general and directed medical information. Most ask for registration to use features such as email alerts on specific medical topics, or health assessment, or medical records organizers. While each of these sites offers excellent information, be cautious about maintaining your own privacy. Give only the required data and feel very free to change your name or some other identifier. It's a good idea to withhold a key identifier such as your Social Security Number or mother's maiden name. While the web sites say they are secure, computer experts recommend caution.

Several of these useful web sites are listed below:

America's Doctors
http://www.americasdoctors.com

This very popular site offers a dialogue feature stating that they have "real doctors-real answers-real time."

Dr. Susan Love's web site
http://www.susanloveMD.com

Sponsored by Susan Love, MD, a web site for women's health issues. Offers weekly live chats and a special in-depth women's health topic each week.

drkoop.com
http://www.drkoop.com

The best prescription is knowledge, according to C. Everett Koop, MD.

Ferguson Report
http://www.fergusonreport.com

From Tom Ferguson, MD, one of the pioneers in online health information, this free newsletter has excellent links and recommendations.

Health Central
http://www.healthcentral.com

From Dean Edell, MD.

Journey of Hearts.
http://www.journeyofhearts.org

From Kirsti Dyer, MD, MS, a healing place in cyberspace for enhancing physical and mental well-being...for anyone who has ever experienced a loss.

Mayo Health
http://www.mayohealth.org

From the Mayo Clinic.

Medscape
http://www.medscape.com

George Lundberg, MD, Editor in Chief.

Legal and financial issues

Affording Care
429 East 52nd Street, Suite 4G
New York, NY 10022-6431
(212) 371-4740
http://www.thebody.com/afford/affordix.html

Financial information for those with serious illnesses. Publishes a free newsletter, "The Affording Care Bulletin."

Cancer Treatment Centers of America
http://www.cancercenter.com

A list of national cancer organizations, advocacy groups, and other valuable resources.

The Center for Medical Consumers
237 Thompson Street
New York, NY 10012
(212) 674-7105

Provides information referrals to other organizations and maintains a medical consumer's library.

Consumer Credit Counseling
(800) 388-2227

Provides help getting expenses under control.

Federal Trade Commission
(202) 326-3650

Can provide information about the Federal Consumer Credit Protection Act, a landmark series of laws passed in 1968 to protect debtors.

Health Care Cost Hotline
(900) 225-2500

Can furnish the median fee and range of fees charged by doctors for various services and procedures. The call is $2.00 to $4.00 per minute.

Health Insurance Association of America (HIAA)
555 13th Street NW
Washington, DC 20004
(202) 824-1600
http://www.hiaa.org/index.html

Has more than 250 members consisting of insurers and managed care companies. HIAA can supply booklets on disability income, health insurance, long-term care, medical savings accounts, and general insurance information, including a directory of state insurance departments.

Patient Advocate Foundation (PAF)
780 Pilot House Drive, Suite 100-C
Newport News, VA 23606
(800) 532-5274
http://www.patientadvocate.org/paf/welcome.html

Provides education and legal counseling to cancer patients concerning managed care, insurance and financial issues.

Professional research organizations—fee-based

American Society for Information Science (ASIS)
8720 Georgia Avenue, Suite 501
Silver Spring, MD 20910
(301) 495-0900
http://www.asis.org

Association of Independent Information Professionals (AIIP)
7044 South 13th Street
Oak Creek, WI 53154-1429
(414) 766-0421
http://www.aiip.org

Medical Search Services
http://www.cancerguide.org/search_service.html
From Steve Dunn's *CancerGuide,* a list of services, as well as guidelines for evaluating these services.

Books and articles

General

Daus, Carol. *Past Imperfect: How Tracing Your Family Medical History Can Save Your Life.* Santa Monica, CA: Santa Monica Press, 1999.

Morse, Janice M., and Joy L. Johnson, eds. *The Illness Experience: Dimensions of Suffering.* Newbury Park, CA: Sage Publications, 1991.

Oxman, Andrew D., MD, David L. Sackett, MD, and Gordon H. Guyatt, MD. "Users' Guides to the Medical Literature: I. How to Get Started." *Journal of the American Medical Association* 270, no.17 (3 November 1993): 2093–7.

Spiegel, David. *Living Beyond Limits.* New York: Fawcett Columbine, 1993.

"Users Guides to the Medical Literature." *Journal of the American Medical Association's* "Users'Guides" is a continuing series, each article addressing a particular aspect of the medical literature. At the time of this writing, the series contained over twenty articles. Search on the title in the PubMed database under "Users' Guides to the Medical Literature" to locate the full collection of articles.

Medical dictionaries

American Heritage. *Compact American Medical Dictionary*. Boston: Houghton Mifflin, 1998.

Dorland's Illustrated Medical Dictionary. Philadelphia: W. B. Saunders Co., 2000.

Jablonski, Stanley. *Dictionary of Medical Acronyms & Abbreviations*. 3rd ed. Philadelphia: Hanley & Belfus, 1998.

Magalini, Sergio and Sabina Magalini. *Dictionary of Medical Syndromes*. 4th ed. Philadelphia: Lippincott, Williams & Wilkins, 1997.

MEDLINEPlus (*medlineplus.gov*). A web site with links to medical dictionaries and encyclopedias.

Mosby's Medical, Nursing & Allied Health Dictionary. 5th ed. St. Louis: Mosby, 1998.

Tabers Cyclopedic Medical Dictionary. 18th ed. Philadelphia: F. A. Davis, 1997. (New edition planned for 2001.)

Standard treatment

Standard treatment may be viewed as the traditional treatments taught in medical schools and provided in hospitals. The list of resources below can help you determine which treatments are considered "standard" for your condition. The information may also be useful in understanding that standard treatment may vary from place to place.

Books and articles

Coleman, C. Norman. *Understanding Cancer: A Patient's Guide to Diagnosis, Prognosis, and Treatment*. Baltimore, MD: Johns Hopkins University Press, 1998.

Dambro, Mark R. *Griffith's 5-Minute Clinical Consult, 2000*. Philadelphia: Lippincott, Williams & Wilkins, 2000.

Dudley, R. A., and others. "Selective Referral to High-Volume Hospitals: Estimating Potentially Avoidable Deaths." *Journal of the American Medical Association* 283, no. 9 (March 2000): 1159–66.

Justice, Amy C., MD, Kenneth E. Covinsky, MD, and Jesse A. Berlin. "Assessing the Generalizability of Prognostic Information." *Annals of Internal Medicine*, 130, no.6 (16 March 1999): 515–24.

Payer, Lynn. *Medicine and Culture: Varieties of Treatment in the United States, England, West Germany, and France*. New York: Henry Holt and Company, 1996.

Rakel, Robert E., MD. *Conn's Current Therapy: Latest Approved Methods of Treatment for the Practicing Physician, 2000*. Philadelphia: W. B. Saunders, 2000.

Root-Bernstein, Robert and Michele Root-Bernstein. *Honey, Mud, Maggots, and Other Medical Marvels: The Science Behind Folk Remedies and Old Wives Tales*. Boston: Houghton Mifflin, 1997.

Stevens, Larry. "Medical Megasites: One-stop Shopping?," *Medicine On the Net*, July 1999, 9–10.

Tierney, Lawrence. *Current Medical Diagnosis and Treatment 2000*. 39th ed. New York: McGraw-Hill, 2000.

Clinical trials

Clinical trials are highly regulated processes used to test the quality, value, safety, and usefulness of certain procedures, drugs, or medical devices. The information below is useful in finding trials and evaluating them as treatment options for your own medical situation.

Organizations and web sites

Clinical Trials in the United States
http://www.clinicaltrials.gov

Sponsored by the National Institutes of Health and the National Library of Medicine, this web site makes information available on both privately and publicly funded clinical trials.

European Organization for Research and Treatment of Cancer (EORTC)
http://www.eortc.be/protoc/default.htm

A European cancer clinical trials database.

University of Pennsylvania Oncolink Clinical Trials Information
http://www.oncolink.org/clinical_trials

From the well known "Oncolink" database, this section explains clinical trials and lists many key trials and links to clinical trial information.

Books and articles

Assendelft, William J., and others. "Scoring the Quality of Clinical Trials." *Journal of the American Medical Association* 283, no.11 (15 March 2000): 1421.

Finn, Bob K. *Cancer Clinical Trials: Experimental Treatments and How They Can Help You.* Sebastopol, CA: O'Reilly & Associates, 1999.

Geisler, R. Brian, and Stephen D. Williams. "Opportunities and Challenges: Assessing Quality of Life in Clinical Trials." *Journal of the National Cancer Institute,* 90, no. 20 (21 October 1998): 1498–9.

Kalb, Claudia. "To Be A Guinea Pig: How to Decide On Entering a Clinical Drug Research Trial." *Newsweek* (19 October 1998): 86.

Macbeth, Fergus and Richard Stephens. "Marketing Clinical Trials." *Lancet* 348, no. 9020 (13 July 1996): 111–2.

Mathews, N. S. "Sponsored Trials Do Not Necessarily Give More Favourable Results." *British Medical Journal* 318, no. 7200 (26 Jun 1999): 1762.

"Testing New Drugs: Joining a Study Can Be Rewarding—But Risky," *Consumer Reports*, December 1998: 54–64.

Complementary and alternative therapies

Complementary and alternative medicine (CAM) involves a wide range of healing philosophies and therapies. Generally, it is considered to be those treatments not usually taught in medical schools or used widely in hospitals. As complementary and alternative therapies have become more widely accepted, they have begun to be seen as "Integrative Therapies," i.e., integrating traditional treatment with other valuable healing techniques. The resources listed below can assist you in finding more information about this growing field of medicine.

Organizations and web sites

General

American Holistic Medical Association (AHMA)
http://www.holisticmedicine.org

Focuses on the art and science of healing that addresses the whole person—body, mind and spirit. There is also an AHMA student section.

NAPRALERT
http://www.info.cas.org/ONLINE/DBSS/napralerts.html

Natural Products Alert is a fee-based database maintained by the University of Illinois. It includes profiles on various natural products and adds approximately 600 articles per month.

University of Texas Center for Alternative Medicine
http://www.sph.uth.tmc.edu/utcam/resink.htm

National Center for Complementary and Alternative Medicine (NCCAM)

NCCAM Clearinghouse
P.O. Box 8218
Silver Spring, MD 20907-8218
(888) 644-6226
TTY/TDY: (888) 644-6226
FAX: (301) 495-4957
http://nccam.nih.gov

The NCCAM has funded Specialty Research Centers for focusing on specific conditions. The Aging Center at Stanford is no longer listed with the NCCAM, nor is the Cancer Center at University of Texas—funding and personnel changes may impact research sites. Each year the NCCAM sites may change.

Center for Addiction and Alternative Medicine Research (CAAMR)
Minneapolis Medical Research Foundation
914 South Eighth Street, Suite D917
Minneapolis, MN 55404
Phone: (612) 347-7670
Fax: (612) 337-7367
http://www.mmrfweb.org/caamrpages/caamrcover.html

CAAMR specializes in addictions. Its principal investigator is Thomas J. Kiresuk, PhD.

Center for CAM Research in Aging & Women's Health
Columbia University
College of Physicians & Surgeons
630 West 168th Street, Box 75
New York, NY 10032
Fax: (212) 543-2845
http://cpmcnet.columbia.edu/dept/rosenthal

The center's specialties are aging and women's health. The principal investigator is Fredi Kronenberg, PhD.

Center for Alternative Medicine Research on Arthritis
University of Maryland School of Medicine
Division of Complementary Medicine
2200 Kernan Drive
Baltimore, MD 21207-6693
http://www.compmed.ummc.umaryland.edu

The center's specialty is arthritis. Its principal investigator is Brian M. Berman, MD.

CAM Research Center for Cardiovascular Diseases
715 East Huron Street
Suite 1W
Ann Arbor, MI 48104
Phone: (734) 998-7715
Fax: (734) 998-7720

This center specializes in cardiovascular diseases. Its principal investigator is Steven F. Bolling, MD.

Center for Natural Medicine and Prevention
College of Maharishi Vedic Medicine
Fairfield, IA 52557
Phone: (515) 472-1129
Fax: (515) 472-1167
http://www.mum.edu/CNMP

This center specializes in aging, minority health, and cardiovascular disease. Its principal investigator is Robert H. Schneider, MD.

Consortial Center for Chiropractic Research
Palmer Center for Chiropractic Research
741 Brady Street
Davenport, IA 52803
http://www.c3r.org

This center's specialty is chiropractic. Its principal investigator is William C. Meeker, DC, MPH.

Oregon Center for Complementary and Alternative Medicine Research in Craniofacial Disorders
Center for Health Research
Kaiser
3800 North Interstate Avenue
Portland, OR 97227-1110

The center's specialty is craniofacial disorders. Its principal investigator is B. Alexander White, DDS, DPh.

Oregon Center for Complementary and Alternative Medicine in Neurological Disorders
Oregon Health Sciences University
3181 SW Sam Jackson Park Road, Mail Stop CR-120
Portland, OR 97201
http://www.ohsu.edu/orccamind

This center's specialty is neurological disorders. Its principal investigator is Barry S. Oken, MD.

Pediatric Center for Complementary and Alternative Medicine
University of Arizona Health Sciences Center
Department of Pediatrics
1501 N. Campbell Avenue
P.O. Box 245073
Tucson, AZ 85724-5073
Phone: (520) 626-5170
Fax: (520) 626-3636

This center specializes in pediatrics. Its principal investigator is Fayez K. Ghishan, MD, DCH.

Books and articles

Blumenthal, Mark, ed. *The Complete German Commission E. Monographs: Therapeutic Guide to Herbal Medicines.* Austin, TX: American Botanical Council, 1998. On the web at *http://www.herbalgram.org.*

Eisenberg, David M., MD. "Advising Patients Who Seek Alternative Medical Therapies." *Annals of Internal Medicine* (1 July 1997): 61–9.

Fugh-Berman, Adriene. *Alternative Medicine: What Works: A Comprehensive Easy-To-Read Review of the Scientific Evidence Pro and Con.* Baltimore: Williams & Wilkins, 1997.

"Going Online to Find Alternative Medicine and Treatment." *Medicine on the Net,* September 1999, 9–12. On the web at *http://www.mednet-i.com.*

Graedon, Joe, and Teresa Graedon. *Dangerous Drug Interactions: How to Protect Yourself from Harmful Drug/Drug, Drug/Food, Drug/Vitamin Combinations.* New York: St. Martin's Press, 1999.

Goleman, Daniel and Joel, Gurin, eds. *Mind Body Medicine: How to Use Your Mind for Better Health.* Yonkers, NY: Consumers Reports Books, 1993.

Joyce, Christopher. *Earthly Goods: Medicine Hunting in the Rainforest.* Boston: Little Brown & Co., 1993.

"The Mainstreaming of Alternative Medicine," *Consumer Reports*, May 2000, 17–25.

PDR for Herbal Medicines. Montvale, NJ: Medical Economics, 1998.

Pelletier, Kenneth R. *The Best Alternative Medicine: What Works? What Does Not?* New York: Simon & Schuster, 2000.

Review of Natural Products. St. Louis: Facts and Comparisons, 2000. Updated monthly, a comprehensive source of evaluated scientific information about natural products including toxicity, interactions and pharmacology.

Tyler, Varro E. *The Honest Herbal: A Sensible Guide to the Use of Herbs and Related Remedies*. New York: Pharmaceutical Products Press, 1993.

"Web Resources: Alternative Medicine." *Medicine on the Net*, September 1999, 13–6.

Wolfe, Sidney M., MD, and others. *Worst Pills, Best Pills: A Consumer's Guide to Avoiding Drug-Induced Death or Illness*. New York: Pocket Books, 1999.

Evaluating and using statistics

Statistics are routinely used in making medical decisions and yet they are not always clearly explained or understood. The additional resources listed below can help you understand the use of statistical information and assist you in making your own decisions based on a better understanding of statistics.

Organizations and web sites

STATS
http://www.cmh.edu/stats/journal.htm
"How to Read a Medical Journal Article," by Steve Simon from Children's Mercy Hospital in Kansas City.

An excellent tutorial and in-depth guide to reading and evaluating a medical article.

Harvard Center for Risk Analysis
http://www.hsph.harvard.edu/Organizations/hcra/hcra/html
Launched in 1989 by the Harvard School of Public Health, the mission of the Center for Risk Analysis is to promote reasoned public responses to health, safety, and environmental hazards.

Books and articles

Cohn, Victor. *News & Numbers: A Guide to Reporting Statistical Claims and Controversies in Health and Other Fields*. Ames, IA: Iowa State University Press, 1989.

Dewdney, A. K. *200% of Nothing: An Eye-Opening Tour Through the Twists and Turns of Math Abuse and Innumeracy*. New York: John Wiley & Sons, 1993.

Gordis, Leon, MD. *Epidemiology*. Philadelphia: W. B. Saunders, 1996.

Gould, Stephen Jay. "The Median Isn't the Message," *Discover* June 1985, 40–42.

Huff, Darrell. *How to Lie With Statistics*. New York: W. W. Norton, 1993.

Kelly, Patricia T. *Understanding Breast Cancer Risk*. Philadelphia: Temple University Press, 1991.

Lauden, Larry. *Danger Ahead: The Risks You Really Face on Life's Highway*. New York; John Wiley & Sons, 1997.

Lauden, Larry. *The Book of Risks: Fascinating Facts About the Chances We Take Every Day.* New York: John Wiley & Sons, 1994.

Lewis, H. W. *Why Flip a Coin? The Art and Science of Good Decisions.* New York: John Wiley & Sons, 1997.

McKibbon, Ann, with Angela Eady and Susan Marks. *PDQ: Evidence-Based Principles and Practice.* Hamilton, Ontario: B. C. Decker, 1999.

Pitkin, Roy M., MD, and others. "Accuracy of Data in Abstracts of Published Research Articles." *Journal of the American Medical Association,* (24/31 March 1999): 1110–1.

Sackett, David L., and others. *Clinical Epidemiology: A Basic Science for Clinical Medicine.* 2nd ed. Boston: Little Brown, 1991.

Walsh, James. *True Odds: How Risk Affects Your Everyday Life.* Santa Monica, CA: Merritt Publishing, 1996.

Weaver, Jefferson Hane. *Conquering Statistics: Numbers Without the Crunch.* New York: Plenum Press, 1997.

Whittelsey, Frances Cerra. "Red Flags in Journal Articles: Learn to Spot Research Studies that Don't Measure Up." *MAMM* (September/October 1999): 28–9.

Making your decision

Books and articles

Eddy, David M. *Clinical Decision Making From Theory to Practice: A Collection of Essays from the Journal of the American Medical Association.* Sudbury, MA: Jones and Bartlett, 1996.

Sox, Harold C., Jr., MD. *Medical Decision Making.* Newton, MA: Butterworth-Heineman, 1988.

Glossary

Absolute risk
Measures the difference in risk between two groups. Used for describing the clinical impact of a treatment.

Acid reflux
Gastric fluids that travel back up the esophagus from the stomach.

Accrual
Process of recruiting patients into a trial. Also refers to number of patients in trial.

Adenoma
A polyp; an initially benign growth that forms in the colon from the innermost layer of mucin-producing epithelial cells.

Advance directives
Written statements made prior to a serious illness that explain your treatment preferences and who you would like to make treatment decisions if you become unable to make them yourself. Living wills and durable powers of attorney for healthcare are examples of advance directives.

Adjuvant treatment
Treatment that occurs after potentially curative primary treatment. Usually given in expectation of preventing recurrence.

Alzheimer's disease
A neurological form of dementia which includes the progressive loss of memory, thinking skills, and coordination.

Anecdotal evidence
A physician's case report or an individual patient's story illustrating a particular outcome. Not as reliable for predicting outcomes as a reports substantiated by studies treating large numbers of people.

Anemia
A lack of adequate numbers of oxygen-carrying red blood cells.

Anesthesia
A medical technique that reduces or eliminates consciousness, pain, and voluntary movements by administering medications that create a sleeplike state.

Anesthesiologist
A physician who studies and administers anesthesia.

Angiogram
A diagnostic x-ray that tracks the flow of blood through the blood vessels. An injection of dye enhances the image of the vessels.

Angioplasty
Repair of a damaged blood vessel through widening (usually via a small balloon-tipped instrument which is inflated in the vessel) or reconstruction.

Anonymous remailer
> A computer service that forwards an email message with a dummy return address so that the sender's identity is not revealed.

Antiangiogenesis
> Prevention of the growth of new blood vessels into a solid tumor, restricting the blood supply to the tumor.

Antihypertensive
> Drugs used for high blood pressure.

Antiretroviral
> A drug that inhibits the activity of a retrovirus. The Human Immunodeficiency Virus (HIV) that causes AIDS is a retrovirus.

Arm of a clinical trial
> Trial subgroup. All trials have at least two arms, the control group and the treatment group. Some compare multiple treatment options, so they will have multiple arms.

Arthroscopic
> Use of a tubular viewing device to examine the inside of a joint.

Ataxia-telangiectasia
> A rare genetic disorder that includes progressive neurological problems and immune system abnormalities that begin in childhood.

Atherosclerosis
> Accumulation of fat and other materials in the artery that can restrict the flow of blood through the artery.

Autistic
> Mental disorder characterized by withdrawal from interaction with other people.

Autoimmune
> When the immune system begins to attack the body's own healthy tissue.

Autologous
> Coming from your own body. An autologous blood transfusion is done using blood that was drawn from an individual prior to surgery.

AZT
> An antiviral drug used in the treatment of AIDS.

Bile duct
> Duct that carries wastes from the liver through the gall bladder to the small intestine.

Bioelectromagnetic
> The effects of electromagnetic fields on living beings.

Bio-markers
> Substances identified in the body fluids such as the blood or in tissues. These markers may indicate an increased likelihood of some types of disease.

Biologic
> A serum, toxin, antitoxin, or analogous microbial product used for prevention, cure, or treatment of disease or injury. A vaccine is a biologic.

Biomedical

Referring to the use of engineering methods and instrumentation to increase the understanding of and to help solve medical problems.

Biopsy

The removal and examination of fluid or tissues for study under a microscope for characteristics of a disease.

Biotechnology

Biological approaches and use of living organisms for research and product development. Antibiotics and insulin are the result of biotechnology as are bread making, cheese making, and beer brewing.

Bone marrow transplant (BMT)

Treatment which involves the use of higher dose chemotherapy than can normally be tolerated by a person's bone marrow. After the treatment, the bone marrow is replenished using donor bone marrow or the person's own immature bone marrow, removed prior to the high dose chemotherapy (autologous bone marrow transplant).

Calcium channel blocker

Drug used to treat high blood pressure, chest pain, and irregular heartbeat.

Cardiologist

Heart specialist.

Carpal tunnel syndrome

Numbness, soreness, or tingling in fingers caused by nerve pressure in the wrist.

Case control study

A group of people with the disease is compared to a group of people without the disease to study for exposures which might contribute to the development of the disease being studied.

Case study

A physician's report on an unusual case.

Cataplexy

Sudden loss of muscle tone.

Celiac disease

Improper digestion caused by sensitivity to the protein in grains like wheat and rye.

Chemotherapy or chemo

Use of drugs to treat disease; usually refers to cancer.

Chiropractor

Practitioner who uses spinal manipulation as a therapy to correct disorders of the nervous system.

Cholectcystectomy

Surgical removal of the gallbladder.

Cholelithiasis

Severe abdominal pain occurring in spasms. Caused by a gall stone lodged in the bile duct.

Clear margins
    Removal of healthy tissue surrounding the diseased tissue to ensure that all diseased tissue has been found and removed.

Cocci
    A type of bacteria.

Colitis
    Inflammation of the large intestine.

Colectomy
    Surgical removal of the colon.

Colonoscopy
    The examination of the entire length of the colon, up to its juncture with the small intestine, using a flexible tube that has a camera and a light source attached.

Complete blood count or CBC
    A count of the red, white, and platelet cells in peripheral blood.

Complete remission
    The disappearance of all signs of disease for a period of time.

Computed tomography (CT)
    A scan used for examining the soft tissues and internal structures of the body, using low doses of ionizing radiation to do the imaging and computer technology to interpret and produce the images. A head CT scans the head in thin slices. (Also known as computed axial tomography CAT.)

Confidence interval (CI)
    The range within which the true results might fall if multiple studies of the same size were performed. The standard interval is based on a 95 percent confidence range.

Contraindication
    Caution about the increased risk of use of a drug or therapy in patients with particular conditions or characteristics.

Control group
    The group of people in a trial that does not receive the experimental treatment. Compares those treated experimentally to those not treated or those being treated with the most effective proven treatment.

Coronary artery bypass graft (CABG)
    A piece of vein or artery from another part of the body is used to bypass a blocked heart artery.

Correlation
    The degree to which one occurrence affects another. A positive correlation predicts that an increase in one variable is associated with the increase in another.

Coumadin
    Drug used to thin the blood to prevent the development of blood clots.

CPT Codebook
    Contains numerical codes assigned to medical procedures, services, and supplies. The codes are used to standardize billing and the ordering of tests. Updated annually by the American Medical Association.

Cyst
Benign sacs or closed cavities that are filled with fluid.

Dapsone
An antibiotic used to treat skin disorders such as leprosy, as well as to prevent or treat a type of pneumonia.

DES (diethylstilbestrol)
A synthetic hormone approved for use in the 1940s to reduce complications of pregnancy. DES was later linked to an increased risk breast cancer in the women who took it and an increased risk of vaginal cancer in the daughters of women who took DES. It was taken off the market in 1971.

Digoxin
Medication that strengthens the heart muscle to prevent congestive heart failure. Also used to correct irregular heartbeat.

Diplomate
A physician who has received certification in a particular specialty.

Diuretic
Any medication that is used to increase the output of urine.

Double-blinded
Neither the patient nor the physician knows which arm of the trial the patient is on. Revealed only at the end of the trial.

Durable power of attorney for healthcare
A signed, dated, and witnessed document which identifies an "agent" or "proxy" to make medical decisions for you if you are not able to make them for yourself.

ECOG Performance Status
Scale developed by the Eastern Cooperative Oncology Group (ECOG) for measuring patient's level of physical disability from fully active and able to work (ECOG 0) to completely bedridden (ECOG 4). Most trials require at least ECOG 1 or ECOG 2.

Efficacy
Effectiveness.

Electrocardiogram (ECG or EKG)
An electrocardiogram produces a graphic record of heart rhythms.

End point
A specific identifiable event or state that is measured by the study (e.g., disease-free survival for five years, death of patient, etc.)

Endometrial
In or on the inner lining of the uterus.

Endoscope
A small camera, used during surgery, which allows the surgeon to observe internal structures of the body on a television monitor.

Endoscopic surgery
Surgery aided by the use of an endoscope.

Epidemiology
The study of populations to find patterns of disease and factors that influence those patterns.

Ethnobotanist
A scientist who studies the traditional use of plants in various cultures. Many of today's most successful medicines have been derived from medical uses described in the traditional lore of indigenous people.

Evaluable disease
Can be deduced, but the physical manifestation is not measurable.

Evidence-based medicine (EBM)
The process of finding and evaluating current research literature to develop a thorough understanding of the strength of evidence for the effectiveness of the available clinical treatment options.

FEC (fluorouracil-epirubicin-cyclophosphamide)
A drug combination used to treat cancer (more commonly used for breast cancer in Europe).

Fen-phen
A drug combination used for weight loss. One of these medications was taken off the market after the discovery that the risk of heart valve damage exceeded the benefits.

Flow chart
A diagram used for project management or decision-making. Identifies the steps needed to reach a particular goal, with decision or evaluation points where a choice must be made between alternate paths.

Fully-sourced
Completely documented and referenced.

Gallbladder
Organ which stores bile, the fluid that breaks down fats and transports wastes from the liver.

Gallstones
Stone-like collections of cholesterol, calcium salt, or bile that are sometimes formed in the gall bladder and pass into the bile duct.

Gastrointestinal
Referring to the digestive system.

Gastroenterologist
Physician who specializes in the problems of the digestive system.

Gleason scale
A grading system for prostate cancer cells. A high Gleason score indicates that the cells are very abnormal.

Granuloma
A mass of tissue that may form in certain disease processes.

Hemoglobin
The iron-containing protein found in a red blood cell that can bind to and transport oxygen.

Herbalism
Medicinal and nutritional uses for plants in their natural form.

HMO (health maintenance organization)
A managed care organization that provides a predetermined periodic prepayment to the contracted healthcare provider on a per patient basis, regardless of the amount of services provided for an individual patient.

Hodgkin's disease
Cancer of the lymphoid tissue, usually found in the lymph nodes or spleen.

Holistic
Looking at how the parts of the body function together as a whole.

Homeopathic remedies
Very small doses of medicine or herbs, which are believed to heal by stimulating the immune system.

Homogeneous
Composition is the same through the structure or group.

H-pylori (helicobacter pylori)
Bacteria found to be the cause of many gastrointestinal ulcers.

Hyperbolic
Exaggerated.

Hyper-irritable
Easily irritated and excessively irritable.

Hypertension
High blood pressure.

Hydrocephalus
Accumulation of fluid in the cranium. Sometimes called "water on the brain."

Hypoglycemia
Low blood sugar.

Hypothesis
Expected response of a disease to a proposed treatment, or theory of disease cause and development.

Hysterectomy
Surgery to remove the uterus.

ICD (International classification of diseases)
International numeric categorization of diseases or conditions requiring medical treatment. The first three digits before the decimal point represent the disease category. The numbers following the decimal point represent the disease sub-category.

Idiopathic
Unknown cause.

In situ cancer
Non-invasive. An in situ tumor has not grown into surrounding tissue. Not all *in situ* cancers spread.

In vitro
Medical research done in test tubes or petri dishes, not in a living organism.

In vivo
> Medical research done to study the response in living tissue, such as research on laboratory animals.

Inapparent disease
> No observable symptoms of disease.

Inborn error of metabolism
> Disorder of a chemical process of the body, present at birth.

IND (Investigational New Drug) application
> Request to the FDA to begin testing new drug on human subjects.

Informed consent
> Acknowledgement that the patient understands the risks, benefits, possible complications, and alternatives before agreeing to have the treatment or procedure.

Internist
> A physician who manages a general variety of medical conditions for adults. A specialist in internal medicine sometimes also has other subspecialty areas.

Intervention
> Treatment or therapy.

Interventional study
> A study comparing two matched groups where participants in one group receive the treatment or intervention and those in the other group do not.

Invasive
> A disease that has spread into other tissues of the body, or a treatment which penetrates body tissues.

Investigational
> Still under study.

IRB (Investigational Review Board)
> Committee that reviews clinical trial proposals and procedures to ensure that they provide sufficient protection of the well-being of trial participants and disclosure of potential risks to the participants.

ISP (Internet service provider)
> Commercial company which provides Internet access to individuals or companies.

Interlibrary loan
> Library network that allows libraries to borrow resources from each other for their patrons.

Karnofsky Performance Status
> Rates severity of symptoms and degree of disability from 100 percent (no symptoms) to 0 percent (deceased).

Laparoscope
> A fiber-optic device inserted into the body to view areas within the body for diagnostic and surgical procedures.

Leprosy

A chronic disease that affects the skin, mucous membranes, and parts of the nervous system. It is caused by bacteria, but is not highly contagious. Can lead to loss of sensation and, in its most serious form, deformation.

Leukemia

The uncontrolled growth of white bloods cells in bone marrow, often overflowing to the circulating blood.

Listserver

An Internet mailing list or discussion group. Mailing list software at the subscription site sends all subscribers any email sent to the mailing list address.

Living will

A written statement of your treatment preferences should you become too ill to express those preferences.

Lyme disease

Disease caused by bacteria transmitted through the bite of some ticks.

Lymphedema

Swelling caused by restricted flow of the lymphatic system.

Magnetic resonance imaging (MRI)

A computerized body-imaging process that uses non-ionizing radiofrequency waves and powerful magnets to provide three-dimensional images of the body.

Managed care

Healthcare delivery program designed to control price, volume, location, and extent of healthcare services with the goal of making healthcare more cost-effective.

Mandate

Require.

Markers

See bio-markers.

Mean

The average.

Measurable disease

Disease response that can be accurately measured, like a clearly defined tumor that can be seen on an x-ray and measured

Median

The midpoint. If eighty-one patients were treated with drug x, and the time for white blood cell counts to recover following this treatment ranged from 2 to 60 days, after you rank the patients by the number of days required for their white blood cells to recover, the median is the number of days that it took patient number 41's white blood cells to recover.

MEDLINE

The most complete database of medical journal article abstracts.

Megasites

A major clearinghouse for information on a topic usually featuring a collection of links to other sites offering additional information.

Mesothelioma
Cancerous tumor in the lining of the lungs or chest cavity, sometimes related to exposure to asbestos.

Meta-analysis
Report which combines results from multiple smaller studies to try to get a more reliable overview than the smaller trials can offer. Adjustments have to be made for variations between the study groups and treatments.

Metabolic
Relating to the body's chemical processes.

Metabolic acidosis
Excessive acids in the body associated with a decreased capacity of the blood's ability to buffer the acids.

Metastasis
The spread of cancer to other tissues.

Micrometastasis
Less than 2 millimeters of detectable cancer at a site other than the original tumor.

Misinformation
Information that is misleading or misunderstood.

Monograph
A scholarly essay or book length explanation of a single topic.

Morbid or morbidity
Illness, as opposed to mortality (death). A treatment may result in 20 percent low-level morbidity (illness) but only 2 percent mortality (death). Likewise, comorbidity indicates the person has an illness in addition to another illness, such as high blood pressure or diabetes in addition to cancer.

MRI (magnetic resonance imaging)
Diagnostic imaging procedure using a magnetic field and radio frequencies.

Multicenter trial
Study offering treatment at more than one location.

Multiphasic screening
Use of multiple tests in one screening for indications of abnormalities.

Multiple sclerosis (MS)
Chronic, usually progressive, disorder of nervous system.

Narcolepsy
A sleep disorder characterized by unexpectedly falling asleep during daily activities and by disturbed sleep at night.

NDA (new drug approval) application
Request for FDA for approval to market a medical product or new procedure.

Non-Hodgkin's lymphoma (NHL)
Cancer found in lymph system that is not Hodgkin's disease.

Norm
Normal range of response.

Nutraceuticals
Food products promoted for their healing or protective qualities.

Neurologist
A doctor who specializes in the study of the structure and function of the body's nervous system. This includes the brain, spinal cord, and the peripheral nerves.

Number needed to treat (NNT)
The number of people who would need to be treated for one additional person to be helped by the treatment.

OB/GYN (obstetrician/gynecologist)
Specialist in women's reproductive health.

Observational study
Study that involves observation only; no treatment is given or restrictions applied to the population studied.

Odds ratio
Used in the same way as the relative risk but compares the extent of the exposure or intervention in one group to the extent of the exposure or intervention in the other group. Usually used in case-control studies or for rare disease where the number of cases in the control group is zero or almost zero.

Off-label prescription
A drug prescribed for a use that shows promise in preliminary studies but has not been added to the FDA-approved list of uses yet.

Oncologist
Cancer specialist.

Orthopedist
A physician who specializes in the bone structure of the body.

Osteoarthritis
Stiffening and pain in joints caused by deterioration of the cartilage in those joints.

Outcomes
Results.

Overall survival
The total amount of time that a patient survives following treatment, including relapses that were successfully retreated.

Pancreatitis
Inflammation of the pancreas.

Parkinson's disease
Progressive disorder of the central nervous system characterized by muscle rigidity and tremors.

Partial response
Describes a tumor's response to treatment that is 50 percent smaller or more, but still remains. It's not unusual to see a partial response on imaging halfway through treatment and a total response by the end of treatment.

Pathologist
Physician who specializes in studying cells and tissues under a microscope to identify and classify extent of disease.

Peer-reviewed journal
   A magazine where all articles are read and evaluated by one or more physicians or scientists with expertise in the field covered in the article.

Performance status
   Evaluation of a patient's mobility, functionality, and severity of symptoms. Usually rated on a numerical scale from normal to nonfunctional.

Petri dish
   Round glass or plastic dish with a lid. Used for tissue cultures and growing microorganisms in the laboratory.

Pharmacognocist
   A scientist who studies the medicinal use of plants.

Phenylalanine
   An amino acid.

Pheochromocytoma
   A very rare adrenal gland tumor.

PKU (phenylketonuria)
   A hereditary lack of the enzyme that converts phenylalanine into another amino acid. Requires rigid dietary restriction of phenylalanine.

Placebo
   Inactive substance designed to look like an active substance. Usually in pill form.

Placebo effect
   Response to treatment that occurs as a result of the expectation that treatment will be effective when, in fact, the treatment given only simulated effective treatment but had no effective properties.

Platelet
   A blood cell called a thrombocyte, important in the blood clotting process.

Pleura
   Lining of the lungs and chest cavity.

Prednisone
   A steroid used to treat cancer and other disorders by inhibiting the body's immune response.

Premed
   In preparation for medical school.

Presymptomatic
   Before the symptoms are apparent.

Primary tumor
   The original tumor. Metastases may spread from certain malignant primary tumors.

Primary care physician (PCP)
   Your primary or family doctor.

Prognosis
   The expected or probable outcome.

Proliferative therapy
Injection of an anesthetic irritant into the area where there is joint, ligament, or tendon damage with the intent of stimulating connective tissue growth (scarring) in the damaged area.

Prospective study
Subjects are followed into the future.

Prostate
Organ located under the bladder that contributes to the production of semen.

Prostate-specific antigen (PSA)
A substance found in the blood, which may indicate a prostate cancer if levels are elevated. Benign conditions can also elevate the PSA.

Prostatectomy
Removal of the prostate.

Prosthesis
Artificial replacement.

Protease inhibitor
Drug that reduces a virus' ability to replicate itself.

Protocol
Design of project. Includes enrollment requirements and restrictions, trial objectives, treatment plan, and review of scientific literature leading to current hypothesis.

Pseudocyst
A cavity resembling a cyst but which does not have a membrane lining like a true cyst, often the result of pancreatitis. Sometimes requires surgical drainage.

Psoriasis
A chronic skin condition characterized by the patches of dry scaly skin.

Psychologic
Relating to the processes of the mind.

Psychotherapist
Specialist in mental and social disorders.

P-value (probability value)
The measure of statistical confidence that the trial results did not occur by chance only. A p-value of less than .05 means there is a less than 5 percent chance that the results are due to chance. Less than 5 percent is the acceptable standard.

Qi Gong
A Chinese healing system which includes breathing and movement to help restore the patient's flow of *qi* (life energy).

Radiologist
Specialist who uses x-ray images to diagnose disease.

Raloxifene
Drug approved for the prevention and treatment of osteoporosis.

Randomization
Assignment of patients randomly to control or treatment groups. Usually done by computer to guarantee unbiased selection.

Recalibration
Redefining the standard range on lab tests.

Reimbursement
Insurance payment for medical services.

Relative risk
Compares the proportional level of risk between two groups. Used to indicate the proportional strength of a risk factor.

Remission
The tumor-free time period, dated from the first, not the last, therapy session. Patients with tumors that recur within one month of treatment ending are considered to have had no remission. Disappearance of all disease is complete remission; reduction of tumor size by more than 50 percent is considered partial remission.

Response
Regression of disease. Complete response means disease is undetectable. Partial response means disease has regressed, but not disappeared.

Response duration
Duration of positive response.

Retrospective study
Subjects' past history is examined to try to find out what factors might have led to their development of particular diseases.

Revascularization
Restoration of the flow of blood, usually through surgical techniques.

Review article
Article which includes a historical review of a treatment and a description of currently accepted modes of therapy, often with reviews of specific cases. Written by an expert in the field.

Salk vaccine
Vaccine used to prevent polio.

Sensitivity of a medical test
Ability of the test to detect true disease (true positive test results).

Shaman
Spiritual healer, traditionally in a tribal setting.

Side effects
Conditions that occur as the result of treatment that are not part of the intent of the treatment.

Single-blinded
The trial personnel know, but the patient does not know whether he is in the control group or the treatment group.

Sound bite
Very quick comment on a much more complex topic.

Specificity of a medical test
Ability to rule out disease (true negative test results).

Stable disease
One or more tumors, still visible on imaging, that are not growing.

Staging
Categorization of the extent of the disease, most often used for evaluation of a cancer.

Statistically significant
The size of the group studied is large enough to provide an acceptable level of confidence that the results are not likely to be due just to chance.

Stem cells
Young blood cells from which all blood cells develop.

Strep
A throat infection caused by streptococci (a type of bacteria).

Subject
Trial volunteer.

Tamoxifen
Drug used to reduce the risk of recurrence of breast cancer, more recently being offered to reduce the risk of initial occurrence.

Taxanes
Drugs made from the Pacific yew tree. Used to treat breast cancer.

Taxol
A drug for breast cancer made from the bark of the Pacific yew tree.

Thalidomide
A drug removed from the market as the result of birth defects in the children of the women who used it. Currently being studied as an antiangiogenesis treatment for cancer.

Time frame
Period of time being considered.

Total response or total remission
Describes a tumor's response to treatment. The tumor has either completely disappeared, or is so small and stable it may just be scar tissue. See also Partial response, and Remission.

Treatment group
The group in a study who receives the experimental treatment (intervention).

Treatment IND
Emergency use protocol for compassionate use of an unapproved drug that might offer benefit to a patient in a desperate situation.

Tumor
An abnormal growth of tissue that grows independently of the normal rate. This tissue may be benign or malignant.

Ultrasound
Diagnostic imaging tool that uses sound waves.

URL (uniform resource locator)
Web site location or address.

Urologist
Physician who specializes conditions of the urinary tract as well as male reproductive organs.

Ventricles
Small cavity. The heart, for example, has two ventricles that pump the blood
through the body.

Vinblastine
An anticancer drug that inhibits cancer growth by preventing cell division.

Vincristine
An anticancer drug that inhibits cancer growth by preventing cell division.

Visceral angiogram
Also called celiac and mesenteric arteriography. Used to detect blood vessel
abnormalities and to detect gastrointestinal bleeding.

Voltaren
Nonsteroidal anti-inflammatory medication used sometimes for arthritis pain.

Web site
A location on the Internet. Offers information about a business, organization, or
individual. Anyone can create a web site on any topic.

Workup
Physician's evaluation of the current state of a patient's health, which includes
history, symptoms, test results, and observations.

Notes

Chapter 1: *Preparing for Research*

1. Nancy Keene, *Working With Your Doctor: Getting the Healthcare You Deserve* (Sebastopol, CA: O'Reilly & Associates, 1998), 19–44.

Chapter 2: *Knowing Your Rights*

1. Joint Commision on the Accreditation of Healthcare Organizations, *Comprehensive Accreditation Manual for Hospitals: The Official Handbook* (Oakbrook Terrace, IL: JCAHO, 2000), Section RI 1.2.1.
2. George J. Annas, *The Rights of Patients: the Basic ACLU Guide to Patient Rights,* 2nd ed. (Totowa, NJ: Humana Press, 1992), 171.
3. American Medical Association, *Current Procedural Terminology: CPT 2000* (Chicago: American Medical Association, 1999).
4. *ICD-9-CM: International Classification of Diseases,* 9th Revision, Millennium Edition (Los Angeles, CA: Practice Management Information Corporation, 1999).

Chapter 4: *Identifying Information Resources*

1. Robert E. Rakel, ed., *Conn's Current Therapy: Latest Approved Methods of Treatment for the Practicing Physician, 2000.* (Philadelphia: Saunders, 2000).
2. Anthony S. Fauci et al., eds. *Harrison's Principles of Internal Medicine,* 14th ed. (New York: McGraw-Hill, 1998).
3. *Medical and Health Care Books and Serials in Print, 2000* (New Providence, NJ: Bowker, 2000).
4. "The Gag Clause in Pharmaceutical Research," *60 Minutes.* CBS Television. New York, December 19, 1999.
5. Sandra Steingraber, *Living Downstream* (New York: Vintage Books, 1998).
6. Marcia Angell et al., "Disclosure of Authors' Conflicts of Interest: A Follow-Up," *New England Journal of Medicine* 342, no. 8:(24 February 2000) 586–7.
7. Norman Cousins, *Anatomy of an Illness as Perceived by the Patient: Reflections on Healing and Regeneration* (New York: W. W. Norton, 1979).
8. Alan M. Rees, *Consumer Health Information Sourcebook,* 6th ed. (Phoenix, AZ: Oryx Press, 2000).
9. *A.D.A.M. Interactive Physiology CD-ROM* (New York: ADAM Software, Inc., 1997).
10. Vladimer Lange, *Be a Survivor: Your Guide to Breast Cancer Treatment*, Interactive CD-ROM (Los Angeles, CA: Lange Productions, 1998).

Chapter 5: *Gaining Access to Information Resources*

1. Joint Comission on the Accrediation of Healthcare Organizations, *Comprehensive Accreditation Manual for Hospitals: The Official Handbook* (Oakbrook Terrace, IL: JCAHO, 2000), Section PF 4.
2. Dorothy R. Hill, "Brandon/Hill selected list of books and journals for the small medical library," *Bulletin of the Medical Library Association* 87, no. 2 (April 1999): 145–69.
3. *Merck Manual of Diagnosis and Therapy*, 17th ed. (Rahway, NJ: Merck Sharpe and Dohme, 1999). Also in CD-ROM format and Internet version, *http://www.merck.com*.
4. Lynn M. Pearce, ed., *Medical and Health Information Directory: Organizations, Agencies, and Institutions*, 11th ed. (Farmington Hills, MI: GALE Group, 2000).
5. Peter Wehrwein, "Strong Medicine (The New England Journal of Medicine)," *American Journalism Review* 20, no. 3 (April 1998): 38.
6. Medical Research Centers, *A World Directory of Organizations and Programmes*, 11th ed., (New York: Stockton Press, 1995).
7. Paul Kim et al., "Published criteria for evaluating health related web sites: review," *BMJ* 318 (6 March 1999): 647–9. The table can be found at *http://www.bmj.com/cgi/content/full/318/7184/647/T2* and was reprinted by permission of BMJ.

Chapter 6: *Effective Search Strategies*

1. *Merck Manual of Diagnosis and Therapy*, 17th ed. (Rahway, NJ: Merck Sharpe and Dohme, 1999). (Also CD-ROM format and Internet version: *http://www.merck.com*.)
2. *PDR/Physicians Desk Reference*, 54th ed. (Montvale, NJ: Medical Economics, 2000). Published annually. Also available in CD-ROM and other formats.
3. *Merriam Webster's Medical Desk Dictionary* (New York: Merriam-Webster, Inc., 1993). Also available in Internet version, *http://www.intelihealth.com*.
4. S. Terry Canale, ed., *Campbell's Operative Orthopaedics*, 9th ed., 4 vols. (St. Louis: Mosby, 1998). Also available in CD-ROM version.
5. Charles H. Epps, *Complications in Orthopaedic Surgery*, 3rd ed., 2 vols. (Philadelphia: Lippincott, 1997).
6. Vincent T. DeVita et al., *Cancer: Principles and Practice of Oncology*, 5th ed., 2 vols. (Philadelphia: Lippincott-Raven, 1997).
7. James F. Holland et al., *Cancer Medicine*, 4th ed., 2 vols. (Baltimore: Williams & Wilkins, 1997).

Chapter 7: *Understanding Standard Treatment Options*

1. David L. Sackett et al., "Evidence based medicine: what it is and what it isn't: It's about integrating individual clinical expertise and the best external evidence," *BMJ* 312, no. 7023 (13 January 1996): 71–2.
2. Louise Williams, "Framingham Heart Study Celebrates 50 Years" from the National Institute of Health website at *http://www.nih.gov/NIH-Record/11_17_98/story06.htm*. November 17, 1998.

3. Robert E. Rakel, ed., *Conn's Current Therapy: Latest Approved Methods of Treatment for the Practicing Physician, 2000.* (Philadelphia: Saunders, 2000).

4. Mark R. Dambro, *Griffith's 5 Minute Clinical Consult, 2000* (Philadelphia: Lippincott, Williams & Wilkins, 2000).

5. Lawrence M. Tierney, ed., *Current Medical Diagnosis and Treatment 2000,* 39th ed. (New York: McGraw-Hill, 2000).

6. Dorothy R. Hill, "Brandon/Hill selected list of books and journals for the small medical library." *Bulletin of the Medical Library Association* 87, no. 2 (April 1999): 145–69.

7. Mark E. Frisse and Valerie Florance, "A Library for Internists IX: Recommendations from the American College of Physicians," *Annals of Internal Medicine* 126, no.10 (15 May 1997): 836–46.

8. Daniel Doody, ed., *Doody's Rating Service: A Buyer's Guide to the 250 Best Health Sciences Books* (Oak Park, IL: Doody Publishing Inc., 1993 to date).

9. Institute of Medicine, *Clinical Practice Guidelines: Directions for a New Program* (Washington, D.C: National Academy Press, 1990).

10. Dean Ornish et al., "Can lifestyle changes reverse coronary heart disease? The Lifestyle Heart Trial," *Lancet* 336, no. 8708 (21 July 1990): 129–33.

Chapter 8: *Researching Clinical Trials*

1. This story came from multiple sources. Katie Hafner, "Can the Internet cure the common cold?" *New York Times* (9 July 1998):D1. *NBC Healthcheck 10,* "Ganglioside: New drug for paralysis," *http://nbcin.nbc10wjar.com/health/ganglio.html.* Media Relations, Children's Hospital San Diego, telephone: (858) 576–5801.

2. "Trials of War Criminals before the Nuremburg Military Tribunals under Control Council Law No. 10," Washington, DC: US Government Printing Office 2 (1949): 181–2.

3. Department of Health and Human Services. "Federal Policy for the Protection of Human Subjects; Notices and Rules." *Federal Register 56,* no. 117 (18 June 1991): 28016–7.

4. Robert Finn, *Cancer Clinical Trials: Experimental Treatments & How They Can Help You* (Sebastopol, CA: O'Reilly & Associates, 1999), 142–3.

Chapter 9: *Complementary and Alternative Therapies*

1. David M. Eisenberg et al., "Unconventional Medicine In The United States. Prevalence, Costs, And Patterns Of Use," *New England Journal of Medicine* 328, no. 4 (28 January 1993): 246–52.

2. Carola Burroughs, "Alternative AIDS Therapies: An Historical Review," *Gay Men's Health Crisis: Treatment Issues* 7, no. 11 (Nov 1993): *http://www.critpath.org/newsletters/ti/TI.11.txt.*

3. "Classification of CAM Practices," National Center for Complementary and Alternative Medicine web site, *http://nccam.nih.gov/nccam/fcp/classify.*

4. William Fair, MD, "Complementary Therapy is an Essential Part of Cancer Treatment," Center for Mind-Body Medicine's Integrating Complementary & Alternative Therapies Conference in Arlington, VA (12–14 June 1998), *http://www.cmbm.org.*

5. David M. Eisenberg et al., "Unconventional Medicine In The United States. Prevalence, Costs, And Patterns Of Use," *New England Journal of Medicine* 328, no. 4 (28 January 1993): 246–52.

6. David M. Eisenberg et al., "Trends In Alternative Medicine Use In The United States, 1990–1997," *Journal of the American Medical Association* 280 (11 January 1998): 1569–75.

7. M. Wetzel et al., "Courses Involving Complementary And Alternative Medicine At US Medical Schools," *Journal of the American Medical Association* 280, no. 9 (2 September 1998): 784–7.

8. John A. Astin, PhD, et al., "A Review Of The Incorporation Of Complementary And Alternative Medicine By Mainstream Physicians," *Archives of Internal Medicine* 158 (1998): 2303–10.

9. The National Center for Complementary and Alternative Medicine, "The Unconventional Timeline," (November 1998), *http://altmed.od.nih.gov/nccam.*

10. Lynn Payer, *Medicine and Culture: Varieties of Treatment in the United States, England, West Germany, and France* (New York: Henry Holt and Company, 1996), 125.

11. Edward W. Campion, MD, "Why Unconventional Medicine?" *New England Journal of Medicine* 328 (28 January 1993): 282–3.

12. John A. Astin, PhD, "Why Patients Use Alternative Medicine," *Journal of the American Medical Association* 279 (20 May 1998): 1548–53.

13. "Acupuncture Effective for Certain Medical Conditions, Panel Says," *Complementary and Alternative Medicine Newsletter* 5, no. 1 (January 1998): 1–2, *http://nccam.nih.gov/nccam/ne/newsletter/1998/jan/1.htm.*

14. William Fair, MD, "Complementary Therapy is an Essential Part of Cancer Treatment," Center for Mind-Body Medicine's Integrating Complementary & Alternative Therapies Conference in Arlington, VA (12–14 June 1998), *http://www.cmbm.org.*

15. Charles B. Wessel et al., "Complementary And Alternative Medicine (CAM): Selected Internet Resources For HIV/AIDS," *Health Care on the Internet* 2, no. 2/3 (1998): 105–9.

16. Yashar Hirshaut, MD, "Re: Objecting to Alternative Post—Why?" *listserv@morgan.ucs.mun.ca*, April 18, 1996. Used with permission.

17. David M. Studdert et al., "Medical Malpractice Implications Of Alternative Medicine," *Journal of the American Medical Association* 280 (11 November 1998): 1551.

18. Peter Montague, "Another Kind Of Drug Problem," *Rachel's Environment & Health Weekly* (7 January 1999), *http://www.rachel.org.*

19. David M. Eisenberg et al., "Trends In Alternative Medicine Use In The United States, 1990–1997," *Journal of the American Medical Association* 280 (11 January 1998): 1569–75.

20. Ralph Moss, PhD, "Providing Good Information to People with Cancer," Center for Mind-Body Medicine's Integrating Complementary & Alternative Therapies Conference in Arlington, VA (12–14 June 1998): 13, *http://www.cmbm.org.*

21. Ralph Moss, PhD, "Providing Good Information to People with Cancer," Center for Mind-Body Medicine's Integrating Complementary & Alternative Therapies Conference in Arlington, VA (12–14 June 1998): 13, *http://www.cmbm.org.*

22. John Greenwald, "Herbal Healing," *Time* (23 November 1998): 59–68.

23. Michael Lerner, *Choices In Healing: Integrating The Best Of Conventional And Complementary Approaches To Cancer* (Cambridge, MA: MIT Press, 1994).

24. Miriam S. Wetzel et al., "Courses Involving Complementary And Alternative Medicine At US Medical Schools," *Journal of the American Medical Association* 280, no. 9 (2 September 1998): 784–7.

25. David M. Eisenberg et al., "Trends In Alternative Medicine Use In The United States, 1990–1997," *Journal of the American Medical Association* 280 (11 January 1998): 1569–75.

26. David M. Eisenberg et al., "Trends In Alternative Medicine Use In The United States, 1990–1997," *Journal of the American Medical Association* 280 (11 January 1998): 1569–75.

27. "Complementary Services: Consumer Demand Outplaces Research, Insurance," *Stanford (online) Report* (29 April 1998), *http://www.stanford.edu/dept/news/report/news/april29/demand429.html*.

28. M. Stano and M. Smith, "Chiropractic and Medical Costs of Low Back Care," *Medical Care* 34, no. 1 (1996): 191–204.

29. "Acupuncture Effective for Certain Medical Conditions, Panel Says," *Complementary and Alternative Medicine Newsletter* 5, no. 1 (January 1998): 1–2, *http://nccam.nih.gov/nccam/ne/newsletter/1998/jan/1.htm*.

30. "Acupuncture Effective for Certain Medical Conditions, Panel Says," *Complementary and Alternative Medicine Newsletter* 5, no. 1 (January 1998): 1–2, *http://nccam.nih.gov/nccam/ne/newsletter/1998/jan/1.htm*.

31. Landmark Healthcare, "Health Maintenance Organizations and Alternative Medicine: A Closer Look" Landmark Healthcare report. Sacramento, CA (1996), *http://www.landmarkhealthcare.com/96hmo.htm*.

32. Landmark Healthcare, "The Landmark Report II on HMOs and Alternative Care," Landmark Healthcare report. Sacramento, CA (1996), *http://www.landmarkhealthcare.com/99tlrIIm.htm*.

Chapter 10: *Support: Learning from Others*

1. Leonard Berkman and S. L. Syme, "Social networks, host resistance, and mortality: a nine-year follow-up study of Alameda County residents," *American Journal of Epidemiology* 109, no. 2 (February 1979): 186–204.

2. F. V. Wenz, "Marital status, anomie, and forms of social isolation: a case of high suicide rate among the widowed in an urban sub-area," *Diseases of the Nervous System* 30, no. 11 (November 1977): 891–5.

3. David Spiegel et al, "Effect of Psychosocial Treatment on Survival of Patients with Metastatic Breast Cancer," *Lancet* 2, no. 8668 (14 October 1989): 888–91.

4. Harold G. Koenig and David B. Larson, "Use of Hospital Services, Religious Attendance, and Religious Affiliation," *Southern Medical Journal* 91, no. 10 (October 1998): 925–32.

5. Fred F. Sicher, et al., "A Randomized Double-Blind Study of the Effect of Distant Healing in a Population With Advanced AIDS," *Western Journal of Medicine* 169, no. 6 (December 1998): 356–63.

6. Tom Ferguson, *Health Online: How to Find Health Information, Support Groups, and Self-Help Communities in Cyberspace* (Reading, MA: Addison Wesley Publishing Co., 1996).

Chapter 11: *Evaluating and Using Statistics*

1. National Safety Council, Accident Facts® (Itaska, IL, 1997): "Leading Causes of Death," 10, 16–7, 26. Table compiled using cited number of deaths in 1994 from these specific causes. The total number of deaths for that year was 2,278,994.

2. Nancy Keene, *Working With Your Doctor: Getting the Healthcare You Deserve* (Sebastopol, CA: O'Reilly & Associates, 1998), 206.

3. Victor Cohn, *News and Numbers: A Guide to Reporting Statistical Claims and Controversies in Health and Other Fields* (Ames, IA: Iowa University Press, 1989), 65.

4. W. S. Browner, "Diagnostic Dilemma," *American Journal of Medicine* 104, no. 4 (April 1998): 406–7. Reprinted with permission from Excerpta Medica Inc.

5. Centers for Disease Control and Prevention, "Cancer Registries: The Foundation for Comprehensive Cancer Control," *http://www.cdc.gov/nccdphp/dcpc/npcr/register. htm*, April 2, 2000.

6. Lorraine Johnston, *Non-Hodgkin's Lymphomas: Making Sense of Diagnosis, Treatment & Options* (Sebastopol, CA: O'Reilly & Associates, 1999), 53.

7. Nancy Keene, *Working with Your Doctor: Getting the Healthcare You Deserve* (Sebastopol, CA: O'Reilly & Associates, 1998, 87.

8. NCI Surveillance, Epidemiology, and End Results (SEER) Program, and American Cancer Society, 1993. National Cancer Institute website, "Lifetime Probability of Breast Cancer in American Women," *http://rex.nci.nih.gov/INFO_CANCER/Cancer_ facts/Section5/FS5_6.html*, April 3, 2000.

9. American Cancer Society, "Breast Cancer Facts and Figures 1999–2000," *http:// www.cancer.org/statistics/99bcff/risk.html*, April 3, 2000.

10. US Department of Health and Human Services. "Health United States 1996–97 and Injury Chartbook," Hyattsville, MD, DHHS Publication No. (PHS) 96–1232. GPO stock number 017-022-01377, *http://www.cdc.gov/nchs/data/hus96_97.pdf*, April 3, 2000.

11. American Cancer Society, "1999 Cancer Facts and Figures," Atlanta, GA, American Cancer Society, 1998. *http://www.cancer.org/statistics/cff99/selectedcancers.html*, April 4, 2000.

12. American Heart Association, "2000 Statistical Heart and Stroke Update," *http:// www.americanheart.org/statistics/03cardio.html*, April 4, 2000.

13. Ann McKibbon et al., *PDQ Evidence-Based Medicine Principles and Practice* (Hamilton, Ontario: B.C. Decker, Inc., 1999), 40.

14. Stephen Jay Gould, "The Median Isn't the Message," *Discover*, June 1985: 40–2.

15. US Department of Health, Education and Welfare. "Smoking and Health: Report of the Advisory Committee to the Surgeon General." Washington, DC: Public Health Service, 1964.

16. Musa Mayer, *Advanced Breast Cancer: A Guide to Living with Metastatic Disease,* 2nd ed.(Sebastopol, CA: O'Reilly & Associates, 1998), 84–5.

17. R. M. Pitkin et al., "Accuracy of Data in Abstracts of Published Research Articles," *Journal of the American Medical Association* 281, no. 12 (24–31 Mar 1999): 1110–1.

18. Lorraine Johnston, *Non-Hodgkin's Lymphomas: Making Sense of Diagnosis, Treatment and Options* (Sebastopol, CA: O'Reilly & Associates, 1999), 53.

19. Andy Oxman, "Science of Reading," *Pediatrics* 83, no. 4 (April 1989): 617–9.

20. Henry D. Weaver, *Confronting the Big C: A Family Faces Cancer* (Scottdale, PA: Herald Press, 1984), 74–5.

Chapter 12: *Reviewing Information with Your Doctor*

1. Nancy Keene, *Working with Your Doctor: Getting the Healthcare You Deserve* (Sebastopol, CA: O'Reilly & Associates, 1998), 75.
2. Susan Love, MD. Personal correspondence, March 22, 2000.

Chapter 13: *Making Your Decision*

1. David M. Eddy, *Clinical Decision Making From Theory to Practice: A Collection of Essays from The Journal of the American Medical Association* (Sudbury, MA: Jones and Bartlett, 1996), 8.
2. W. Scott Richardson and Allan S. Detsky, "Users' Guides to the Medical Literature VII.: How to Use a Clinical Decision Analysis." *Journal of the American Medical Association* 273, no. 20 (24–31 May 1995): 1610–3.
3. George M. Burnell. *Final Choices: To Live or to Die in an Age of Medical Technology* (New York: Insight Books, 1993), 90.

Index

doctors (*continued*)
  clinical trials, asking about, 173
  communicating with, 4–8, 51
  cooperation from, 302
  expertise a factor in choosing
        treatments, 125
  giving referrals, 275
  informed consent and, 24–26
  preparing for visits to, 6, 281–283
  professional associations, 82
  role and contribution, 273–277
  selecting treatments, 122
  training and experience, 273
  as treatment coordinators, 276
  treatment options, asking
        about, 129
  web sites, 321
Doody's Rating Service, 137
dosages, maximum safe, 161
double-blind studies, 159
drugs
  for chronic conditions, 106
  interactions with alternative
        therapies, 201
  overseas availability only, 180
  researching specific, 99–102
  using unapproved, 181
Durable Power of Attorney for Health
        Care, 55

E

Eisenberg, Dr. David, 183, 186, 191
emergency treatment options, 153
estimated life expectancy, 248
ethics, research, 155
European Organization for Research and
        Treatment of Cancer
        (EORTC) database, 179
evidence-based medicine (EBM), 143
  evaluating, 144
  publishers of, 144
experimental treatment options, 14
experts, finding, 108, 133

F

family members
  carrying out your medical
        decisions, 306–309

doing research for the
        patient, 40–56
  medical backgrounds, 55
  using patient
        questionnaire, 313–316
federal health agencies, 81
Ferguson, Dr. Tom, 224
financial issues, resources, 322
Food and Drug Administration
        (FDA), 81, 148
  pre-approval clinical trial
        phases, 161–163
Framingham Heart Study, 122
friends
  carrying out your medical
        decisions, 306–309
  doing research for the
        patient, 40–56
  providing support, 228–231
  using patient
        questionnaire, 313–316

G

genetic links to diseases, 55
glossary, 331–346
Gould, Stephen Jay, 254
government agencies, health
        information, 80–82
guidelines. *See* clinical practice
        guidelines

H

Harrison's Principles of Internal
        Medicine, 58
Health and Human Services
        agencies, 81
Health Care Financing Administration
        (HCFA), 243
health history programs, 37
Health Profiler, 38
healthcare agents, 54
Healthcare Proxy, 55
Healthminder, 38
hearsay bias, 264
hospitals
  clinical trials at, 174, 179
  consent policies, 24
  libraries in, 77

I

ICD (International Classification of
     Diseases), 36
importing unapproved drugs, 182
incidence rates, 243–245
INDs (Investigational New Drugs), 153
information
     about alternative
          therapies, 210–212
     accessing resources, 74–94
     identifying resources, 57–73
     resources, 319–324
     reviewing with your
          doctor, 269–292
     sharing with your
          doctor, 283–286
information brokers. *See* professional
          researchers
informed consent, 24–26
     clinical trials and, 156
informed decision making. *See* decision
          making
Institutional Review Boards (IRBs), 157
insurance
     coverage of
          alternative therapies, 208
          clinical trials, 166
          therapy, 219
     getting second opinions, 131
     restrictions, 13, 126
          billable time, 289
          physician referrals, 288
International Classification of Diseases
          (ICD), 36
Internet
     access, 90–94
     online services, 93
     subscription services, 94
Internet resources, 317–329
     alternative therapies, 210
     bookstores, 79
     clinical practice guidelines, 63
     clinical trials, 173, 175, 178–180
     discussion groups, 112, 180,
          224–228
     evaluating health information, 92
     government agencies, 81
     health history programs, 37
     medical databases, 70
     medical school locations, 77

NIH cancer trials, 175
positives and negatives, 90–93
professional medical
          associations, 82
research studies, 87
reviewing medical textbooks, 137
specialists, 133
interpretation bias, 263
interventional studies, 260

K

Karnofsky scale, clinical trial
          acceptance, 164

L

lab technicians, 15
Landmark Healthcare, Inc., 209
language, medical, 9
law of large numbers, 247
legal issues, resources, 322
Lexis-Nexis, 94
librarians, helping with research, 116
libraries
     academic, 75
     consumer health, 78
     hospital, 77
     medical school, 76
     public, 74
licensing, alternative practitioners, 199
life expectancy, estimated, 248
LifeForm, 38
lifetime risk, 247
listening to the patient, 49
listservers, Internet, 112, 180,
          224–228
local health agencies, 81
Login Books, 137

M

magazines
     alternative therapies, 211
     consumer health, 64
managed care, patient rights and, 22
managing time, 19
manufacturers
     drugs, clinical trials, 175
     medical products, 88

MDConsult, 94
mean/median survival rate, 245
media reports, clinical trial
   information, 177
Medical and Health Care Books and
   Serials in Print, 60
Medical and Healthcare Marketplace
   Guide, 88
medical decisions
 components of, 295
  assessing risks and
   uncertainty, 301
  complementary/alternative
   treatments, 299
  cooperation from
   caregivers, 302
  diagnosis, 296
  disruption of life, 299
  personal preferences, 298
  treatment options, 296–298
  treatment trade-offs, 300
 difficulties of, 293
 your right to make
   choices, 309–311
 See also decision making
medical dictionaries, 324
medical experts, finding, 108, 133
medical genealogy, 55
medical journals
 how to read, 258–267
 non-reviewed, 61
 peer-reviewed, 60
medical librarians, helping with
   research, 116
medical libraries, 98
medical newsletters, 66
medical products, 88
medical records
 access
  limitations to, 32, 54
  troubleshooting, 38
 accessing another's, 53–55
 deciphering, 35
 finding older, 27, 53
 information in, 31
 ownership question, 28
 privacy of, 33
 requesting copies of, 29–31
 test results and, 34
 used in medical genealogy, 55

medical research papers. *See* studies;
   research, papers
medical schools
 bookstores, 79
 libraries, 76
 research centers, 86
medical statistics. *See* statistics
medical studies. *See* studies; research,
   papers
medical team, getting to know, 15–17
medical terms, 9
medical tests. *See* test results; tests
medical textbooks, 58
 as research tools, 98
 cost of, 79
 guidelines, 134
  evaluating, 136
  publishers of, 136
medications. *See* drugs
meditation support groups, 223
Medline, 94, 98
 access to abstracts, 258
 alternative therapy
   information, 210
 clinical trial information, 179
MEDLINEplus, 98–103
 medical expert information, 108
 surgical procedures, 111
Medscape, 37
mortality rates, 244
Moyers, Bill, 72

N

National Board for Certified
   Counselors, 219
National Cancer Institute, 116
National Cancer Registry, 80
National Center for Complementary and
   Alternative Medicine
   (NCCAM), 211, 326
 classification listing, 184
National Institutes of Health (NIH), 81
 assistance for treatment costs, 166
 clinical study database, 178
 clinical trials sponsor, 149, 175
National Library of Medicine, 70, 320
 medical library information, 77,
   98

National Network of Libraries of
Medicine, 117
National Patient Air Transport
Helpline, 165
National Self-Help Clearinghouse, 221
Netwellness, 107
New Drug Approval (NDA), 154
New England Journal of Medicine, 61
new therapies, searching for, 107
news reports, medical, 71–73
newsletters
    alternative therapies, 211
    medical, 66
newspapers, medical stories in, 71
NNT (number needed to treat), 252
nonprofit organizations, 83
non-reviewed medical journals, 61
nonstandard treatments. See CAM
number needed to treat (NNT), 252
Nuremberg Code, 155
nurses/nurse practitioners, 16

O

observational studies, 254, 260
observing the patient, 49
odds ratios, 251
office visits
    asking comprehensive
        questions, 285
    discussing risks and benefits, 284
    preparing for, 6, 281–283
off-label prescriptions, 152
online services, Internet, 93
options. See standard treatments;
        treatment options
organizations
    nonprofit, 83
    professional, 177, 323
overseas clinical trials, 180
Ovid subscription service, 94

P

pamphlets, medical, 67
panels of tests, 242
pathologists, 15
patient questionnaire, 313–316
patient records. See medical records
patient resource centers, 85

patient rights
    informed consent, 24–26
    making medical choices, 309–311
    medical records, copies of, 26–34
    participating in decision
        making, 21–23
    understanding, 37–39
patient support groups. See support,
        groups
peer-reviewed medical journals, 60
Pharmaceutical Research and
        Manufacturers of America
        (PhRMA), 176
    product development costs, 189
pharmacists, 16
phases of clinical trials, 161–163
physician guidelines. See clinical
        practice guidelines
Physician's Desk Reference, 88
physicians. See doctors
pilot studies, 161
placebo reaction to alternative
        therapies, 202
population averages and risk
        calculation, 251–253
practitioner licensing, 199
predicting risk, 246–250
prescriptions
    off-label, 152
    potential toxicity, 200
press releases, 72
prevalence rates, disease, 244
prioritizing research, 12
privacy
    of medical records, 33
    respecting patient, 41
probability
    risk and, 246
    value (p-value), 261
Prodigy online service, 93
professional associations, 82
professional organizations, 177, 323
professional researchers
    information to give, 120
    qualifications, 118
    what to look for when hiring, 119
    when to use, 117
prospective studies, 260
protocol documents, 159
Public Broadcasting Service, 72

About the Authors

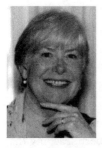

Nancy Oster is a medical writer, healthcare activist, Internet expert, and educator. She received her bachelor's degree from the University of California at Santa Barbara and has written several articles for medical and healthcare journals. Recently, Nancy was honored in the US House of Representatives for her role as the founding president of the Breast Resource Center of Santa Barbara. Nancy is also one of the founders of the South Coast Telecommunications Alliance, a forum for networking and information sharing on the central coast of California. Nancy has long been active in support of open and free information and access to healthcare and health information.

When Nancy is not writing, she is busy preparing gourmet meals, practicing yoga, creating numerous web sites, gardening, working on a designer quilt with friends, or traveling with her husband, Dave. Nancy and Dave have two grown children and two very active puppies. Nancy and Dave live in Santa Barbara, California.

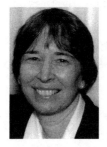

Lucy Thomas, MLS, is currently the director of the Reeves Medical Library in Cottage Hospital, Santa Barbara, California. She completed her bachelor's and master's degrees at the University of Illinois in Champaign-Urbana, Illinois, before moving to California. She is a distinguished member of the Academy of Health Information Professionals of the Medical Library Association and is on the editorial board for Medicine on the Net. Lucy has written numerous articles for professional journals and has been a speaker at professional conferences. She has long been an advocate for free access to information and for the rights of the healthcare consumer.

When she is not working, you can find Lucy skiing in the Sierra Mountains, sailing, hiking, gardening, attending a meeting of her book club, or taking a long beach walk with her husband, Bill, and their golden retriever, Brig. Lucy and her husband live in Santa Barbara, California.

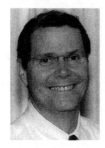

Darol Joseff, MD, is a board certified nephrologist and internist. He completed his medical degree at the University of Cincinnati School of Medicine and his fellowship and residency training at Harbor UCLA Medical Center, and at Santa Barbara Cottage Hospital. Dr. Joseff has written numerous articles for medical journals. He is also on the faculty of the University of Southern California Medical School and is active in teaching for the residency programs at Cottage Hospital. Recently, Dr. Joseff was named "Teacher of the Year" by the resident staff at Cottage Hospital. Dr. Joseff has a private practice specializing in nephrology in Santa Barbara and is on the medical staff at several hospitals. Dr. Joseff communicates with his patients and colleagues via telephone, email, listservs, and the Web.

When Dr. Joseff is not practicing medicine, teaching residents, or attending a Mac users' convention, he is at home with his beautiful wife, Janet, who is also a physician. They have two lively children and their free time is filled with activities such as soccer, hiking, beach walks, and travel.

Nancy, Lucy, and Darol teach an Internet Health Information course for the Santa Barbara Community College Adult Education program. They've been teaching the class for several years and have taken the class on the road as far as the First World Conference on Breast Cancer in Kingston, Ontario, Canada and to other communities in California.

Colophon

Patient-Centered Guides are about the experience of illness. They contain personal stories as well as a combination of practical and medical information. The faces on the covers of our Guides reflect the human side of the information we offer.

Edie Freedman and Ellie Volckhausen designed the cover of *Making Informed Medical Decisions: Where to Look and How to Use What You Find,* using Adobe Photoshop 5.5 and QuarkXPress 3.32 with Berkeley fonts from Bitstream. The cover photos are from Photodisc and are used by permission. Emma Colby prepared the cover mechanical.

Alicia Cech and David Futato designed the interior layout for the book based on a series design by Nancy Priest and Edie Freedman. The interior fonts are Berkeley and Franklin Gothic. Mike Sierra prepared the text using FrameMaker 5.5.6.

The book was copyedited by Sarah Jane Shangraw and proofread by Kate Wilkinson. Maureen Dempsey and Claire Cloutier conducted quality assurance checks. Judy Hoer wrote the index. The illustrations that appear in this book were produced by Robert Romano and Rhon Porter using Macromedia Freehand 8.0 and Adobe Photoshop 5.5. Interior composition was done by Ann Schirmer, Molly Shangraw, Sarah Jane Shangraw, and Nancy Williams.

Patient-Centered Guides™

Questions Answered
Experiences Shared

We are committed to empowering individuals to evolve into informed consumers armed with the latest information and heartfelt support for their journey.

When your life is turned upside down, your need for information is great. You have to make critical medical decisions, often with information that seems little to go on. Plus you have to break the news to family, quiet your own fears, cope with symptoms or treatment side effects, figure out how you're going to pay for things, and sometimes still get to work or get dinner on the table.

Patient-Centered Guides provide authoritative information for intelligent information seekers who want to become advocates for their own health. The books cover the whole impact of illness on your life. In each book, there's a mix of:

- **Medical background for treatment decisions**
  We can give you information that can help you to work with your doctor to come to a decision. We start from the viewpoint that modern medicine has much to offer and we discuss complementary treatments. Where there are treatment controversies, we present differing points of view.

- **Practical information**
  Once you've decided what to do about your illness, you still have to deal with treatments and changes to your life. We cover day-to-day practicalities, such as those you'd hear from a good nurse or a knowledgeable support group.

- **Emotional support**
  It's normal to have strong reactions to a condition that threatens your life or that changes how you live. It's normal that the whole family is affected. We cover issues such as the shock of diagnosis, living with uncertainty, and communicating with loved ones.

Each book also contains stories from both patients and doctors — medical "frequent flyers" who share, in their own words, the lessons and strategies they have learned while maneuvering through the often complicated maze of medical information that's available.

We provide information online, including updated listings of the resources that appear in this book. This is freely available for you to print out and copy to share with others, as long as you retain the copyright notice on the printouts.

www.patientcenters.com

Other Books in the Series

Cancer

Advanced Breast Cancer
A Guide to Living with Metastatic Disease, Second Edition
By Musa Mayer
ISBN 1-56592-522-X, Paperback, 6" x 9", 544 pages, $24.95 US, $36.95 CAN

"An excellent book...if knowledge is power, this book will be good medicine."
—David Spiegel, MD, Stanford University, Author, Living Beyond Limits

Cancer Clinical Trials
Experimental Treatments and How They Can Help You
By Robert Finn
ISBN 1-56592-566-1, Paperback, 5" x 8", 232 pages, $14.95 US, $21.95 CAN

"I highly recommend this book as a first step in what will be for many a difficult, but crucially important, part of their struggle to beat their cancer."
—From the Foreword by Robert Bazell, Chief Science Correspondent for NBC News
Author, Her-2: The Making of Herceptin, a Revolutionary Treatment for Breast Cancer

Colon & Rectal Cancer
A Comprehensive Guide for Patients & Families
By Lorraine Johnston
ISBN 1-56592-633-1, Paperback, 6" x 9", 556 pages, $24.95 US, $36.95 CAN

"I sure wish [this book] had been available when I was first diagnosed. I wouldn't change a thing: informative, down-to-earth, easily understandable, and very touching."
—Pati Lanning, colon cancer survivor

Non-Hodgkin's Lymphomas
Making Sense of Diagnosis, Treatment & Options
By Lorraine Johnston
ISBN 1-56592-444-4, Paperback, 6" x 9", 584 pages, $24.95 US, $36.95 CAN

"When I gave this book to one of our patients, there was an instant, electric connection. A sense of enlightenment came over her while she absorbed the information. It was thrilling to see her so sparked with new energy and focus."
—Susan Weisberg, LCSW, Clinical Social Worker, Stanford University Medical Center

Patient-Centered Guides
Published by O'Reilly & Associates, Inc.
Our products are available at a bookstore near you.
For information: 800-998-9938 • 707-829-0515 • info@oreilly.com
101 Morris Street • Sebastopol • CA • 95472-9902
www.patientcenters.com

Child/Adolescent Health

Adolescent Drug & Alcohol Abuse
How to Spot It, Stop It, and Get Help for Your Family
By Nikki Babbit
ISBN 1-56592-755-9, Paperback, 6"x 9", 304 pages, $17.95 US, $26.95 CAN

"The clear, concise, and practical information, backed up by personal stories from
people who have been through these problems with their own children or clients,
will have readers keeping this book within easy reach for use on a regular basis."
> —James F. Crowley, MA President, Community Intervention, Inc.
> Author, Alliance for Change: A Plan for Community Action on Adolescent
> Drug Abuse

Bipolar Disorders
A Guide to Helping Children & Adolescents
By Mitzi Waltz
ISBN 1-56592-656-0, Paperback, 6" x 9", 464 pages, $24.95 US, $36.95 CAN

"As bipolar disorders are becoming more commonly diagnosed in children and adolescents, a readable, informative guide for these youths and their families is certainly
needed. This book certainly fits the bill. It covers all of the major topics that are of
greatest importance to guide parents and families on the topic of pediatric bipolarity."
> —Robert L. Findling, MD, Director, Division of Child and Adolescent
> Psychiatry, Co-director, Stanley Clinical Research Center, Case Western
> Reserve/University Hospitals of Cleveland

Childhood Cancer
A Parent's Guide to Solid Tumor Cancers
By Honna Janes-Hodder & Nancy Keene
ISBN 1-56592-531-9, Paperback, 6"x 9", 544 pages, $24.95 US, $36.95 CAN

"I recommend [this book] most highly for those in need of high-level, helpful
knowledge that will empower and help parents and caregivers to cope."
> —Mark Greenberg, MD, Professor of Pediatrics, University of Toronto

Childhood Cancer Survivors
A Practical Guide to Your Future
By Nancy Keene, Wendy Hobbie & Kathy Ruccione
ISBN 1-56592-460-6, Paperback, 6" x 9", 512 pages, $27.95 US, $40.95 CAN

"Every survivor of childhood cancer should read this book."
> —Debra Friedman, MD, Assistant Professor of Pediatrics, Division of
> Hematology/Oncology, Children's Hospital and Regional Medical Center,
> Seattle, WA

Patient-Centered Guides
Published by O'Reilly & Associates, Inc.
Our products are available at a bookstore near you.
For information: **800-998-9938** • **707-829-0515** • **info@oreilly.com**
101 Morris Street • Sebastopol • CA • 95472-9902
www.patientcenters.com

Child/Adolescent Health

Childhood Leukemia
A Guide for Families, Friends, and Caregivers, Second Edition
By Nancy Keene
ISBN 1-56592-632-3, Paperback, 6" x 9", 520 pages, $24.95 US, $36.95 CAN

"What's so compelling about *Childhood Leukemia* is the amount of useful medical information and practical advice it contains. Keene avoids jargon and lays out what's needed to deal with the medical system."
—The Washington Post

Hydrocephalus
A Guide for Patients, Families & Friends
By Chuck Toporek and Kellie Robinson
ISBN 1-56592-410-X, Paperback, 6" x 9", 384 pages, $19.95 US, $28.95 CAN

"In this book, the authors have provided a wonderful entry into the world of hydrocephalus to begin to remedy the neglect of this important condition. We are immensely grateful to them for their groundbreaking effort."
—Peter M. Black, MD, PhD, Franc D. Ingraham Professor of Neurosurgery, Harvard Medical School, Neurosurgeon-in-Chief, Brigham and Women's Hospital, Children's Hospital, Boston, Massachusetts

Obsessive-Compulsive Disorder
Help for Children and Adolescents
By Mitzi Waltz
ISBN 1-56592-758-3, Paperback, 6" x 9", 408 pages, $24.95 US, $36.95 CAN

"More than a self-help manual...a wonderful resource for patients and professionals alike. Highly recommended."
—John S. March, MD, MPS, Author, OCD in Children and Adolescents: A Cognitive-Behavioral Treatment Manual

Pervasive Developmental Disorders
Finding a Diagnosis and Getting Help
By Mitzi Waltz
ISBN 1-56592-530-0, Paperback, 6" x 9", 592 pages, $24.95 US, $36.95 CAN

"Mitzi Waltz's book provides clear, informative, and comprehensive information on every relevant aspect of PDD. Her in-depth discussion will help parents and professionals develop a clear understanding of the issues and, consequently, they will be able to make informed decisions about various interventions. A job well done!"
—Dr. Stephen M. Edelson, Director, Center for the Study of Autism, Salem, Oregon

Patient-Centered Guides
Published by O'Reilly & Associates, Inc.
Our products are available at a bookstore near you.
For information: **800-998-9938** • **707-829-0515** • **info@oreilly.com**
101 Morris Street • Sebastopol • CA • 95472-9902
www.patientcenters.com

Disabilities

Choosing a Wheelchair
A Guide for Optimal Independence
By Gary Karp
ISBN 1-56592-411-8, Paperback, 5" x 8", 140 pages, $9.95 US, $14.95 CAN

"I love the idea of putting knowledge often possessed only by professionals into the hands of new consumers. Gary Karp has done it. This book will empower people with disabilities to make informed equipment choices."
—*Barry Corbet, Editor,* New Mobility Magazine

Life on Wheels
For the Active Wheelchair User
By Gary Karp
ISBN 1-56592-253-0, Paperback, 6" x 9", 584 pages, $24.95 US, $36.95 CAN

"Gary Karp's *Life On Wheels* is a super book. If you use a wheelchair, you cannot do without it. It is THE wheelchair-user reference book."
—*Hugh Gregory Gallagher, Author,* FDR's Splendid Deception

General Interest

Organ Transplants
Making the Most of Your Gift of Life
By Robert Finn
ISBN 1-56592-634-X, Paperback, 6" x 9", 336 pages, $19.95 US, $29.95 CAN

"This book is factual, easy to read and intelligently written...a wonderful job."
—*Joan Miller, RN, Department of Cardiothoracic Surgery, Stanford University School of Medicine*

Working with Your Doctor
Getting the Healthcare You Deserve
By Nancy Keene
ISBN 1-56592-273-5, Paperback, 6" x 9", 384 pages, $15.95 US, $22.95 CAN

"*Working with Your Doctor* fills a genuine need for patients and their family members caught up in this new and intimidating age of impersonal, economically driven health care delivery."
—*James Dougherty, MD, Emeritus Professor of Surgery, Albany Medical College*

Patient-Centered Guides
Published by *O'Reilly & Associates, Inc.*
Our products are available at a bookstore near you.
For information: **800-998-9938** • **707-829-0515** • **info@oreilly.com**
101 Morris Street • Sebastopol • CA • 95472-9902
www.patientcenters.com

General Interest

Your Child in the Hospital
A Practical Guide for Parents, Second Edition
By Nancy Keene and Rachel Prentice
ISBN 1-56592-573-4, Paperback, 5" x 8", 176 pages, $11.95 US, $17.95 CAN

"When your child is ill or injured, the hospital setting can be overwhelming. Here is a terrific 'road map' to help keep families 'on track.'"
> —*James B. Fahner, MD, Division Chief, Pediatric Hematology/Oncology, DeVos Children's Hospital, Grand Rapids, Michigan*

Inspiration/Human Interest

The Nicholas Effect
A Boy's Gift to the World
By Reg Green
ISBN 1-56592-860-1, Paperback, 6" x 9", 272 pages, $12.95 US, $18.95 CAN

"This book is a story of grace, dignity, and how one family turned senseless tragedy into a life-affirming gesture."
> —*Robert Kiener,* Reader's Digest

Patient-Centered Guides
Published by O'Reilly & Associates, Inc.
Our products are available at a bookstore near you.
For information: **800-998-9938 • 707-829-0515 • info@oreilly.com**
101 Morris Street • Sebastopol • CA • 95472-9902
www.patientcenters.com